MOSBY'S

Paramedic Refresher

AND

Review

A Case Studies Approach

Visit our website at **www.mosby.com**

MOSBY'S

Paramedic Refresher AND Review

A Case Studies Approach

ALICE "TWINK" DALTON, RN, MS, CNS

EMS Education Coordinator
Omaha Fire and Rescue Department
Omaha, Nebraska

with

RICHARD A. WALKER, MD

Associate Professor, Section of Emergency Medicine
Department of Surgery
University of Nebraska Medical Center
Physician Medical Director
Life Net Omaha
Rocky Mountain Helicopters
Omaha, Nebraska

with 59 illustrations

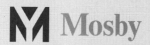

St. Louis Baltimore Boston Carlsbad Chicago Naples New York Philadelphia Portland
London Madrid Mexico City Singapore Sydney Tokyo Toronto Wiesbaden

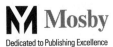
Mosby

Dedicated to Publishing Excellence

Editor: Claire Merrick
Developmental Editor: Kellie White
Project Manager: Patricia Tannian
Senior Production Editor: Melissa Lastarria
Design Manager: Gail Morey Hudson
Cover Design: Teresa Breckwoldt

NOTICE

Pharmacology is an ever-changing field. Standard safety precautions must be followed, but as new research and clinical experience broaden our knowledge, changes in treatment and drug therapy may become necessary or appropriate. Readers are advised to check the most current product information provided by the manufacturer of each drug to be administered to verify the recommended dose, the method and duration of administration, and contraindications. It is the responsibility of the treating physician, relying on experience and knowledge of the patient, to determine dosages and the best treatment for each individual patient. Neither the publisher nor the editor assumes any liability for any injury and/or damage to persons or property arising from this publication.

Mosby, Inc.
A Harcourt Health Sciences Company
11830 Westline Industrial Drive
St. Louis, Missouri 63146

Printed in United States of America

International Standard Book Number: 0-8151-1729-9

99 00 01 02 03 TG/RRD 9 8 7 6 5 4 3 2 1

Introduction

One of my responsibilities at our training program was to organize and teach the paramedic refreshers. To determine the details of subject matter, I always consulted the service program medical director and the chief of EMS. I then adjusted the DOT curriculum to include the areas they had deemed necessary for "refreshing." Class preparation, however, was the most difficult part. To have paramedics back in a classroom setting, after receiving extensive field experience, was always tough. From my experience with remediation, I knew that the traditional lecture format, although sufficient for introducing new concepts, didn't really work to enhance memory or memory cues. I also knew that if the subject matter was going to mean anything, the paramedics had to be able to relate class information to patient situations and that meant teaching in context. To do a refresher "in context" meant using case studies. Because I had recently returned to the training program from being assigned to our fire department, I had four years of case studies to reference. My experience had also taught me that caregivers need closure; in other words, they need to know the outcome of their patients. Outcomes are necessary not only for helping medics relate assessment findings and treatment to severity and results of care, but also to help in-hospital personnel relate to the field report (run reviews included ED staff). Outcomes are also very important for remediation. For these reasons I had already determined the outcomes for most of the cases I had collected.

When I started teaching refreshers using case studies, I used a method of questioning that helped assess knowledge base and develop a more thorough understanding of physiology, pathophysiology, and recognition of a degree of seriousness of the patient situation. Once that was established, treatment options could then be more readily related to the priorities of care. The method of questioning followed the model of critical thinking produced here:

Critical Thinking Process for Prehospital Care Providers

MOI/Scene + Assessment + Chief Complaint + Patient Affect + Diagnostic Tests

↓

Data Gathered + Knowledge of A&P and Pathophysiology + Attitude + Experience

↓

Field Impression + Protocol + Treatment

↓

Reassessment + Reflection-In-Action + Experience

↓

Revision of Impression + Protocol + Revision of Treatment

↓

Reflection-On-Action (Run Critique) + Experience

Illustration from Dalton, A. (1996). Enhancing critical thinking in paramedic continuing education. *Journal of Prehospital and Disaster Medicine* (11) 4:246-253.

Class discussions were guided by moving the medics through the model of critical thinking. Resulting discussions often stimulated further questions from the medics, as well as stimulating comparisons to other patient experiences by medics in the class. The cumulative effect was one of continual sharing of information and building on the experiences of the medics who participated. By asking questions that forced the medics to relate signs and symptoms to pathophysiology, degree of seriousness, and treatment modalities chosen, I could ensure that memory cues were accurate and that future actions, based on this information, had a better chance of being correct.

I have used case studies in teaching for many years. When sharing the cases with fellow instructors, I kept getting the request for supplying questions with answers. When I finally sat down to do so, the idea of publishing them so they were available and affordable was suggested. Because there was currently no book on the market for paramedic refreshers, and these case studies had been used for refreshers, as well as primary training, a paramedic refresher book seemed the perfect avenue.

When preparing a book with case studies, based on actual cases, the issue of patient confidentiality became a major issue. To maintain confidentiality, certain identifying characteristics have been changed or altered but not in a manner that changes the patient's problem or the seriousness of the situation. Each case study provides actual physical assessment information and as much as possible, the actual historical data.

Some situations or patient/family explanations may seem bizarre, but the unusual are truly representative of the situations we run into in the field. Every effort was made to keep those intact, without violating confidentiality, to add to the contextual feel for the cases.

I hope this text provides instructors and participants with an enjoyable, as well as an educational, exercise in satisfying the requirements for a paramedic refresher. Any comments for future editions would be welcome. I certainly learned a tremendous amount putting it together.

How To Use This Book

The cases in this book are intended to provide enough didactic material to complete any subject matter that a program might want to include in a paramedic refresher. The subject matter follows the subject matter in the new paramedic curriculum. There are two tables of contents; the first is by specific body system, and the second is by patient chief complaint. This will enable the user to have a choice in how to review cases. A "chief complaint" approach will help avoid tunnel vision; for instance, not every complaint of difficulty breathing is a primary respiratory problem.

Each chapter begins with a chapter summary. It is not so much organized around a particular diagnosis as it is organized around the anatomy, physiology, and pathophysiology of that system, assessment findings when that system is involved, and specific treatment. Details of drug dosage and options are dealt with in more detail in the specific cases. The exception is the chapter summary on challenging patients. That summary is more general.

Case studies follow the chapter summary. The cases are organized as if the reader were actually dispatched and reporting what is first seen on arrival. This is followed by the initial physical, focused history, and focused physical. Questions are provided that are designed to assess the knowledge base of the first step of the model of thinking. These questions encourage the reader to think of the physiology and pathophysiology involved and the relationship between that and the patient's signs and symptoms. This helps in concept formation and thus the recognition of the seriousness or potential seriousness of the patient situation. Questions about treatment and treatment options are also included. By moving through the questions as they are posed, the reader will be led through the model. Depending on how the cases are used, some questions will have more importance than others and should be answered before others. However, if the order is kept intact, a specific thinking process will be enhanced and enforced. Answers to the questions are supplied. These answers are referenced and sources are at the back of each chapter.

As the reader moves through the questions, other questions may be stimulated and should be asked and answers explained. The reference list is a good place to obtain further information on the subject matter. All instructors using this text are encouraged to add to the answers or explanations as necessary for student needs.

Current patient care controversies are included when appropriate. As much as possible I tried to include all aspects of the controversy, utilizing information supplied by my physician advisor/reviewer/friend, Rick Walker. I also took care to point out current recommendations and where those recommendations originated. Patient care would, however, always follow local protocols and local medical direction.

A comprehensive index is included in the back of the book to aid providers and instructors in specifically locating a subject of interest.

Twink Dalton

Dedication

This book is dedicated to all those who taught me so well:

Dr. Melvin Bechtel, Dr. Donald Harvey, Dr. Dean Magee, Chief Chester Guinane, Forrest Dalton, Bill Howell, Bill Gentleman, Dave Hajek, Perry Guido, Corky Janing, Jim Love, Brian Sorenson, Jack Diesing, Red Barbee, Ole Cherko, Vic Bochek, Jim Schenkelberg, Mark Lloyd, Bill Rytych, Mike Buscher, Doug Lloyd, John Herman, Ron Wiley, John Goessling, Bob Moon, Dale Fausset, Jim Hendricksen, Kevin Carritt, Scott Muschall, Tony Lang, Lee Dunbar, Dave Linnell, Ron Benak, Dave Hawley, Rick Walker, Mick Jadlowski, and all the other early paramedics I learned so much from and whose names I don't have room to mention. God bless you.

Acknowledgment

No book would be complete without the numerous people who worked so hard behind the scenes. Throughout the reviews and editing of this book there were numerous people who helped tremendously by encouraging the best out of those who reviewed the material and supported me when I got discouraged. Among these were Claire Merrick, Nancy Peterson, Carla Goldberg, Kathleen Scogna, Deb Lejeune, Jennifer Roche, Kellie White, Jeanne Murphy, and Melissa Lastarria. I couldn't have done it without the support of all those in the beginning and the calm and consistent support of Kellie.

Richard Walker, a dear friend and colleague, gave invaluable insights regarding the medical accuracy of the explanations for each case study. The reviewers were invaluable for pointing out phrases that were regional, explanations that didn't make sense, and potential controversies that should be either explained or avoided. When I got sidetracked on pathophysiology, they always got me back on track. For that, the readers should be grateful.

Preface

This book came about because of a group of students who just "didn't get it." The students were smart enough and read the books but couldn't tie together all the loose ends. In many cases these were students who had already made it through the class, and some had even passed the National Registry examination and were practicing paramedics. I had encountered students like this many times before. Early in my teaching career my co-worker, Jeanne O'Brien, and I would discuss ways to teach by the hour and would continually try different methods. Sometimes a method seemed to work, but more times than not, the method didn't. Because of student self-doubt and our observations, we rode with them. Almost from the beginning, when we reviewed the run in terms of what we taught in the classroom, we noticed the light bulbs going on. The key seemed to be relating pathophysiology to patient history and physical findings. A connection was made for the students that helped them for the rest of the class. Thus was born my awareness of the absolute importance of contextual learning. From this beginning came an insatiable curiosity and lifelong interest in critical thinking. Jeanne and I developed many strategies from this early discovery. We used scenarios (patient situations) constantly and in many different ways throughout the class. Most of the time scenarios were used in the form of case studies (written patient situations). Eventually, at the end of class we would introduce scenarios in the form of simulations the students planned, acted out, and required two fellow classmates to respond. These were video-taped and critiqued. What a learning environment!

It was not until much later that I realized what we were actually doing. In 1989, I was assigned to the Omaha Fire Department to do in-house continuing education and to ride along evaluating patient care. I was also given the task of remediating, whenever it was needed. But to remediate appropriately, I had to figure out where the problem was. I fell back to what I had previously done; I started asking questions to force the medics to relate pathophysiology to patient presentations. I made another discovery. Not all the medics made the same connections. Even though they came from the same class, and in most cases I had taught them originally, something had happened from the time I had them in class until now. There were differences in recognizing the significance of findings, identifying pathophysiologic processes, and choosing appropriate treatment. Sometimes the problem was in past experiences. If an observation was made and an inappropriate conclusion reached, then similar patient situations were affected from that time on. Sometimes the problem was due to an incomplete assessment, lack of knowledge of treatment options, or, more often, a lack of adequate knowledge of pathophysiology, which then led to an inability to recognize the significance of the patient's presentation. As I observed practicing paramedics, those who were novice medics, those who were excellent at their practice, and all those in between, a distinct thinking process became evident. As I worked more with remediation, a model took form. But I wasn't the first to discover this model or the process.

Hilda Taba (1966) developed a model of concept formation that she applied to improve the thinking skills of grade school social studies students. That model was surprisingly close to the process that I observed in my medics. It was, however, missing some aspects of the process I noted. Eventually I discovered Schon (1987) and his work with the concept of reflection-in-action and reflection-on-action and Benner (1984) and her work describing the process of expert thinking. About this time I shared my thoughts, and the model that I developed, with another colleague, Judy Janing. She took the model, which by this time we called a model of critical thinking, and worked with it in the classroom, adding to my observations. After she improved on the model, I took it back out in the field and continued to refine it.

Eventually I was reassigned to the classroom, but I had learned much. My earlier experiences with Jeanne had been validated and confirmed. Never again would I leave a classroom without relating subject matter to a patient situation. I developed questioning techniques, based on the model of critical thinking, to ensure that memory cues were accurate and patterns of organization were correct. I published my experience with the model in the *Journal of Prehospital and Disaster Medicine* (1996).

During my time with the Omaha Fire Department, I had collected a bank of case studies, based on actual patients that I either took care of or had intimate knowledge of and whose outcomes I knew. I used those case studies everywhere and shared them with anyone who asked. I especially used them with paramedic refreshers. It was at this point that I was encouraged to publish the case studies so that other students and other instructors could use them.

This book is a collection of those case studies, complete with questions and answers. References are included so the reader can see where the explanations came from and perhaps, if curious enough, look for further information. It is my hope that these case studies stimulate thought, explain observations, invite treatment considerations, add to vicarious experience, and, eventually, lead to better patient care. If so, their purpose has been achieved.

REFERENCES

Benner, P. (1984). *From novice to expert.* Menlo Park, CA: Addison-Wesley Publishing.

Dalton, A. (1996). Enhancing critical thinking in paramedic continuing education. *Journal of Prehospital and Disaster Medicine* (11) 4: 246-253.

Schon, D. (1987). *Educating the reflective practitioner.* San Francisco, CA: Jossey-Bass.

Taba, H. (1966). *Teaching strategies and cognitive functioning in elementary school children.* Cooperative Research Project No. 2404. Palo Alto, CA: San Francisco State College.

Contents

Contents *by Nature of Condition*

1

Respiratory Emergencies

OVERVIEW

Caring for a patient with a respiratory complaint can be one of the greatest challenges that a pre-hospital care provider can face. Treatment is determined by a basic knowledge of anatomy, physiology, and pathophysiology; accurate history and physical findings; thorough understanding of disease processes and pharmacology; and an intuitive grasp of the acuity of the situation.

Anatomy, Physiology, and Pathophysiology

The airway is divided into two main parts, an upper airway and lower airway, separated by the vocal cords contained in the larynx. The upper airway consists of the mouth and nasal passages, the tongue, throat, epiglottis, and surrounding soft tissues. The soft tissues are very vascular, and prone to profuse bleeding when traumatized and extreme swelling when irritated (especially in cases of infection, trauma, or allergic reaction).

The lower airway consists of the trachea, mainstem bronchi, bronchioles, and alveoli. The lower airway passages are lined with a mucous membrane that secretes mucus for trapping foreign particles, such as dust, bacteria, or viruses. The mucus, along with trapped particles, is moved, by way of cilia, up to the throat to be coughed or swallowed. If anything interferes with the movement of the cilia, the mucus tends to collect and settle, thus blocking the smaller airways. This predisposes the patient to atelectasis, as well as infection.

The mucous membrane is sensitive to irritation (chemical, inflammation, allergens, foreign material) and will increase secretions or swell in response. The bronchioles, bronchi, and, to a lesser extent, the trachea, all have a muscle layer that has the ability to constrict and dilate. The muscle layer is responsive to beta 2 stimulation (dilation) and irritation that can cause constriction and/or stimulate further mucus production.

The alveoli are one-cell-layer thick and function as the actual exchange membrane for oxygen and carbon dioxide. The alveoli are kept open, dry, and with a minimum of surface tension by surfactant, which is secreted by specialized cells in the walls of the alveoli. Anything that interferes with the secretion of surfactant (such as prolonged shock) or washes it away (as in a fresh water near-drowning) will significantly interfere with the alveoli's ability to exchange gases.

Alveoli are also kept dry by a balance between air pressure from the inhaled atmosphere and hydrostatic pressure in the capillary beds. Anything that disrupts the balance of pressure (congestive heart failure), the permeability of the capillary bed (allergic reactions, septic shock), or the permeability of the alveoli (allergic reactions, sepsis, chemical exposure, certain poisons) can lead to fluid leakage into the interstitial space and the alveoli.

Assessment

A common source of respiratory distress is a foreign body. The tongue is a frequent source of upper airway obstruction in the unconscious patient. Snoring is an audible result. However, a complete airway obstruction does not result in any sound. Careful observance of the absence of air exchange will alert the provider to the problem and appropriate airway clearing methods should be done. Basic maneuvers should be done first while advanced maneuvers are being prepared.

Observable signs of respiratory distress include the presence of accessory muscle use. The primary muscle of respiration is the diaphragm. Secondary muscles include the intercostal muscles. When the diaphragm is working hard, abnormal muscle use can be noticed in the abdominal wall. Intercostal muscles normally contract to expand the chest wall. When the contractions become noticeable (outlining the ribs), the term is *intercostal retractions*, they are an indicator of labored breathing. Other accessory muscles include the neck muscles and nasal flaring.

Abnormal lung sounds are another sign of respiratory distress. Normally lung sounds are clear. The presence of wheezing, crackles or rales, and/or bubbles or rhonchi also suggest difficulty with exchange of oxygen and carbon dioxide. Wheezing indicates bronchoconstriction. Crackles or rales indicate the presence of a watery fluid, whereas bubbles or rhonchi suggest mucus or thicker secretions.

Observation of the patient's ability to speak in complete sentences is a particularly useful indication of the adequacy of minute volume. Since minute volume equals tidal volume times respiratory rate, a conscious patient who has a respiratory rate within normal limits should be able to talk in complete sentences. If that is not the case, inadequate tidal volume is likely. A useful assessment tool includes pulse oximetry. Although the device does not replace a good physical assessment, it can point the caregiver in a direction.

Causes of Respiratory Emergencies and Review of Treatment

Bronchoconstriction, which causes wheezing, can be caused by irritants, allergens, infection, or temperature extremes. Irritants include body water (e.g., pulmonary edema), chemicals (e.g., a toxic inhalant), a foreign body, or an environmental irritant (e.g., dust). Wheezing that is unilateral may be caused by a foreign body or an infection. If a patient has been in one position for an extended time, wheezing may be heard in the dependent parts of the chest as a result of a collection of secretions. This is more likely in the elderly or those with a history of congestive heart failure or when recreational drug use is involved.

Wheezing is usually treated by a bronchodilator. In the case of wheezing resulting from body water, a diuretic can be useful. Occasionally the use of a bronchodilator will relax the bronchospasm enough to enable you to hear the crackles.

In the case of an allergic reaction, a bronchodilator or even epinephrine may be appropriate. However, careful history taking and assessment is necessary since treatment for one condition may be contraindicated for another. For example, epinephrine is appropriate for a severe allergic reaction but contraindicated in congestive failure.

Another cause of difficulty breathing is a primary cardiac cause. In the case of congestive heart failure, the left ventricle may not be strong or efficient. Blood backs up into the left atria and the backflow creates a pressure in the capillary beds. This disrupts the hydrostatic pressure leading to body water leaking out of the capillary bed into the interstitial space, irritating the terminal bronchioles, thus causing wheezing. In cases where ventricular muscle is involved and the blood pressure is low, dopamine or dobutamine are helpful pharmacologic agents. In cases where the blood pressure is normal or too high, a vasodilator such as nitroglycerine and/or a diuretic such as furosemide can be helpful.

Cardiac rhythm can also cause a similar effect, especially rhythms that are too fast. When the rhythm is too fast to support perfusion, then pharmacologic agents, such as adenosine or cardioversion, are appropriate.

Bubbles or rhonchi are usually caused by thick mucus. A common cause is infection. Bronchodilators help to open the bronchial passages and aid in air exchange.

Common chronic conditions that cause dyspnea include COPD (emphysema and chronic bronchitis) and asthma, as well as congestive heart failure. COPD is a permanent chronic condition, whereas asthma is temporary but recurring. Between attacks the asthmatic patient is normal.

Beta agonists are appropriate pharmacologic agents for both a person with asthma and a COPD patient with an exacerbation. COPD is a common term that refers to two degenerative lung diseases: emphysema and chronic bronchitis.

Emphysema gradually destroys the alveolar wall and capillary bed, whereas chronic bronchitis results in hypersecretion of mucus and structural changes in the bronchi. One disease process generally leads to the other. Eventually COPD will lead to chronic bronchitis; right-sided heart failure (cor pulmonale); cardiac dysrhythmias, such as atrial fibrillation; and congestive heart failure.

Other less common sources of respiratory problems include, degenerative muscle diseases (such as myasthenia gravis, post-polio syndrome, and amyotrophic lateral sclerosis [ALS]), inflammation or infection (such as pneumonia, tuberculosis), pulmonary emboli, allergic reactions and sepsis.

Dyspnea with hypoxia is the end result of most respiratory conditions. The concept of hypoxia is sometimes difficult to understand. When changes are slow, and over a long period of time, the body will compensate with changes in stimulus to breathe (from levels of CO_2 to levels of O_2) and increases in RBC production. Slow but progressive changes also stimulate the steady release of epinephrine and norepinephrine that increase cardiac contraction, speed up heart rate and blood pressure, but also, paradoxically, increase the cardiac oxygen demand. When hypoxia occurs rapidly, changes in mentation can profoundly vary (lethargy to combativeness) and epinephrine and norepinephrine responses can be extreme resulting in noticeable skin color changes. Cyanosis, however, does not usually occur until 5% of the total hemoglobin is saturated. Cyanosis is a late sign of hypoxia.

Keys to Assessment

Keys to history taking include previous illness, medications and previous occurrence. Keys to physical examination include assessment of lung sounds, cardiac rhythm, presence of pitting edema, barrel chest, fever, and effect of position on breathing. It is extremely important to discriminate between dyspnea of cardiac origin and dyspnea of noncardiac origin.

Use of a pulse oximeter can be very helpful if the device is used appropriately. Keeping in mind when results can be misleading (states of shock, CO_2 poisoning, anemia, and vasoconstrictive states) and used in conjunction with a complete respiratory assessment, pulse oximetry can guide the use of oxygen and oxygen adjuncts.

Treatment

Treatment of patients with the complaint of dyspnea includes: obstructed airway maneuvers, positioning, use of oxygen, use of pharmacologic agents (e.g., beta agonists, diuretics, vasodilators), analgesics (e.g., morphine), and catecholamines (e.g., epinephrine, dopamine, dobutamine).

CASE 1

Dispatch: 20:00 hrs; 67 y/o male with difficulty breathing

On Arrival: You find 67 y/o Fred sitting in a tripod position with a nasal cannula hooked to home oxygen. He is awake, appears dusky, and is using accessory muscles to breathe. His wife is present.

Initial Assessment Findings

Mental Status—Awake and obeys command, GCS 15
Airway—Open and clear
Breathing—R 22, shallow and labored, talking in 1- to 2-word sentences; lung sounds reveal wheezing in all lobes
Circulation—Skin cool, dusky, and diaphoretic
Radial pulse rapid and irregular at 120
BP 164/92
Disability—Pupils are equal and reactive, moving all extremities
Chief Complaint—Difficulty breathing

History

Events—Sudden onset after having a cigarette
Previous Illness—Emphysema for 10 years, "water in lungs," high blood pressure
Current Health Status—Has been on home oxygen, 1 to 2 lpm, for last 5 years. Has been doing well lately with last hospitalization for exacerbation 3 months ago.
Allergies—Pollen, dust, and penicillin
Medications—Furosemide (Lasix), digoxin (Lanoxin), spironolactone (Aldactone), theophylline (Theo-Dur), metaproterenol (Alupent) inhaler

Focused Physical

Current set of VS—P 120, R 20, BP 158/88
Other Pertinent Findings—Thin and barrel-chested, no pitting edema noted, oxygen per nasal cannula at 2 lpm, pulse oximetry 85%
Diagnostic Tests—None done

ECG

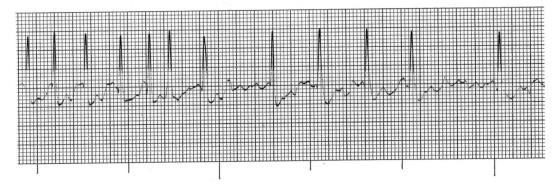

Figure 1-1

QUESTIONS

1. What is significant about Fred's history?

2. What body system(s) is/are affected?

3. What is the significance of the patient's tripod position?

4. What does talking in 1- to 2-word sentences indicate?

5. What is the relationship between Fred's cigarette smoking and his current problem?

6. What area or anatomic part of the lung is primarily affected in emphysema and what is that effect?

7. What is the relationship between emphysema and chronic bronchitis?

8. What is Fred at risk for?

9. What are some possible causes of Fred's current condition?

10. How severe is Fred's situation, and how do you determine this?

11. What immediate actions are appropriate?

12. What treatment is appropriate?

13. Why is low flow oxygen often the best initial approach for the COPD patient?

14. What is the relationship between Fred's emphysema and his history of "water in lungs"?

15. What is Fred's cardiac rhythm?

16. What is the connection between Fred's cardiac rhythm and his previous illness?

17. What is the significance of Fred's assessment finding of bilateral wheezing?

18. Are there any other aspects of Fred's history or physical examination that would help you?

19. What is significant about Fred's focused physical?

20. How would you continue treatment?

QUESTIONS AND ANSWERS

1. **What is significant about Fred's history?**

   On home oxygen at 1 to 2 lpm; previous diagnosis of emphysema; medication combination of furosemide, digitalis, and antihypertensive suggests congestive heart failure; current complaint began after having a cigarette.

2. **What body system(s) is/are affected?**

   Respiratory—bilateral wheezing, talking in 1 to 2 word sentences, presence of accessory muscle use, dusky skin

   Cardiovascular—cool, clammy skin; tachy pulse; hypertensive

3. **What is the significance of the patient's tripod position?**

   The tripod position maximizes muscle excursion and space within the chest cavity. Patients who assume the tripod position are trying to get the most out of every respiratory effort and usually have the complaint of difficulty breathing. This patient is in respiratory distress, if not respiratory failure, and has assumed this position since it is the most advantageous for breathing.

4. **What does talking in 1- to 2-word sentences indicate?**

   Inadequate tidal volume.

5. **What is the relationship between Fred's cigarette smoking and his current problem?**

   The majority of emphysema cases in the United States are caused by cigarette smoking. It is likely that Fred is addicted to cigarettes and the inhalation of smoke acutely exacerbates his emphysema.

6. **What area or anatomic part of the lung is primarily affected in emphysema, and what is that effect?**

   The alveoli. The effect is damage to the delicate cellular membranes of the alveolar sacs, thus expanding a cluster of alveoli into one big sac. The cellular damage also affects supporting structures of the terminal bronchiole and alveoli, as well as the elasticity of the alveoli itself. This causes air trapping. Even if the patient stops smoking, cellular damage continues because it is mediated by inflammatory cell enzymes that remain active.

7. **What is the relationship between emphysema and chronic bronchitis?**

   When the cellular damage from emphysema extends to the terminal bronchioles and mucus producing cells, chronic bronchitis will develop in addition to the emphysema. This is why most emphysema patients develop chronic bronchitis to some degree. A similar process also occurs in chronic bronchitis patients, and eventually, chronic bronchitis patients will also get emphysema.

8. **What is Fred at risk for?**

   Rupture of blebs, worsening of respiratory failure leading to myocardial ischemia, cardiac dysrhythmias and/or myocardial infarction, and respiratory arrest.

9. **What are some possible causes of Fred's current condition?**

   Causes of exacerbations include infections (bronchitis, pneumonia), pulmonary emboli, and congestive heart failure (CHF). Smoking a single cigarette may cause bronchoconstriction, but that, in and of itself, usually does not trigger a full exacerbation.

10. **How severe is Fred's situation and how do you determine this?**

    Fred's wife can better tell you how he currently compares to his usual state. This will help you determine the severity of this episode. Fred's situation could be worse. He is still able to talk, even though he is compromised. His pulse oximetry is only 85%. Chronic obstructive pulmonary disease (COPD) patients will normally have a low pulse oximetry reading (about 89%); however, this episode is bad enough for him to call you. He is hypoxic.

11. **What immediate actions are appropriate?**

    Check his oxygen tank, since it may be empty or not set on the correct liter flow. Check the patency of the oxygen tubing. Smoking with oxygen on causes very hot ash. Hot ashes can burn holes in the tubing allowing the oxygen to escape into the room instead of flowing to the patient.

12. What treatment is appropriate?

Increase Fred's oxygen to 4 to 6 lpm while preparing a bronchodilator. The goal is to supply enough oxygen to raise his pulse oximetry to at least 90%.

13. Why is low flow oxygen often the best initial approach for the COPD patient?

In patients whose normal stimulus to breathe (levels of carbon dioxide) has been overtaxed, the body will no longer respond. The remaining stimulus (level of oxygen) is weaker and operates on the concentration of arterial oxygen. Thus the lack of oxygen, or hypoxia, becomes the stimulus to breathe. The resulting effect is called "hypoxic drive." High oxygen flow rates give high arterial O_2 concentrations, which interfere with this stimulus.

However, resources point out that it takes time (as much as 30 to 45 minutes in some patients) to interfere with hypoxic drive. The short-term use of supplemental oxygen at the highest FiO_2 needed to improve oxygenation (pulse oximetry >90%) usually does not adversely effect respiratory drive. Should respiratory depression occur, assist with a bag-valve-mask. If pulse oxymetry does not improve, assess your patient and titrate oxygen to affect as you would do with any other drug. Some medical directors recommend adjusting FiO_2 to obtain pulse oximetry of 90% to 92%.

14. What is the relationship between Fred's emphysema and his history of "water in lungs"?

Emphysema destroys the capillary beds surrounding affected alveoli. This not only decreases the amount of surface area available for exchange of oxygen and carbon dioxide but also decreases the size of the "container" in the lungs. This decrease in the number of capillaries, in the presence of the same amount of blood, leads to an increase in pulmonary capillary pressure, ultimately causing pulmonary hypertension. Pulmonary hypertension eventually causes hypertrophy of the right ventricle. An increase in central venous pressure is the eventual result. This is evident by presence of jugular venous distention (JVD) and, as a long-term effect, peripheral edema. These findings of JVD and peripheral edema are the hallmarks of right-sided heart failure (cor pulmonale). Eventually the back up of venous pressure leads to left ventricular failure and the better known pattern of congestive heart failure.

15. What is Fred's cardiac rhythm?

Atrial fibrillation. There is no identifiable P wave, QRS is ≤0.10, and the ventricular response is irregular.

16. What is the connection between Fred's cardiac rhythm and his previous illness?

His cardiac rhythm is atrial fibrillation with a rapid ventricular response. Atrial fib is a common finding in patients with congestive heart failure. As the pressure in the left ventricle spreads to the left atrium, the left atrium enlarges to accommodate the buildup of blood. When emphysema is also present, right atrial enlargement is common because of pulmonary hypertension. Atrial enlargement contributes to the development of atrial fibrillation. Lack of coordinated contraction of the atria results in two things. First, ventricular cardiac output is reduced due to ineffective pumping by the atria; this triggers a sympathetic response (vasoconstriction and tachycardia). Second, ineffective pumping by the atria may cause blood to back up into the pulmonary vasculature, thus disrupting the hydrostatic pressure balance in the capillaries, causing fluid to leak out, which results in pulmonary edema, especially at higher heart rates.

The net effect of the sympathetic response is to increase preload, increase the contractility of the ventricles, and increase the oxygen demand on the heart. When this occurs in the presence of previously existing pulmonary hypertension and ineffective atrial pumping, congestive heart failure is exacerbated.

17. What is the significance of Fred's assessment finding of bilateral wheezing?

Wheezing results from a narrowing of the bronchioles and occurs in conditions such as asthma, congestive heart failure, and COPD. Narrowing of the bronchioles can occur from smooth muscle contraction (irritation) or obstruction (pus, mucus, or foreign bodies). Irritation can occur inside the bronchioles (inhalation of smoke or an allergen) or outside the bronchioles (fluid collecting in the interstitial spaces).

18. Are there any other aspects of Fred's history or physical examination that would help you?

Does Fred take his medication regularly? When was the last time he took his blood pressure medication? When was the last time he took his Lasix and Lanoxin?

19. ***What is significant about Fred's focused physical?***

Fred has no evidence of peripheral edema.

20. ***How would you continue treatment?***

Monitor response to O_2 and bronchodilator closely. Increase the oxygen flow as indicated by the response and pulse oximetry values. Choose a bronchodilator with fewer cardiac side effects, such as metaproterenol. Monitor respiratory effort closely for a pneumothorax. Start an IV crystalloid at KVO rate or saline lock.

OUTCOME

Fred was admitted to the local hospital with an acute exacerbation of COPD with pulmonary edema. Chest x-rays showed pulmonary edema that significantly improved with nitroglycerine SL and furosemide (Lasix) 40 mg. However, even after three nebulizer treatments and diuretic therapy, Fred remained in respiratory distress and was admitted. Ten days later he was dismissed to home.

CASE 2

Dispatch: 15:30 hrs; 16 y/o male with difficulty breathing

On Arrival: You find 16 y/o Bob sitting on a chair in his kitchen. He is leaning forward and bracing his arms on the table. He appears pale and you note he is using accessory muscles in his neck. He is awake but sleepy, and his mother is present.

Initial Assessment Findings

Mental Status—Awake, obeys command, GCS 15
Airway—Open and clear
Breathing—R 16 and extremely labored, unable to talk; lung sounds very faint and only heard in apices
Circulation—Skin pale, cool, and clammy; his lips are dusky
          Radial pulse rapid at 136 and irregular
          BP 168/92
Chief Complaint—Difficulty breathing

Focused History

Events—Bob woke up with wheezing but took his inhaler and went to school. When he got home he was worse and now has no relief from inhaler.
Previous Illness—Asthma since early childhood
Current Health Status—Good
Allergies—Pollens, dust, and cats
Medications—Beclomethasone dipropionate (Beconase) nasal inhaler

Focused Physical

Current set of VS—P 136, R 16 and labored with intercostal retractions, BP 168/92
Other Pertinent Findings—Cyanotic nail beds, pulse oximetry 82%
Diagnostic Tests—None performed

ECG

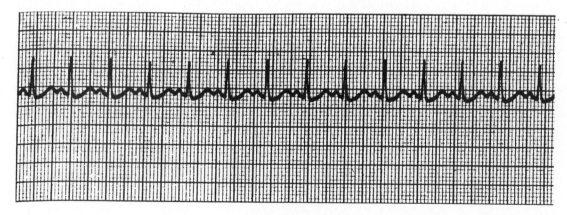

Figure 1-2

QUESTIONS

1. What is significant about Bob's history?

2. What body systems are affected?

3. What is the significance of Bob's fatigue?

4. What is the significance of Bob's lung sounds?

5. Is Bob's ability to talk related to his lung sounds? Why or why not?

6. How severe is Bob's situation, and how do you determine this?

7. Bob's pulse is rapid and irregular but his rhythm strip shows a regular sinus tachy. Why?

8. Why is Bob pale, cool, and clammy?

9. There are at least two reasons for Bob's tachycardia. What are they?

10. What is Bob in immediate danger of?

11. What is the immediate priority for Bob?

12. What are possible causes of Bob's condition?

13. What treatment is appropriate for Bob?

14. Once the airways start to open and the hypoxia begins to resolve, patients with severe asthma, such as Bob, have another problem that should be treated. What is the problem and how should it be treated?

15. Is there a difference in the treatment of known asthma in a child versus treatment of known asthma in an adult?

16. When an asthmatic is tachycardic, and a sympathomimetic is given, is there not a risk of increasing the tachycardia and thereby increasing the workload of the heart?

17. What are the contraindications to giving epinephrine to an asthmatic?

18. If epinephrine is not indicated, what are additional options?

19. If an asthmatic loses consciousness and needs to be intubated in the field, it is often very difficult to ventilate the patient. It is also true that forceful ventilation can be hazardous. What is the biggest risk to assisted ventilation in the asthma patient?

20. Bob was sleepy. What is the possible cause and the significance of sleepiness in an asthmatic?

QUESTIONS AND ANSWERS

1. **What is significant about Bob's history?**

   Asthma began this morning, Bob has used inhaler all day, and has no relief now.

2. **What body systems are affected?**

   Respiratory—Abnormal lung sounds, dusky lips

   Cardiovascular—Tachycardic and irregular rhythm; hypertension; cool, clammy skin, dusky lips

3. **What is the significance of Bob's fatigue?**

   It is a serious sign of impending respiratory failure. Bob is getting so tired from the effort of breathing that he may soon quit.

4. **What is the significance of Bob's lung sounds?**

   There is so much bronchoconstriction with resultant air trapping that there is very little air exchange.

5. **Is Bob's ability to talk related to his lung sounds? Why or why not?**

   Yes. There is so little air exchange that tidal volume is inadequate for speech. In fact the air exchange is so limited that lung sounds are almost absent.

6. **How severe is Bob's situation, and how do you determine this?**

   Bob's condition is life threatening. Tidal volume is so inadequate that his lung sounds are almost absent and he is unable to speak.

7. **Bob's pulse is rapid and irregular but his rhythm strip shows a regular sinus tachy. Why?**

   There is so much air trapping that every time Bob attempts to inhale, intrathoracic pressure is increased to the point that cardiac output is inhibited. This is detected as an irregular radial pulse in the presence of a regular monitored rhythm. This is a paradoxical pulse and is typical of conditions that cause increased pressure on the heart.

8. **Why is Bob pale, cool, and clammy?**

   Bob is hypoxic. The body perceives hypoxia as a significant stressor and releases stores of epinephrine and norepinephrine. Anxiety does the same thing. The result of epi/norepi release causes peripheral vasoconstriction and diaphoresis, thus leading to pale, cool, and clammy skin.

9. **There are at least two reasons for Bob's tachycardia. What are they?**

   His epi/norepi release and his hypoxia. Both will stimulate tachycardia.

10. **What is Bob in immediate danger of?**

    Respiratory arrest.

11. **What is the immediate priority for Bob?**

    Breathing. Bob can't breathe adequately on his own and is rapidly losing energy to maintain respiratory drive. He needs to be assisted. Assisted breathing with supplemental oxygen would be the ideal but may be almost impossible to do. The ideal airway would be intubation.

12. **What are possible causes of Bob's condition?**

    Status asthmaticus is the most likely cause of his current problem.

13. **What treatment is appropriate for Bob?**

    Bob needs supplemental O_2 and immediate bronchodilation. Supplemental O_2 can be given in any way Bob will accept it. This includes assisting with a BVM, using a mask non–rebreather at 15 lpm or applying a nasal cannula at 4 to 6 lpm. (Adjust the flow rate for patient comfort).

    In some systems this patient would be a candidate for rapid sequence intubation or nasal tracheal intubation. If Bob loses consciousness, intubation should be accomplished in any case.

    Immediate bronchodilation can be done in two ways. An attempt to deliver a nebulized bronchodilator, such as albuterol, metaproterenol, or terbutaline by mask or hand-held device at 5 to 7 lpm O_2, may be tried at the same time as a subcutaneous injection of epinephrine 1:1,000, 0.3 to 0.5 mg.

14. *Once the airways begin to open and the hypoxia begins to resolve, patients with severe asthma, such as Bob, have another problem that should be treated. What is the problem and how should it be treated?*

> Dehydration. An IV should be started and a bolus of crystalloid such as normal saline should be given. In younger children with asthma, dehydration is of greater concern. In Bob's case it is probably an incidental concern.

15. *Is there a difference in the treatment of known asthma in a child versus treatment of known asthma in an adult?*

> Not really, the treatment is essentially the same. However, you must be more cautious in adults where an exaggerated tachycardic response to sympathomimetics may be detrimental. Most bronchodilators are sympathomimetic. Some, such as albuterol (Ventolin), metaproterenol (Alupent), terbutaline (Brethine), and isoetharine (Bronkosol), are B2 selective, whereas others, such as aerosolized epinephrine, are not. The difference has to do with cardiac side effects. In adults, especially, cardiac side effects (such as tachycardia) can aggravate left ventricular failure leading to a worsening of asthmalike symptoms. In left ventricular failure, asthmalike wheezing is a consequence of fluid irritating the smooth muscles in the bronchioles triggering bronchoconstriction. The cause requires a different pharmacologic treatment.

16. *When an asthmatic is tachycardic, and a sympathomimetic is given, is there not a risk of increasing the tachycardia and thereby increasing the workload of the heart?*

> Yes, however, the tachycardia in the severe asthmatic is due to hypoxia and the increased work of breathing. When the bronchodilation occurs and the hypoxia resolves, the tachycardia usually slows. Depending on the particular sympathomimetic used, heart rates usually decline with treatment but may not drop below 90.

17. *What are the contraindications to giving epinephrine to an asthmatic?*

> The contraindications are related to the cardiac effects of this nonselective catecholamine. Epinephrine's beta$_1$ effects increase contractility, rate, automaticity, and irritability thus increasing oxygen demand along with the workload of the heart. If an asthmatic has a history of a myocardial infarction within the last year or angina, epinephrine is not indicated. For most adults, a beta$_2$ selective bronchodilator is preferred (albuterol, metaproterenol, or terbutaline). Some systems caution against use of certain bronchodilators, such as isoproterenol (Isuprel) or isoetharine (Bronkosol) in adults over the age of 40.

18. *If epinephrine is not indicated, what are additional options?*

> There are a number of nebulized selective beta$_2$ bronchodilators that can be used in the field, among them are albuterol (Ventolin) and metaproterenol (Alupent).

19. *If an asthmatic loses consciousness and needs to be intubated in the field, it is often very difficult to ventilate the patient. It is also true that forceful ventilation can be hazardous. What is the biggest risk to assisted ventilation in the asthma patient?*

> Causing a pneumothorax. The pathophysiology of asthma is prolonged expiratory phase resulting in excessive air trapping and eventual rupture of alveoli, especially if adequate time for expiration is not allowed. Forcing additional air into the lungs can contribute to air trapping and, without adequate expiratory time, may result in a pneumothorax.

20. *Bob is sleepy. What is the possible cause and the significance of sleepiness in an asthmatic?*

> High levels of PaCO$_2$ are narcotic, causing somnolence and clouding of consciousness that is often perceived as sleepiness. High levels of PaCO$_2$ also accelerate the onset of fatigue in a patient who already has an increased workload of breathing. Thus a vicious cycle occurs. Together these two conditions may result in respiratory arrest.

OUTCOME

Bob lost consciousness shortly after being given epinephrine 0.5mg, 1:1,000 SQ. He was intubated and ventilated with a metaproterenol nebulizer adapter for the ET tube. On arrival at the hospital, Bob started to exhibit audible wheezes. He was admitted to the pediatric ICU with the diagnosis of status asthmaticus. In the ICU he was maintained on a continuous metaproterenol treatment by ventilator and prednisone. He was weaned off the ventilator in 2 days and was dismissed to home on day 3.

CASE 3

Dispatch 19:30 hrs; 35 y/o female with difficulty breathing

On Arrival You find 35 y/o Susan sitting at her kitchen table. There are pens, stationery, and letters scattered about the table. Your patient is awake, appears slightly pale, and is very anxious and restless.

Initial Assessment Findings
Mental Status—Alert, oriented, and anxious; obeys commands; GCS 15
Airway—Open and clear
Breathing—R 36 and shallow, unable to talk in complete sentences
       Lung sounds clear in upper lobes, diminished in bases
Circulation—Skin pale, cool, dry
       Radial pulse strong and irregular at 124
       BP 150/98
Chief Complaint—Can't catch her breath

Focused History
Events—Sudden onset of shortness of breath while writing letters, felt like she was going to die
Previous Illness—None
Current Health Status—No recent colds or infections; noticed tenderness 2 days ago in right calf but denies trauma to area
Allergies—None known
Medications—Birth control pills, denies recreational drug use

Focused Physical
Current set of VS—P irregular at 124, RR 36 and shallow, BP 150/98
Other Pertinent Findings—Right calf tender to palpation, no bruising, good range of motion. She is also complaining of numbness and tingling around her nose and mouth, and chest pressure. Pulse oximetry 90% on room air. Attempts to "talk her down" are unsuccessful.
Diagnostic Tests—None performed

ECG

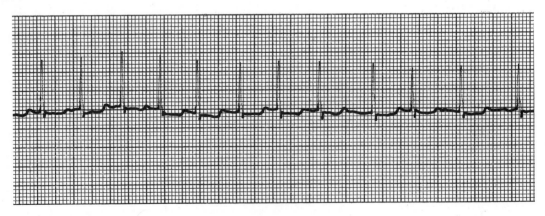

Figure 1-3

QUESTIONS

1. What is significant about Susan's history?

2. What body systems are affected?

3. What is the significance of Susan's impending sense of doom?

4. How can one tell the difference between uncomplicated anxiety and a true sense of impending doom?

5. What is the significance of Susan's inability to talk in complete sentences? What is a contributing cause?

6. What is the relationship, if any, of her tachycardia, hypertension, and cool, pale skin to her pulse oximetry of 90% on room air?

7. How severe is Susan's situation, and how do you determine this?

8. What is the immediate priority for Susan?

9. What is Susan's cardiac rhythm?

10. What is the significance of her rhythm?

11. How would you treat Susan?

12. What are possible causes of Susan's condition?

13. In the ED Susan's first set of blood gases showed a PaO_2 of 85, $PaCO_2$ of 30, pH of 7.5, and an O_2 sat. of 95%. What do these findings suggest regarding her field treatment? What do they suggest about her condition?

14. Is there a relationship between Susan's complaint of right calf pain, the use of birth control pills, and her present complaint; or are these unrelated?

15. What is the pathophysiology of the circumoral numbness and tingling caused by hyperventilation?

16. What is the difference, if any, between Susan and a patient who is suffering from hyperventilation syndrome?

17. Is there a relationship between Susan's cardiac rhythm and her pulmonary emboli?

18. Susan closely resembles a patient with hyperventilation syndrome. What is the worst thing that can happen if the possibility of pulmonary emboli is overlooked in the hyperventilating patient?

19. Are there any clear cut indicators of pulmonary emboli in the conscious patient?

QUESTIONS AND ANSWERS

1. What is significant about Susan's history?

Sudden onset of shortness of breath without exertion, associated with the feeling she was going to die; presence of "chest pressure;" on birth control pills; previous history of right calf tenderness in absence of trauma.

2. What body systems are affected?

Respiratory—R 36 and shallow, unable to talk in complete sentences, pulse oximetry 90% on room air

Cardiovascular—Tachycardic; skin cool and pale; hypertensive

CNS—anxiety (impending sense of doom)

3. What is the significance of Susan's impending sense of doom?

It may indicate the presence of a threat to life.

4. How can one tell the difference between uncomplicated anxiety and a true sense of impending doom?

It may be difficult, given the fact that many hyperventilation syndrome patients and those with panic attacks may also have a sense of impending doom. However, the ease with which the care provider can "talk the patient down" indicates a lesser probability for the presence of a life threatening problem. Of most help to the care provider is a careful and complete history and physical assessment along with the presence of an index of suspicion.

5. What is the significance of Susan's inability to talk in complete sentences? What is a contributing cause?

An inability to talk in complete sentences indicates an inadequate minute volume (minute volume = tidal volume × respiratory rate). A contributing cause is the rapid respiratory rate of 36. The rate is too fast to allow good tidal volume.

6. What is the relationship, if any, of her tachycardia, hypertension, and cool, pale skin to her pulse oximetry of 90% on room air?

A pulse oximetry value of 90% on room air in a 35 y/o with no history of chronic lung problems is an indicator of hypoxemia. Susan's hypoxemia is triggering a release of epinephrine and norepinephrine. This response is causing peripheral vasoconstriction, which increases preload, thereby increasing cardiac output. Additional effects include an increased heart rate and increased cardiac contractility, which further increase cardiac output, raising her blood pressure. Because there is no volume problem, the increase in cardiac output results in hypertension. The peripheral vasoconstriction is also responsible for her cool, pale skin.

7. How severe is Susan's situation and how do you determine this?

Susan is very hypoxic. Her vital signs, skin color, pulse oximetry value of 90% on room air, and sense of impending doom are all indicators of the severity of the situation.

8. What is the immediate priority for Susan?

Apply oxygen by mask, non–rebreather with reservoir at 15 lpm and recheck pulse oximetry to see if O_2 sats improve.

9. What is Susan's cardiac rhythm?

Atrial fibrillation with a rapid ventricular response. There is no discernible P wave, QRS is <0.10, and the ventricular response is >100.

10. What is the significance of her rhythm?

Atrial fib in a previously healthy, young person is unusual and needs to be explored. Her cardiac rhythm, as well as presence of hypoxemia, hypertension, and abnormal skin vitals, indicate the seriousness of Susan's situation.

11. **How would you treat Susan?**

Continue high flow oxygen; start an IV of crystalloid, either KVO or saline lock; and continue to monitor during transport. Some systems would allow use of sublingual nitro in an attempt to relieve the sensation of chest pressure.

12. **What are possible causes of Susan's condition?**

Pulmonary emboli, cardiac ischemia or hyperventilation syndrome are three possibilities. However, atrial fibrillation is unlikely in hyperventilation syndrome.

13. **In the ED Susan's first set of blood gases showed a PaO_2 of 85, $PaCO_2$ of 30, pH of 7.5, and an O_2 sat. of 95%. What do these findings suggest regarding her field treatment? What do they suggest about her condition?**

The high flow oxygen helped increase her O_2 saturation. She has a respiratory alkalosis (pH 7.5 and $PaCO_2$ of 30). However, her PaO_2 of 85 is low considering she is on high flow oxygen. This suggests that there is a perfusion (of alveoli) problem versus a ventilation (diffusion of oxygen and carbon dioxide) problem.

14. **Is there a relationship between Susan's complaint of right calf pain, the use of birth control pills, and her present complaint; or are these unrelated?**

Yes, there is a relationship. Calf pain in the absence of trauma may indicate the presence of a deep venous thrombosis (DVT). A piece of this thrombus (blood clot) can break off (an embolus) and travel to the lungs, resulting in pulmonary embolus. Use of birth control pills predisposes to DVT.

15. **What is the pathophysiology of the circumoral numbness and tingling caused by hyperventilation?**

Because hyperventilation causes excessive loss of carbon dioxide (referred to as "blowing off" CO_2), an increase in blood pH occurs, called respiratory alkalosis. Respiratory alkalosis causes a drop in ionized calcium (hypocalcemia), which is irritating to both the central and peripheral nevous systems. The irritation is marked by dizziness, confusion, tingling of extremities (paresthesias), and carpopedal spasms. A sensation of pressure in the chest may also occur. Hyperventilation resulting in an increase in blood pH, regardless of the underlying cause, will provoke these signs and symptoms.

The signs and symptoms of hyperventilation can occur in any condition with an increased respiratory rate—benign conditions such as panic attack, or life threatening conditions such as pulmonary emboli.

16. **What is the difference, if any, between Susan and a patient who is suffering from hyperventilation syndrome?**

A patient suffering from hyperventilation syndrome may appear to be very anxious and may have similar vital signs; however, pulse oximetry values are typically 99% to 100% and the cardiac rhythm is usually sinus tachycardia. Their anxiety is frequently managed by removing them from the environment and taking the time to "talk the patient down." The situation is often one where anxiety has been triggered, such as during an argument or any incident with extreme emotion. It may also be associated with recreational drug use, including use of alcohol.

Susan's episode was sudden and occurred when she was writing letters. There was no evidence of recreational drug use. Her pulse oximetry was 90% and Susan's anxiety is such that she cannot be talked down. Her cardiac rhythm is unusual for a person of her age with no previous history. Susan does have numbness and tingling in the circumoral area and has chest pressure that is consistent with respiratory alkalosis. Susan also has a history that is compatible with thrombus formation, for example, the use of birth control pills and calf tenderness in the absence of acute trauma.

17. **Is there a relationship between Susan's cardiac rhythm and her pulmonary emboli?**

Yes. Although ECG results are usually normal in early PE, the infarcted pulmonary area develops an inflammatory response that releases chemicals that can be irritating to cardiac muscle resulting in dysrhythmias. The more infarcted areas that are present, the greater the amount of chemicals of inflammation is present, and the greater the potential for cardiac irritation.

18. **Susan closely resembles a patient with hyperventilation syndrome. What is the worst thing that can happen if the possibility of pulmonary emboli is overlooked in the hyperventilating patient?**

   The patient will not get transported. Potential consequences of PE are sudden death, right-sided heart failure (cor pulmonale), pulmonary hypertension, and pulmonary infarction.

19. **Are there any clear-cut indicators of pulmonary emboli in the conscious patient?**

   No. Presenting signs/symptoms vary according to the age of the patient, preexisting respiratory condition, number and character of emboli, and area of lung infarcted. Pulmonary emboli can be mild, moderate, or severe. Thus a wide variety of presentations can occur. The most consistently common symptoms include: pleuritic chest pain, dyspnea, and anxiety. The most common signs include tachycardia, tachypnea, cough, syncope, hemoptysis and diaphoresis. The patient does not always have a complaint of chest pain. Shortness of breath or syncope may be the only symptom. Approximately 10% die within the first hour of onset of symptoms.

OUTCOME

Susan was admitted to the local hospital with the diagnosis of acute pulmonary emboli. Admission vital signs were unchanged. A 12-lead ECG confirmed the presence of atrial fibrillation. Anticoagulant therapy was started in the ED. A V/Q scan strongly suggested the presence of pulmonary emboli. A doppler study of her right calf showed evidence of deep vein thrombosis. Susan was admitted to the ICU and eventually had a full recovery with complete resolution of atrial fibrillation.

CASE 4

Dispatch: 08:00 hrs; Unconscious female, possible stroke

On Arrival: You find 76 y/o Margaret in bed. She appears pale and asleep. There are half-filled glasses of juice on her bed stand and a plate of half-eaten toast. Her daughter is present.

Initial Assessment Findings

Mental Status—She awakens to her name, is confused but obeys commands, and moves all extremities

Airway—Open and clear

Breathing—R 24, able to speak in complete sentences but seems out of breath
　　　Lung sounds rhonchi and wheezes R midaxillary line

Circulation—Skin pale, very warm, poor turgor
　　　Radial pulse irregular at 100 to 110
　　　BP 106/72

Chief Complaint—"I feel rotten"

Focused History

Events—Daughter called and there was no answer so she came over to check. She found her mother unresponsive in bed and called EMS.

Previous Illness—Cataract surgery a year ago, hypertension, and "heart problems"

Current Health Status—Has had a cough and has not been feeling well for about 5 days

Allergies—Morphine, sulfa

Medications—Furosemide (Lasix), digoxin (Lanoxin), hydrochlorothiazide, 1 aspirin per day, and Dimetapp (OTC for cough)

Focused Physical

Current set of VS—P 110 and irregular, R 24, BP 106/72

Other Pertinent Findings—Tenting of skin mid forehead and forearms, pulse oximetry 95%

Diagnostic Tests—Blood sugar 88, sitting up produced dizziness, and BP 86 systolic

ECG

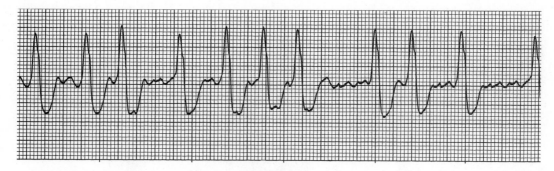

Figure 1-4

QUESTIONS

1. What is significant about Margaret's history?

2. What body systems are affected?

3. What is the significance of Margaret's being out of breath when she talks?

4. What is the significance of localized rhonchi and wheezes?

5. What is the most probable reason for Margaret's being out of breath?

6. Is there a relationship between her pale, very warm skin; poor turgor; tachycardia; and localized rhonchi/wheezing?

7. What is Margaret's Glasgow Coma Score?

8. What is/are the probable reason(s) for Margaret's confusion?

9. What is Margaret's cardiac rhythm?

10. What is significant about Margaret's cardiac rhythm?

11. What is the significance of the types of medication she is taking?

12. What is the significance of her history of hypertension, medications, and her current blood pressure?

13. How serious is Margaret's situation and how do you determine this?

14. Are there additional elements of her history or physical examination that would be useful?

15. What are the possible causes of Margaret's condition?

16. How would you treat Margaret?

17. What are the benefits to delivering a bolus of fluid versus maintaining a continuous drip rate in a patient like Margaret?

18. What part(s) of Margaret's assessment must be continually reassessed?

QUESTIONS AND ANSWERS

1. What is significant about Margaret's history?

She has a history of "heart problems," medications that are consistent with congestive heart failure, has had a cough and "not been feeling well" for 5 days, has been taking an over-the-counter drug containing an antihistamine.

2. What body systems are affected?

CNS—confusion

Respiratory—out of breath when talking, presence of unilateral rhonchi, and wheezes

Cardiovascular—skin pale and very warm, irregular pulse at 100 to 110

Integumentary—poor turgor

3. What is the significance of Margaret's being out of breath when she talks?

Inadequate tidal volume at rest. It is necessary to find out if this is normal or abnormal for her. For a patient at rest, always assume it is abnormal unless you find information to the contrary.

4. What is the significance of localized rhonchi and wheezes?

Localized rhonchi and wheezes are unlikely with pulmonary edema (if pulmonary edema is present sounds are usually bilateral) and may indicate aspiration, a site of infection (pneumonia), or that she has been lying on that side for a prolonged period (pooling of secretions).

5. What is the most probable reason for Margaret's being out of breath?

It is likely that the rhonchi and wheezes indicate a process that is narrowing the airways and interfering with her ability to maintain an adequate tidal volume.

6. Is there a relationship between her pale, very warm skin; poor turgor; tachycardia; and localized rhonchi/wheezing?

Her poor turgor is consistent with dehydration. Her pale skin suggests vasoconstriction or pooling of blood, and her very warm skin suggests a fever. Tachycardia is consistent both with fever from an infective process and dehydration. Localized rhonchi/wheezing in the presence of a cough and fever is highly suspicious of pneumonia. Her shortness of breath at rest suggests a hypoxemic process is going on that is causing a compensatory mechanism of increasing the respiratory rate and/or the tidal volume to increase the minute ventilation. The compensation is relatively successful since her pulse oximetry is 95%.

7. What is Margaret's Glasgow Coma Scale?

GCS 13 (3 Eye Opening, 4 Verbal Response, 6 Motor Response)

8. What is/are the probable reason(s) for Margaret's confusion?

Since Margaret is not systemically hypoxemic (pulse ox 95%), other common causes to suspect include fever and/or possible infection. Another possibility is the Dimetapp that, if not physician recommended, may be reacting with her medication or increasing the workload on her heart.

9. What is Margaret's cardiac rhythm?

Atrial fibrillation with a wide QRS and rapid ventricular response.

10. What is the significance of Margaret's cardiac rhythm?

Margaret's rhythm is consistent with her history of "heart problems" and medication. Her tachycardia is consistent with her hydration state, probable fever and hypoxia. It is likely that her rhythm is one that she has lived with for some time.

11. What is significant about the types of medication she is taking?

Furosemide (Lasix) and digoxin (Lanoxin) are typical medications for a person with congestive heart failure. Aspirin interferes with platelet aggregation and is taken as a prophylactic measure to prevent thrombus formation that may cause stroke or heart attack in susceptible patients. All three medications are reasonable to expect in a patient with atrial fibrillation. Hydrochlorothiazide is a common diuretic used to control blood pressure. Margaret's use of this drug is consistent with her history of hypertension. Dimetapp is an OTC antihistamine decongestant commonly taken for upper respiratory infections. It is unwise for cardiac patients to take cold preparations without consulting their physician. Many contain pseudoephedrine (a sympathomimetic) or other drugs that increase the workload of the heart and/or interfere with or compound the effects of prescription medications the patient is already on. OTC preparations that contain antihistamines may also predispose to dizziness and confusion, especially in the elderly.

12. **What is the significance of her history of hypertension, medications, and her current blood pressure?**
Margaret has a relatively low blood pressure for someone with a history of hypertension. This may be explained by the diuretics (Lasix and hydrochlorothiazide), fever and dehydration, which are probably all interrelated. This is further confirmed by the results of her sitting up that produced dizziness and a lower BP. However, the presence of hypotension in an elderly patient with signs and symptoms of infection and pulmonary involvement may indicate the more serious problem of sepsis.

13. **How serious is Margaret's situation, and how do you determine this?**
Margaret is very ill. Her orthostatic changes when she sat up, pulmonary involvement, and presence of fever are all suggestive of a potentially serious problem.

14. **Are there additional elements of her history or your physical that would be useful?**
Is her cough productive? What does her sputum look like? Has she been running a fever? If so, how high and what has she been taking for it? Has she been eating or drinking? How much and when? When was the last time she went to the bathroom to void? When was the last time she saw or talked to her physician? Does she take her medication regularly? Has she been taking it while she hasn't been feeling well?

15. **What are the possible causes of Margaret's condition?**
Pneumonia is highly likely because of localized wheezing and rhonchi, fever, and cough. Sepsis is indicated by orthostatic hypotension in the presence of signs of an infective process. An electrolyte imbalance is indicated by the dehydration, diuretics, and fever. Margaret could just have a URI complicated by dehydration, electrolyte imbalance, and aspiration. The likelihood of a medication reaction is also high.

16. **How would you treat Margaret?**
Oxygen by nasal cannula at 4 to 6 lpm (to increase pulse oximetry to 98% to 99%) in conjunction with a nebulizer treatment to bronchodilate. An IV of crystalloid, such as normal saline with a 200 to 300 cc bolus of fluid to support perfusion. Do not delay transport for administration of a fluid bolus that can be done en route. Continue to monitor her cardiac rhythm during transport.

17. **What are the benefits to delivering a bolus of fluid versus maintaining a continuous drip rate in a patient like Margaret?**
Unless a portable IV maintenance machine is available, maintaining drip rates in the back of a moving vehicle is very difficult. A bolus is more controlled and, in Margaret's case, assessing for immediate changes in pulse, respiratory rate and effort, and BP can be done en route. A bolus will also help to bring Margaret's fever down.

18. **What part(s) of Margaret's assessment must be continually reassessed?**
Margaret's level of consciousness, lung sounds (especially after a fluid bolus), respiratory rate and effort, and BP.

OUTCOME

Margaret was admitted to the hospital with a diagnosis of lobar pneumonia, dehydration, and electrolyte imbalance (low potassium). Her fever in the ED was 102° F. Antibiotics were begun and she was admitted to the ICU. She was dismissed to home seven days later.

BIBLIOGRAPHY

American Heart Association. Cummins R. O. (Ed.). (1994). *Advanced cardiac life support textbook.* Dallas, TX: American Heart Association.

American Heart Association. Chameides L., & Hazinski M. F. (Eds.). (1994). *Textbook of pediatric advanced life support.* Dallas, TX: American Heart Association.

Berkow R., & Fletcher A. J. (Eds.). (1992). *Merck manual of diagnosis and therapy.* Rahway, NJ: Merck Research Laboratories.

Bongard, F. S., & Sue, D. Y. (Eds.). (1994). *Current: Critical care, diagnosis and treatment.* Norwalk, CT: Appleton & Lange.

Callaham, M. (1989). Hypoxic hazards of traditional paper bag rebreathing in hyperventilating patients. *Annals of Emergency Medicine,* 18(6), 622-627.

Davey, S. S., & Huether, S. E. (1994). Alterations of Pulmonary Function. In K. L. McCance & S. E. Huether (Eds.). *Pathophysiology: The biologic basis for disease in adults and children* (2nd ed., pp. 1148-1190). St Louis, MO: Mosby.

DeVito, A. J., & Kleven, M. (1987). Dyspnea: Finding the cause, treating the symptoms. *RN* (6), 41-45.

Janson-Bjerklie, S., Ferketich, S., Benner, P., & Becker, G. (1992). Clinical markers of asthma severity and risk: Importance of subjective as well as objective factors. *Heart & Lung,* 21(3), 265-272.

Gyetvan M. C. (Ed.). (1994). *Nursing timesavers: Respiratory disorders.* Springhouse, PA: Springhouse Corporation.

Kelley, S. J. (1994). *Pediatric emergency nursing* (2nd ed.). Norwalk, CT: Appleton & Lange.

Martini, F. H., & Bartholomew, E. F. (1997). *Essentials of anatomy and physiology.* Upper Saddle River, NJ: Prentice Hall.

Pepe, P. E. (1996). Acute respiratory insufficiency. In A. L. Harwood-Nuss, C. H. Linden, R. Luten, J. A. Shepherd, & A. B. Wolfson (Eds.). *The clinical practice of emergency medicine* (2nd ed., pp. 636-640). Philadelphia, PA: Lippincott-Raven.

Robin, E. D., & McCauley, R. F. (1995). The diagnosis of pulmonary embolism: When will we ever learn? *Chest,* 107, 3-4.

Tierney, L. M., McPhee S. J., & Papadakis M. A. (eds). (1994). *Current: Medical diagnosis and treatment.* Norwalk, CT: Appleton & Lange.

West, J. B. (1992). *Pulmonary pathophysiology: The essentials* (5th ed.). Philadelphia, PA: Williams & Wilkins.

2

Neurologic Emergencies

OVERVIEW

Neurologic emergencies usually involve altered mental status; the exception is the problem that involves the peripheral nervous system. It is not uncommon to find a patient who doesn't realize various complaints are related and may only offer one complaint, downplaying or not recognizing the others. Nor is it unusual to find a patient with a neurologic problem where the paramedic has no idea what the origin of the problem is, but is able to recognize the body system(s) affected and act accordingly. In such cases, it is not important to make a diagnosis; it is more important to recognize the seriousness of the situation and treat appropriately. In any case, the patient with a neurologic problem is challenging and requires close attention to a careful assessment.

Anatomy, Physiology, and Pathophysiology

The central nervous system is composed of the cerebrum, the region where personality, skeletal muscle movement, and conscious thought reside; the cerebellum, where coordination of skeletal muscle and balance reside; the brain stem, where the vegetative functions, temperature regulation, and the origin of several cranial nerves reside; and the spinal cord, which is the connection between the periphery and the brain. Both the brain and spinal cord are covered by three membranes called the meninges—the dura mater, which is the outermost covering; the pia mater, which adheres to the surface of the brain; and the arachnoid membrane, which forms an extensive cushion of capillary vessels. All structures are bathed in cerebrospinal fluid (CSF), secreted by the choroid plexus in the ventricles of the brain. The CSF is reabsorbed by the arachnoid villi in the arachnoid layer of the meninges. If anything interferes with the reabsorption of CSF, it will accumulate, causing pressure to increase on the structures within the skull.

The cerebrum is divided into two hemispheres. The inner layers house the personality, memory, and higher thinking skills. The left hemisphere controls the right side of the body while the right hemisphere controls the left side of the body. This is because the connecting fibers cross in the spinal cord. Conditions that affect the cerebrum usually result in weakness or paralysis of skeletal muscles on the vertical plane, personality changes, changes in cognition, or awareness.

The cerebellum is under the posterior lobes of the cerebrum and regulates coordination, balance, and maintaining posture. Conditions that affect the cerebrum usually result in lack of coordination, ataxia, and loss of balance when posture changes.

The brain stem, consisting of the medulla, pons, and upper spinal cord, maintains the vegetative functions of respiration, blood pressure, digestion, and heart rate. The brain stem is also the origin for many of the cranial nerves. Pressure on the brain stem often results in signs and symptoms that are a result of cranial nerve pathology. Some examples are unequal or unreactive pupils resulting from pressure on the oculomotor nerve, or dysrhythmias, such as bradycardia or junctional rhythms, caused by pressure on the vagal nerve, and so on. Pressure on the brain stem can also result in brain stem reflexes, such as flexion or extension posturing.

The spinal cord serves as a reflex center and a pathway for conduction of impulses. It extends to the second lumbar vertebra. Lesions of the spinal cord may involve nervous deficits of the extremities on the horizontal plane, such as paraplegia or quadriplegia, or on the vertical plane as in lateral cord syndrome (Brown Séquard syndrome). With Brown Séquard syndrome the patient may have feeling present with motor deficit on one side and feeling absent but motor function present on the opposite side.

There are a number of other smaller structures of the brain, all equally important with specific functions. The speech centers are primarily located on the left side of the cerebrum, but for 15% of the population, one of the speech centers is located on the right side of the cerebrum. This is why a right-sided stroke victim frequently has an associated speech deficit.

The vomiting center and temperature-regulating center are in the hypothalamus, just above the brain stem. Pressure on this area can stimulate vomiting. Lesions in this area can also cause changes in body temperature. The temperature-regulating center is also affected by infection and infective processes. Fever is a "resetting of the hypothalamic thermostat" to a higher level. Exogenous pyrogens or endotoxins act on the hypothalamus to raise the set point and a fever occurs. During an infection, the presence of a fever will kill many microorganisms and inhibit the growth and replication of others.

The area that regulates consciousness, the reticular activating centers, sometimes referred to as the reticular activating system (RAS), is located throughout the brain stem and connects to the cerebrum. The RAS is the center of arousal, whereas the cerebrum is the center of awareness. Both must be functioning and connected for a person to be awake and aware. Anything that interferes with the connection between the RAS and the cerebrum will result in a patient who can be aroused but is not aware. Nonpurposeful movement and unintelligible words are usually observed. In some rare instances, the connection between the cerebrum and RAS is intact but not connected to the spinal cord. This is called "locked-in syndrome." Usually a result of head trauma, the only connection may be the cranial nerves. Communication is done through eye movement.

Cellular function in the CNS requires oxygen, glucose and thiamine, and waste removal. Insulin is not required for glucose to cross the cellular membrane of neurons. However, thiamine is required for the neurons to be able to process glucose efficiently for energy. Most people with reasonable diets ingest enough thiamine for normal brain metabolism and do not need supplements. However, those who do not eat regularly or who have poor dietary intake over a long period may need supplements of thiamine to use glucose efficiently. Lack of thiamine over a long period may result in Wernicke's encephalopathy (a temporary state) or Korsakoff's syndrome (a permanent state).

The brain cannot store glucose or glycogen like muscle cells can, nor can it go long periods without adequate oxygen. The first sign of hypoxia or hypoglycemia is altered mental status. The CNS is also very sensitive to pH imbalance. The respiratory centers are stimulated by concentrations of CO_2 in the blood (pH balance) that act on the chemoreceptors in the brain stem. The back-up system is concentration of O_2. When the CO_2 receptors are no longer effective because of prolonged elevations of CO_2, the O_2 system, referred to as hypoxic drive, takes over as the main stimulus to breathe.

The brain also creates its own chemicals for use by the brain cells. To ensure that these specialized chemicals stay within the brain and limit outside chemicals from getting into the brain, there is a blood-brain barrier at both the points of secretion and reabsorption of cerebrospinal fluid. Because the brain is very sensitive to abnormal concentrations and foreign substances, the blood-brain barrier serves as a protective mechanism. Anything that alters the balance of brain chemicals, glucose levels, thiamine levels, electrolyte balance, or levels of oxygen will often be noticed first by an alteration in mental status. Alterations or imbalances are sometimes very irritating to the brain, as is free blood (blood outside the vascular system) or infection. Any of these conditions may result in seizurelike activity in a patient with no history of seizure.

The peripheral nervous system functions as a relay system to and from the CNS. It relays sensory information to the brain, as well as relays messages to internal organs and motor movement to the skeletal muscles. There are three divisions: (1) the 12 cranial nerves that go directly from the brain to the target organs, (2) the somatic system that supplies the voluntary muscles or skeletal muscle, and (3) the autonomic system that supplies the involuntary muscles and most organs. The autonomic system is divided into the sympathetic and parasympathetic system. The sympathetic system has the adrenal glands and chemicals called catecholamines associated with it. Catecholamines are dopamine, norepinephrine, and epinephrine. They act on receptors known as alpha, beta, and dopaminergic receptors. There are two types of alpha receptors and two types of beta receptors. Both alpha and beta receptors are found in almost every organ system and structure in the body. The sympathetic system is the "fight or flight" system. The action of the sympathetic system in times of stress to the body cause many of the signs and symptoms associated with the patient who is in shock or a state of stress.

The parasympathetic system is represented by the vagal nerve. The vagal nerve is one of the cranial nerves that has its origin in the brain stem. It is a cable of nerves that branch off as the vagal nerve descends through the body. It supplies the atrium of the heart, the stomach, and fans out to supply the entire GI tract, as well as many other structures. The parasympathetic system is known as the control or balance to the sympathetic system.

The 12 cranial nerves are also a part of the peripheral nervous system and function as valuable assessment tools in helping isolate a patient problem. For example, the third cranial nerve comes off the top of the brain stem and regulates movement of the pupil of each eye. When pressure is exerted on the brain stem, paralyzing the oculomotor nerve, the resulting unilateral unequal or unreactive pupils in the presence of an altered mental status, is a sign of increased intracranial pressure.

Assessment and Treatment

Assessment of a patient with a nervous system problem focuses on the use of the Glasgow Coma Scale. This is a generic score of mental status. It roughly measures both arousal and awareness. Although not indicating the cause of the problem, it will indicate that a problem is present. Scores of 13 to 15 indicate a minor problem, 9 to 12 a moderate problem and scores of 8 or below indicate a severe problem with the CNS.

Pupil movement and reaction are also invaluable. The observance of unequal, unreactive pupils in the presence of an altered mental status strongly suggests increased intracranial pressure. Deviated pupils in the unresponsive patient indicate a lesion (such as a tumor or site of infection) of some sort. Dysconjugate gaze is associated with trauma to the orbit (commonly an orbital fracture) of the eye or a CNS dysfunction.

Increased intracranial pressure should be suspected when altered mental status exists with any of the following: unequal, unreactive pupils; posturing; and/or bradycardia, hypertension, and/or irregular respirations.

Combative, agitated patients should be evaluated for presence of hypoxia and hypoglycemia. Blood glucose levels should be checked in all patients with an altered mental status, especially if they have a history of diabetes.

Assessment should also include a pulse oximetry value to help assess for hypoxia, but it should not substitute for a good respiratory assessment. A fluid bolus in the case of low or borderline hypotension when combined with clear lung sounds and an altered mental status can help determine altered perfusion.

Assessment findings are also based on a knowledge of normal function and origin of the peripheral nerves. Peripheral nerves have a distinctive type of discomfort associated with them. Complaints of numbness, tingling, "burning" pain, or sensation are descriptive terms often used with peripheral nervous system problems. Movement along with strength and position sense is important assessment parameters of the nervous system. Pain associated with peripheral nerves may extend the length of the nerve, where the path of the nerve can literally be traced or may result in a "stocking-glove" effect with a horizontal line surrounding an extremity where the nervous deficit begins, usually extending to the end of the limb.

Causes of Neurologic Emergencies

Causes of neurologic emergencies are many and varied. A popular mnemonic, AEIOU TIPS, helps to indicate possible causes with the following associations: *A,* acidosis, alcohol; *E,* epilepsy, electrolyte; *I,* infection; *O,* overdose; *U,* uremia; *T,* trauma, tumors; *I,* insulin; *P,* psychosis, poisoning; *S,* stroke.

Treatment of Neurologic Emergencies

Administer oxygen, high flow if hypoxia suspected. Hyperventilation is no longer recommended for treatment of increased intracranial pressure. Good tidal volume between 500 to 800 ml is now stressed at a normal rate of 14 to 16. IV access with crystalloid at KVO rate unless hypotensive then repeated boluses until a systolic of at least 100 mmHg. If status present, diazepam 5 to 10 mg slow IV push until seizures stop. Lorazepam is another alternative for prevention of status. Administer D50W slow IV push if hypoglycemia is present. Glucagon 1 mg IM is an alternative for $D_{50}W$ if an IV is unable to be started. Correct perfusion-altering dysrhythmias if present. Keep the patient warm.

CASE 1

Dispatch: 11:00 hrs; Unconscious male in parking lot

On Arrival: In the parking lot of a local shopping center you find an elderly man, Harold, sitting on the pavement with his back against a car. The store manager is with him. Harold appears pale and seems to be sleeping. You see a rise and fall of his chest.

Initial Assessment Findings

Mental Status—He seems to wake up when you touch him and is verbally responsive but confused
Airway—Open and clear
Breathing—RR 24, talking in complete sentences; lung sounds reveal wheezing in posterior RLL
Circulation—Skin pale, cool, and dry
　　　　　Radial pulse regular and rapid at 150
　　　　　BP 90/62 with patient sitting
Chief Complaint—Just doesn't feel good

Focused History

Events—The store manager tells you Harold was walking to his car when he suddenly slumped to the ground. The store clerk, who was helping carry his purchase, eased him to the pavement and sat him with his back against the car.
Previous Illness—Hypertension
Current Health Status—Has had a "cold" for the last week but has not seen a physician
Allergies—None known
Medications—On Vasotec (enalapril) for hypertension, taking Robitussin for cough

Focused Physical

Current set of VS—P 150, RR 24, BP 90/62
Other Pertinent Findings—Skin has poor turgor and "tents;" pulse oximetry is 90%; Harold denies any pain
Diagnostic tests—Blood Sugar 110; fluid challenge with 300 ml NaCl led to a BP of 110 systolic and no change in lung sounds

ECG

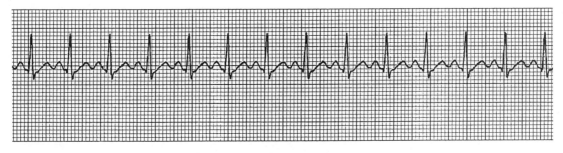

Figure 2-1

QUESTIONS

1. What is significant about Harold's history?

2. What body system(s) is/are affected?

3. What is Harold's Glasgow Coma Score?

4. What is significant about syncope followed by confusion?

5. What is the relationship between tachycardia and hypotension?

6. How does a history of hypertension relate to the findings of tachycardia and hypotension?

7. If the cause of hypotension was primarily cardiac related in nature (congestive failure), what other sign or symptom might you expect to find?

8. What is the significance of a localized area of wheezing?

9. What is the pathophysiology behind this patient's pale, cool, skin?

10. What is the significance of dry skin in the presence of tachycardia and hypotension?

11. Are there any additional parts of the history or physical examination that would help you?

12. What immediate actions, if any, would you take to begin treatment of Harold?

13. What is significant about the findings discovered in the focused physical and the diagnostic tests?

14. How would you describe Harold's ECG?

15. What are common causes of confusion in the elderly?

16. What are the possible causes of Harold's present condition?

17. How serious is Harold's current problem?

18. What is the most likely pathophysiology behind this patient's confusion?

19. How would you continue treatment?

20. How does the patient's age influence your decision making?

21. What should be taken care of before leaving the scene to ease a potential point of anxiety on the patient's part?

QUESTIONS AND ANSWERS

1. ***What is significant about Harold's history?***

   Onset was sudden; Harold has had a week-long "cold" for which he has not seen a physician, and he has a history of hypertension

2. ***What body system(s) is/are affected?***

   CNS—syncopal episode followed by confusion
   Cardiovascular—significant tachycardia that has persisted, hypotension, and skin changes (pale, cool, and dry)
   Respiratory—localized area of wheezing, posterior RLL

3. ***What is Harold's Glasgow Coma Score?***

   GCS 13 (4 confusion, 6 follows command, 3 eye opening on command)

4. ***What is significant about syncope followed by confusion?***

   Syncope followed by confusion suggests that there is another problem present.

5. ***What is the relationship between tachycardia and hypotension?***

   Tachycardia is often a compensatory mechanism for hypotension. However, when the rate becomes too fast to allow for adequate ventricular filling it can actually be the cause of hypotension. Harold's tachycardia is borderline for causing hypotension in a previously healthy person.

6. ***How does a history of hypertension relate to the findings of tachycardia and hypotension?***

   Chronic hypertension causes an increased workload on the heart. Combined with diminished blood flow through coronary arteries (caused by changes in the structure of the vessels themselves), this increased workload leads to left ventricular hypertrophy and myocardial ischemia. The end result is left heart failure eventually becoming congestive heart failure.

   Given this background there are several factors to keep in mind, (1) any change that would normally stimulate an increase in heart rate, may not be tolerated by a heart in failure, thus leading to hypotension; and (2) overdoses of antihypertensives can lead to dehydration and/or hypotension depending on the type of antihypertensive.

7. ***If the cause of hypotension was primarily cardiac related in nature (congestive failure), what other sign or symptom might you expect to find?***

   Evidence of bilateral rales. Wheezing should be present.

8. ***What is the significance of a localized area of wheezing?***

   Localized wheezing is more likely when aspiration of a foreign body has occurred or when an infection, such as pneumonia, is present or a pulmonary emboli has occurred.

9. ***What is the pathophysiology behind this patient's pale, cool skin?***

   Pale, cool skin indicates a lack of normal blood supply to the area. Its presence in this patient is consistent with vasoconstriction secondary to hypotension.

10. ***What is the significance of dry skin in the presence of tachycardia and hypotension?***

    May be a factor of the effect of dehydration or certain medications that interfere with normal sweating mechanisms, or the fact that elderly persons do not always sweat in response to epinephrine/norepinephrine release. Dehydration is a distinct possibility for Harold.

11. ***Are there any additional parts of the history or physical examination that would help you?***

    When do you normally take your medication? Did you take it today? When was the last time you took it? Describe "not feeling good." When did not feeling good start?

12. ***What immediate actions, if any, would you take to begin treatment of Harold?***

    Oxygen by nasal cannula at 2 to 4 lpm and reassess pulse oximetry, adjusting accordingly; initiate an IV of normal saline.

13. ***What is significant about the findings discovered in the focused physical and the diagnostic tests?***

    Harold has evidence of dehydration, which could explain his hypotension and contribute to his tachycardia. The fluid challenge of 300 ml resulting in an increase of systolic pressure, without lung involvement, suggests that lack of fluid volume is at least part of his problem. However, Harold's localized wheezing and relatively low pulse oximetry value are indicators of pulmonary involvement. Hypoxemia together with his dehydration is most likely the causes of his tachycardia.

14. How would you describe Harold's ECG?

This is a sinus tachycardia.

15. What are common causes of confusion in the elderly?

Stroke, hypoxia, infection (pneumonia and urinary tract infections), hypotension, acidosis, low blood sugar, acute MI, seizure, and diabetes-related conditions are all common causes of confusion.

16. What are the possible causes of Harold's present condition?

Harold could have suffered a transient ischemic attack, an episode of cardiac dysrhythmia, have an infection or be septic, be suffering from malnutrition or electrolyte imbalance, or he could just be dehydrated.

17. How serious is Harold's current problem?

Harold is presently compensating and is relatively stable. However, there is no guarantee that he will stay that way.

18. What is the most likely pathophysiology behind this patient's confusion?

Hypoxemia and hypotension could explain the confusion, especially in a patient who is used to higher systolic pressures (history of hypertension). Hypotension leads to lack of perfusion in the brain. The elderly are also very sensitive to hypoxemia. Harold's low oxygen saturations and hypotension are causes for concern.

19. How would you continue treatment?

You should adjust concentration of oxygen according to response, and a bronchodilator for his localized wheezing may be indicated. If you decide to use a bronchodilator, choose one with relatively little cardiac effect. The choice of whether or not to use a bronchodilator will depend on the patient's response to earlier treatment. Monitor boluses of IV crystalloid until BP approaches normal. Maintain with careful assessment of respiratory status.

20. How does the patient's age influence your decision making?

The elderly, like the neonate, do not respond to pathologic processes in the same way as other patients. Because of changes in mental status and changes in nerve conduction, they do not always perceive pain as younger patients do. Age should alert you to specific problems that guide your treatment, specific assessment and choice of diagnostic procedures. For the elderly, "silent" (painless) internal bleeds, stroke, dysrhythmias, and acute MI are causes of syncope.

21. What should be taken care of before leaving the scene to ease a potential point of anxiety for the patient?

Harold's purchases should be placed inside his vehicle and the car locked. His keys should be kept in his possession. The manager of the store should be notified of your actions.

OUTCOME

At the hospital, a detailed history from the family led the physician to suspect aspiration pneumonia. Harold had a fever of 101° F and was severely dehydrated. After receiving an additional liter of crystalloid, his heart rate decreased to 98 by monitor and BP stabilized at 138/86. Harold had swallowing studies done and a swallowing defect was discovered. The defect was likely the result of an unrecognized stroke. He received swallowing and speech therapies and was dismissed to home.

CASE 2

Dispatch: 18:30 hrs; 67 y/o female, dizziness

On Arrival: You find a 67 y/o female, Mavis, lying on the living room couch. She appears to be sleeping and looks pale.

Initial Assessment Findings

Mental Status—No verbal response, flexes R arm to pain, no eye opening
Airway—Open and clear
Breathing—RR irregular at 14
Circulation—Skin normal color and dry
        Radial pulse, slightly irregular at 32
        BP 160/80
Chief Complaint—No verbal response

Focused History

Events—Mavis' husband states she has had a headache for the last several days. Today she complained of a headache also but vomited several times and got so dizzy she just couldn't walk anymore so she lay down. He came to ask her if she wanted dinner and couldn't wake her up.
Previous Illness—Cataract surgery L eye, hypertension
Current Health Status—Healthy except headache for last several days
Allergies—Penicillin
Medications—Hydro Diuril (hydrochlorothiazide)

Focused Physical

Current Set of VS—P 32 and irregular, RR 14 irregular, BP 160/80, pulse oximetry 97%
Other Pertinent Findings—Left pupil unreactive, cataract surgery L eye
Diagnostic Tests—None performed

ECG

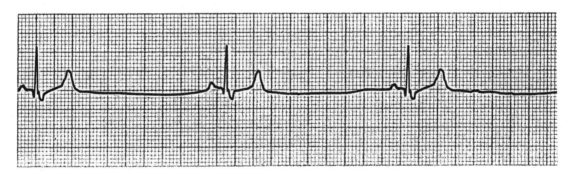

Figure 2-2

1. What is significant about Mavis' history?

2. What body system(s) are affected?

3. What is Mavis' Glasgow Coma Score?

4. What is the significance of posturing (flexing right arm to pain)?

5. What is the relationship between posturing and a history of headache with hypertension?

6. Is there a relationship between the irregular respirations, bradycardia, and blood pressure?

7. What is the most probable cause of Mavis' irregular respirations, bradycardia, and BP?

8. How serious is this patient's situation?

9. What immediate actions would you take, if any, to treat Mavis?

10. What are the pros and cons of hyperventilation in a patient with increasing intracranial pressure?

11. Is there any additional information from the history or physical examination that could help you?

12. What is significant about the findings in the focused physical?

13. How would you describe her ECG?

14. Is any treatment required for her rhythm?

15. How would you continue treatment?

16. What are the possible causes of Mavis' current condition?

17. What is Mavis at risk for?

QUESTIONS AND ANSWERS

1. What is significant about Mavis' history?

Headache for past several days, hypertension, and dizziness leading to present coma

2. What body system(s) are affected?

CNS—coma, posturing
Cardiac—bradycardia
Respiratory—irregular respirations

3. What is Mavis' Glasgow Coma Score?

GCS 5 (1 no eye opening, 3 flexion to pain, 1 no verbal response)

4. What is the significance of posturing (flexing right arm to pain)?

Posturing suggests increased intracranial pressure.

5. What is the relationship between posturing and a history of headache with hypertension?

Chronic hypertension can cause intracranial bleeding, which would lead to increased intracranial pressure (ICP) and posturing.

6. Is there a relationship between the irregular respirations, bradycardia, and blood pressure?

These are classic signs of Cushing's syndrome to increased ICP.

7. What is the most probable cause of Mavis' irregular respirations, bradycardia, and BP?

Pressure on the brain stem (probably from the cerebrum, above the tentorium). The respiratory centers are in the upper portion of the brain stem. Increasing pressure on these respiratory centers causes progressive changes in respiratory patterns, from early Cheyne-Stokes respiration (often recognized as irregular respirations) to central neurogenic hyperventilation to Biot's respiration pattern (clustering) to apneustic or agonal respirations. Eventually respiratory arrest will occur.

Pressure on the brain stem also puts pressure on the vagal nerve. The vagal nerve innervates the atria of the heart. Pressure on the vagal nerve inhibits the SA and AV nodes in the heart causing bradycardias and junctional beats.

As intracranial pressure (ICP) increases beyond normal levels, the body compensates by increasing the mean arterial pressure (MAP) to maintain adequate cerebral perfusion pressure (CPP). (CPP = MAP − ICP.) When ICP increases beyond all compensatory mechanisms, decreasing CPP will reduce blood flow to the brain causing ischemia. Brain death occurs when ICP is approximately equal to the MAP, because CPP approaches zero (i.e., little or no blood flow to the brain).

8. How serious is this patient's situation?

This situation is potentially life threatening.

9. What immediate actions would you take, if any, to treat Mavis?

She needs airway control and ventilatory assistance with a BVM and reservoir at 15 lpm. An IV with either a saline lock or KVO crystalloid can be started en route.

10. What are the pros and cons of hyperventilation in a patient with increasing intracranial pressure?

Hyperventilation used to be the mainstay of treatment for the patient with increasing intracranial pressure. The goal was to decrease the levels of carbon dioxide, which would then cause vasoconstriction, thus reducing volume and therefore intracranial pressure. Hyperventilation also raises the pH, which absorbs the acidosis-causing free radicals produced by injured brain cells. However, the danger of hyperventilation is the same vasoconstriction that reduces volume also reduces circulation to injured brain cells. This reduced circulation promotes ischemia that, in turn, enhances cellular edema.

Currently the goal of treatment is to promote cerebral perfusion, and the goal of ventilation is to provide a good tidal volume. Good tidal volumes ensure adequate oxygenation while providing for maximal exhalation of carbon dioxide. This can be done with a BVM at normal ventilatory rates of 14 to 18.

11. Is there any additional information from the history or physical examination that could help you?

How often does she take her medication? Did she take it today? When did she last see her doctor? Did she describe the location of her headache? Did she have any difficulty walking or standing?

12. What is significant about the findings in the focused physical?

Pupil evaluation of the left eye is not accurate because of her history of cataract surgery

13. How would you describe her ECG?

Sinus rhythm with premature atrial or junctional beats.

14. Is any treatment required for her rhythm?

No, the rhythm is a result of increased ICP and does not require any pharmacologic treatment.

15. How would you continue treatment?

Depending on the response to treatment, continue to ventilate at 14 to 18 per minute with good tidal volume and maintain her IV at KVO or use a saline lock.

16. What are the possible causes of Mavis' current condition?

Mavis' signs and symptoms, together with her history, suggest a hemorrhagic stroke.

17. What is Mavis at risk for?

Vomiting—increased ICP puts pressure on the vomiting center, as well as the vagal nerve, which also innervates the stomach and the rest of the GI tract.

Seizures—free blood in brain tissue is highly irritating, predisposing to seizures.

OUTCOME

Mavis was immediately taken to CT scan where an intracerebral bleed resulting from an aneurysm was discovered. She was taken to surgery where the aneurysm was repaired and the bleed was evacuated. She was sedated, paralyzed, and placed on a ventilator with an ICP monitor. After 3 days she was allowed to wake up, and 10 days later she was transferred to a rehabilitation unit. Three months later she was dismissed to home with weakness in her L hand as her only deficit.

CASE 3

Dispatch: 15:45 hrs, 76 y/o male, possible stroke

On Arrival: You find 76 y/o Ivan sitting on the living room couch. He appears awake and is focusing on your approach. His color looks normal. His wife is present.

Initial Assessment Findings

Mental Status—Awake, verbally responsive and oriented, GCS 15
Airway—Open, speech clear
Breathing—RR 16
Circulation—Skin normal color, dry
   Radial pulse regular at 78
   BP 146/82
Chief Complaint—"I can't get up right"

Focused History

Events—After getting up from an afternoon nap Ivan's wife states he tried to get up but fell; Ivan tells you he can't get up "right."
Previous Illness—Total hip replacement 2 years ago, hypertension
Current Health Status—Relatively healthy
Allergies—None known
Medications—Hydro Diuril (hydrochlorothiazide)

Focused Physical

Current VS—P 78, RR 16, BP 146/82, pulse ox 98%
Other Pertinent Findings—Does not move left leg on command, left arm moves weakly, unable to grasp; states he doesn't know where his left leg and arm came from; moves right arm and leg at will; lung sounds clear
Diagnostic tests—Blood Sugar 110

ECG

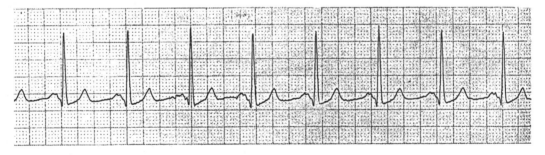

Figure 2-3

QUESTIONS

1. What is significant about Ivan's history?

2. What body system(s) is/are affected?

3. What is the relationship between Ivan's history and his complaint?

4. How serious is Ivan's situation?

5. What additional information from his history or physical examination would be helpful?

6. How would you describe Ivan's ECG?

7. What immediate actions, if any, would you take to treat this patient?

8. What is significant about the findings in the focused physical?

9. What part of Ivan's brain is affected?

10. Why isn't Ivan's speech affected?

11. What are possible causes of Ivan's current condition?

12. What is your treatment?

13. How does hypertension predispose to stroke?

14. What type of stroke did Ivan most likely have and why?

15. What is significant about Ivan's statement that he doesn't know where his left leg and arm came from?

16. What is Ivan at risk for?

17. How does Ivan's stroke compare to Mavis' stroke (Case 2)?

QUESTIONS AND ANSWERS

1. *What is significant about Ivan's history?*

   History of hypertension, unable to walk without falling.

2. *What body system(s) is/are affected?*

   CNS—unable to move left side on command

3. *What is the relationship between Ivan's history and his complaint?*

   Hypertension predisposes to stroke.

4. *How serious is Ivan's situation?*

   Recent studies suggest that there is a 3 hour window between the time of symptom onset until the time of treatment, for treatment to be effective. The onset of symptoms is considered to be the last time the patient was seen and was normal. For Ivan this would be the time he lay down for his nap. While Ivan is in stable condition, timely treatment is important.

5. *What additional information from his history or physical examination would be helpful?*

   What time did he lie down for his nap? Has he taken his medication? How often does he take it? When did he last see his doctor? What is his mental status? Is Ivan confused?

6. *How would you describe Ivan's ECG?*

   Sinus rhythm, normal P wave, normal p-r interval, QRS < 0.10, every QRS has a P wave.

7. *What immediate actions, if any, would you take to treat this patient?*

   Oxygen by nasal cannula at 2 to 4 lpm; cardiac monitor; IV crystalloid KVO or saline lock.

8. *What is significant about the findings in the focused physical?*

   The onset of symptoms was after his nap. Onset of symptoms during or after sleep is typical of an ischemic stroke caused by a thrombus.

9. *What part of Ivan's brain is affected?*

   His right cerebral hemisphere is affected. The left hemisphere controls the right side of the body and the right hemisphere controls the left side of the body.

10. *Why isn't Ivan's speech affected?*

    For 85% of the population the speech centers are located in the left hemisphere. Since Ivan's right hemisphere is affected, he has a greater likelihood that his speech center won't be affected.

11. *What are possible causes of Ivan's current condition?*

    The most likely cause is a stroke, although hypoglycemia can also present in a similar fashion.

12. *What is your treatment?*

    Continue oxygen therapy and maintain IV access.

13. *How does hypertension predispose to stroke?*

    Over time, an increase in systolic pressure produces trauma to the inner layer of blood vessels (tunica intima) and lipid deposits occur, forming plaques. Plaques often break through the intima where their rough surface causes blood clots to develop. Both thrombus or embolus formation can lead to an ischemic stroke.

    Hypertension also weakens vessel walls, predisposing to aneurysm formation and rupture of vessels. Small cerebral penetrating arteries and arterioles are responsible for hemorrhages in these strokes.

14. *What type of stroke did Ivan most likely have and why?*

    Probably ischemic—the onset was after a nap or period of rest. His vital signs and level of consciousness are relatively stable, and he has no complaints of headache or signs of central nervous system irritability (suggestive of intracerebral hemorrhage).

15. *What is significant about Ivan's statement that he doesn't know where his left leg and arm came from?*

Right-sided ischemic strokes may result in a patient not recognizing body parts on the left side. If that is the case, they often try to walk, not recognizing or realizing that their leg doesn't work. They may not recognize that the affected extremity is theirs, but they do recognize that there is a problem.

16. *What is Ivan at risk for?*

By not recognizing his body parts, Ivan is at risk for falling and suffering further injury. As long as his speech is clear, Ivan can swallow. If his speech would become affected he would be at risk for aspiration. He is also at risk for extension of the stroke, and given the relatively small window for treatment, even with treatment he may have some permanent damage unless this is a TIA/RIND (transient ischemic attack/reversible ischemic neurologic deficit).

17. *How does Ivan's stroke compare to Mavis' stroke (Case 2)?*

Ivan's stroke was ischemic, and Mavis' was hemorrhagic. Much about these two types of strokes is similar. Cerebral edema is often present surrounding the area of infarct or hemorrhage. There is increased cellular metabolism resulting in increased acid production and increased production of free radicals. These in turn, disturb calcium ion flow leading to secondary damage and neuronal death. New treatments for the stroke victim are aimed toward alleviating or interrupting these processes.

In terms of presentation, however, there are differences between the two types of stroke. Ischemic strokes usually occur at rest and have no pain. In contrast, hemorrhagic strokes are more frequently related to activity with headache as the chief complaint. Ischemic stroke victims are usually conscious with complaints of weakness, dizziness, paralysis or numbness, sudden blurred or decreased vision of one or both eyes, and difficulty speaking or understanding simple statements. If an ischemic stroke is massive, consciousness may be affected. Hemorrhagic stroke patients frequently present with a history of headache, altered mental status, and signs and symptoms of increasing intracranial pressure. Seizures are more common with hemorrhagic strokes because of the irritation from free blood and toxins from the hematoma itself. To date, however, there is no reliable way to differentiate between the two types of stroke except with a CT scan or MRI.

OUTCOME

Ivan suffered an ischemic stroke. He was admitted to the hospital and was given neuroprotective medications. He was started in physical therapy almost immediately and returned home 10 days later with some residual weakness of the left lower leg and instructions to take aspirin every day.

CASE 4

Dispatch: 16:15 hrs; 35 y/o unconscious female

On Arrival: You find 35 y/o Kiesha in bed. She appears to be somewhat pale and looks like she is sleeping. You notice a strong odor of alcohol.

Initial Assessment Findings

Mental Status—Unresponsive to voice and pain
Airway—Open and clear
Breathing—RR 18 and shallow, lung sounds have rales in both bases
Circulation—Skin warm, dry
        Color pale
        Radial pulse regular at 80
        BP 106/60
Chief Complaint—Unresponsive to all stimuli

Focused History

Events—Kiesha was out with the girls last night, came home around 4:00 AM, told her boyfriend she had too much to drink and to let her sleep in the morning. When he got home from work he discovered that she missed her dialysis treatment and tried to wake her. When he couldn't, he called EMS.
Previous Illness—Insulin dependent diabetic with kidney failure and on hemodialysis, also has hypertension
Current Health Status—Described as "OK," she has dialysis 3 times per week
Allergies—Sensitivity to morphine
Medications—Insulin and Vasotec (enalapril)

Focused Physical

Current VS—P 80, RR 18, BP 106/60
Other Physical Findings—Shunt in R arm, pupils equal and sluggish, abdomen soft, pulse oximetry 91%
Diagnostic Tests—Blood Sugar reads "LOW"

ECG

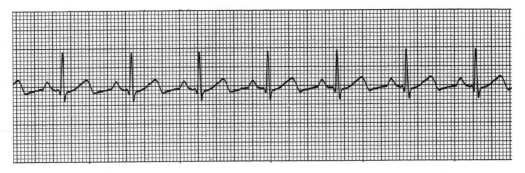

Figure 2-4

QUESTIONS

1. What is significant about Kiesha's history?

2. What body system(s) is/are affected?

3. What is Kiesha's Glasgow Coma Score?

4. What is the relationship between rales, a missed dialysis treatment, and being in a supine or prone position for 12 hours?

5. What effect does alcohol have on the brain, GI tract, renal system, and vascular tone?

6. How would you describe her ECG?

7. What effect does alcohol have on sugar metabolism?

8. What are the effects of kidney failure on kidney function and on the cardiovascular system?

9. How does Kiesha's kidney failure change the normal effect of alcohol on the renal system?

10. What are possible effects of a missed dialysis treatment on the brain? What are the probable effects on the cardiovascular system?

11. How serious is Kiesha's situation?

12. What are the possible causes of Kiesha's current condition?

13. What immediate actions, if any, would you take to treat Kiesha?

14. What is significant about starting an IV in a dialysis patient?

15. What are the potential consequences of a blood sugar that does not register or reads "LOW"?

16. In the absence of an IV, what are the options for treating hypoglycemia?

17. How would you treat her?

18. What is the action of furosemide in a dialysis patient?

19. What is Kiesha at risk for?

20. Kiesha's pulse was not tachycardic nor was her blood pressure very low. What are possible explanations?

QUESTIONS AND ANSWERS

1. What is significant about Kiesha's history?

She is an insulin dependent diabetic who has not eaten or taken insulin. She is on dialysis and missed her treatment today. There has been significant alcohol intake. She has been unresponsive approximately 12 hours.

2. What body system(s) is/are affected?

CNS—unconscious and unresponsive
Respiratory—bilateral rales
Renal—missed dialysis treatment

3. What is her Glasgow Coma Score?

GCS 3 (1 no eye opening, 1 no motor response, 1 no verbal response)

4. What is the relationship between rales, a missed dialysis treatment, and being in a supine or prone position for 12 hours?

Dialysis is a method for eliminating waste products and extra fluid from the body. When a dialysis treatment is missed, extra fluid (along with waste products) continues to build up. When a person is in one position for an extended period, excess fluid tends to gravitate to the lowest point. Kiesha's rales are most likely a result of excess fluid finding a point to settle.

5. What effect does alcohol have on the brain, GI tract, renal system, and vascular tone?

Brain—Alcohol readily crosses the cellular membrane in all body systems including the brain. In the brain it acts as a suppressant and irritant. Cognition is slowed, reaction time delayed and awareness suppressed. Eventually consciousness can be impaired significantly enough to produce coma. The vomiting center may also be stimulated, and along with the GI irritation, places the patient at risk for vomiting with aspiration. The respiratory center is depressed causing respirations to slow in rate and decrease in depth causing inadequate tidal volume. Since the brain stem is affected so is the vagal nerve, causing a slower heart rate. Regular ingestion of alcohol increases the incidence of unprovoked seizures as does withdrawal of alcohol.
GI tract—Alcohol acts as an irritant on the lining of the GI tract often stimulating vomiting. Long-term effects can cause gastritis. Esophageal varices, pancreatitis, and cirrhosis are additional risks of long term use.
Renal system—Alcohol suppresses ADH (antidiuretic hormone or vasopressin) contributing to frequent urination and predisposing to dehydration.
Vascular system—Alcohol promotes vasodilation partly from central vasomotor depression and partly from a direct vasodilating action on blood vessels. This leads to hypotension when at rest and contributes to hypothermia (along with depression of the central temperature-regulating mechanism) in cold weather.

6. How would you describe her ECG?

Sinus rhythm

7. What effect does alcohol have on sugar metabolism?

Alcohol enhances the metabolism of sugar, rapidly depleting stores, especially in the diabetic patient.

8. What are the effects of kidney failure on kidney function and on the cardiovascular system?

Kidney function—Kiesha has chronic renal failure (on dialysis). Because there are two types of renal failure, she may or may not produce much urine.
Cardiovascular system—chronic renal failure predisposes to congestive heart failure as a result of fluid overload. Cardiac dysrhythmias also may occur because of electrolyte imbalances, usually from potassium.

9. How does Kiesha's kidney failure change the normal effect of alcohol on the renal system?

Alcohol may not stimulate urine production.

10. **What are probable effects of a missed dialysis treatment on the brain? What are the probable effects on the cardiovascular system?**

    A missed dialysis treatment will cause waste products to build up along with fluid overload. A build-up in waste products may irritate the brain and/or alter mental status.

    A fluid overload will lead to congestive failure. A build-up in waste products may irritate cardiac muscle leading to cardiac dysrhythmias.

11. **How serious is Kiesha's situation?**

    Very serious, she is comatose and there are several potential causes.

12. **What are the possible causes of Kiesha's current condition?**

    Kiesha most likely has a combination of causes. A build-up of waste products could lead to altered mental status. However, missing just one dialysis treatment is not a likely cause of a comatose state. High alcohol intake could contribute to a comatose state and alcohol poisoning might even be present. Because alcohol is a general body anesthetic, Kiesha could have hit her head and suffered a subdural or subarachnoid bleed. As a known diabetic who has significant alcohol intake, Kiesha is especially prone to hypoglycemia, which could also lead to a coma. This is likely since her blood glucose level reads "LOW." The combination of significant alcohol intake and hypoglycemia are extremely likely possibilities. However, it is also possible that there is another cause, unrelated to her dialysis.

13. **What immediate actions, if any, would you take to treat Kiesha?**

    Secure her airway. Kiesha cannot protect her own. The movement caused by oral intubation may be enough to stimulate a response. Begin ventilating with a BVM with oxygen reservoir at 15 lpm at 16 to 20 breaths/min with good tidal volumes. IV access is also necessary.

14. **What is significant about starting an IV in a dialysis patient?**

    Do NOT start the IV in the shunt. The only exception is in a life-threatening situation. Look for an antecubital vein or an external jugular vein. You decide if this situation would justify using the shunt site given your situation and your transport times.

15. **What are the potential consequences of a blood sugar that does not register or reads "LOW"?**

    The brain cannot function and will die without sugar. The brain stores very little sugar. Therefore the rule of thumb is to consider hypoglycemia, which results in coma, a life-threat.

16. **In the absence of an IV, what are options for treating hypoglycemia?**

    There are two. One is to use glucose gel. Place a teaspoonful in the buccal pouch (between the cheek and gum). It will be directly absorbed through the mucous membrane. Potential consequences include aspiration. This should be controlled if the patient is intubated. The other option is to use glucagon as an intramuscular or subcutaneous injection. To be effective, glucagon depends on adequate liver stores of glycogen. Be aware that alcoholics frequently suffer from depleted glycogen stores. A potential side effect of glucagon is vomiting.

17. **How would you treat her?**

    Oral intubation with hyperventilation at a rate of 26 to 30 (because of the presence of pulmonary edema), IV crystalloid at KVO rate, administer 25 gm of D_{50} and recheck blood sugar. Consider furosemide for pulmonary edema if pulse oximetry did not improve with hyperventilation. Consider repeating 25 gms of D_{50} and naloxone 0.4 to 2.0 mg, slow IV push if no improvement in mental status. Keep in mind that naloxone may have no effect. She may not have taken any narcotics.

18. **What is the action of furosemide in a dialysis patient?**

    In some kidney failure patients, furosemide may actually stimulate urine production, though that is more common with higher doses. Furosemide has two effects: pulmonary capillary bed vasodilation is almost immediate while urine production takes about 15 to 20 minutes for accumulation in the bladder to be perceived. For Kiesha, furosemide would have been an acceptable option for the vasodilatory effect in the lungs.

19. What is Kiesha at risk for?

Kiesha is at risk for aspiration (without intubation), seizures, and cardiac dysrhythmias.

20. Kiesha's pulse was not tachycardic nor was her blood pressure very low. What are possible explanations?

Alcohol does have an irritant effect on the vagal nerve, stimulating bradycardia when at rest. However, hypoglycemia has a definite tachycardic effect, as does hypoxia. It is also possible that the combination of Kiesha's low blood sugar and extremely high blood alcohol (0.145 mg/dl 14 hrs after ingestion) overrode normal tachycardic responses. Because we don't know what Kiesha's normal heart rate was, we can only speculate. The fact that Kiesha was not hypotensive is probably due to her kidney failure. She did not urinate so fluid stayed in the vascular space.

OUTCOME

Kiesha was intubated and hyperventilated with a BVM, an IV was started in the antecubital space of the opposite arm of the shunt, and 25 gms of 50% dextrose given. There was no response to the dextrose. On arrival at the hospital her blood sugar was 20. Two more amps of dextrose were given before Kiesha was responding to pain by withdrawal. Her blood alcohol was 0.145 mg/dl (approximately 14 hours after coming home). She was taken directly to the dialysis unit. After dialysis and 100 gms of D_{50}, Kiesha was alert and oriented. During her stay in the hospital, Kiesha was diagnosed with cirrhosis of the liver. Eventually Kiesha recovered enough to be sent home.

Kiesha's diagnosis of cirrhosis helps explain her extremely low blood sugar. Alcohol causes chronic inflammation of the liver, which stimulates fatty infiltrates known as cirrhosis. The process of cirrhosis depletes existing glycogen stores, predisposing to hypoglycemia. Without adequate stores of glycogen, the body has difficulty maintaining blood sugar levels in states of crisis.

CASE 5

Dispatch: 14:00 hrs; 30 y/o male, possible seizure

On Arrival: You find 30 y/o Henry, fully dressed, lying on his side across his bed in his attic room. He is sitting up on the bed, awake, and looks somewhat disheveled. You note blood-tinged saliva drooling from the corner of his mouth.

Initial Assessment Findings

Mental Status—Verbally responds but is confused, GCS 14
Airway—Open, bloody saliva present, tongue abraded
Breathing—Regular at 18 breaths/min
Circulation—Skin hot and dry
Radial pulse rapid and regular at 124
BP 140/84
Chief Complaint—Headache

Focused History

Events—Was found in active seizure by roommate who then called EMS
Previous Illness—Epileptic
Current Health Status—Has had a "cold" for last several days
Allergies—None known
Medication—Tegretol (carbamazepine)

Focused Physical

Current VS—P 124, RR 18, BP 140/84
Other Pertinent Findings—Lung sounds have basilar wheezes bilaterally
Diagnostic Tests—BS 90

ECG

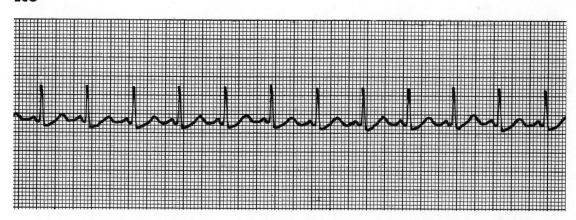

Figure 2-5

QUESTIONS

1. What is significant about Henry's history?

2. What body systems are affected?

3. How would you describe the ECG?

4. What is the relationship between Henry's history of seizure and his vital signs?

5. Henry's roommate states he found Henry in a seizure. How does your physical assessment support the conclusion that a grand mal seizure did occur?

6. After a grand mal seizure, what might you expect the skin temperature, color, and moisture to be? How do Henry's compare?

7. What are the possible causes of wheezing in a post-seizure patient?

8. What is the relationship, if any, between Henry's bilateral wheezing and his history?

9. What additional questions would be especially pertinent?

10. What is the significance of a fever in an epileptic?

11. What are the possible causes of Henry's current condition?

12. How would you treat Henry?

13. What is Henry at risk for?

14. If Henry told you that he was waiting for his disability check to get a refill on his medication, he took his last pill 3 days ago, and his fever was 103° F, how would your treatment change?

QUESTIONS AND ANSWERS

1. **What is significant about Henry's history?**

   A history of epilepsy and a "cold" for last several days.

2. **What body systems are affected?**

   CNS—confusion

   Cardiovascular—tachycardia

3. **How would you describe the ECG?**

   Sinus tachycardia

4. **What is the relationship between Henry's history of seizure and his vital signs?**

   A seizure causes violent cerebral and physical activity. The energy demand increases 250% with a cerebral oxygen consumption that increases by 60%. Although cerebral blood flow also increases approximately 250%, available glucose and oxygen are readily depleted in the brain and skeletal muscle. With a severe seizure, the brain tissue may require more energy (ATP) than can be produced by the available oxygen and glucose. A deficiency of ATP, glucose, and other chemicals then occurs and lactate accumulates within the brain and skeletal muscle. Secondary hypoxia, acidosis, and lactate accumulation contributes to an increase in heart rate, respiratory rate, and blood pressure.

5. **Henry's roommate states he found Henry in a seizure. How does your physical assessment support the conclusion that a grand mal seizure did occur?**

   Presence of tachycardia, slightly elevated systolic pressure, confusion, and an abraded tongue.

6. **After a grand mal seizure, what might you expect the skin color, temperature, and moisture to be? How do Henry's compare?**

   The skin may be flushed, pale or normal color, the temperature is usually normal and diaphoretic. Henry is hot and dry.

7. **What are the possible causes of wheezing in a post-seizure patient?**

   Possible causes include aspiration. Typically aspiration is unilateral unless extensive. Other possibilities include a predisposition to stress-induced asthma or a co-existing upper respiratory infection.

8. **What is the relationship, if any, between Henry's bilateral wheezing and his history?**

   Henry has a history of a "cold" for the last several days and no history of asthma. Consider the possibility of a more serious lower respiratory problem such as pneumonia.

9. **What additional information would be especially pertinent?**

   Has he taken his seizure medication today? Has he had a fever? A cough? When did he have his last seizure? Was his neck stiff? Assess for nuchal rigidity.

10. **What is the significance of a fever in an epileptic?**

    A fever and/or infection predisposes to seizures.

11. **What are the possible causes of Henry's current condition?**

    The most common cause of breakthrough seizures is failure to take medication. However, approximately 10% to 15% of epileptic persons have breakthrough seizures even when taking medication. For these persons, taking their medication limits the number of seizures in a given time period. It is possible that Henry either failed to take his medication or had a breakthrough seizure. Seizures can also be precipitated by other irritants such as fever, infection, extreme stress, acidosis, hypoxia, hypoglycemia, or electrolyte imbalance. Henry may have an infection, such as pneumonia, resulting in a fever, thus triggering this seizure. Another infection to suspect is meningitis. Henry does not have any higher risk for this disease than any other person does; however, meningitis may manifest itself as seizures in the presence of fever. The probability of meningitis is low but not eliminated.

12. How would you treat Henry?

Depending on pulse oximetry values, place him on a nasal cannula at 2 to 4 lpm, and consider administration of a bronchodilator such as terbutaline, metaproterenol, albuterol, or isoetharine.

13. What is Henry at risk for?

Another seizure or status epilepticus. Henry is at risk for seizures because of the fever along with his history of epilepsy.

14. If Henry told you that he was waiting for his disability check to get a refill on his medication, he took his last pill 3 days ago, and his fever was 103° F, how would your treatment change?

The potential seriousness of his situation has just increased. The risk for status epilepticus has increased dramatically. If you elected not to start an IV before, now you definitely should. The saline lock might be changed to a KVO crystalloid such as normal saline.

OUTCOME

On admission to the ED, Henry had another seizure, only this time his seizure was prolonged and status was suspected. Ativan (lorazepam) 6 mg IV push was given. Blood tests showed a subtherapeutic level of his medication and an elevated white count while his chest x-rays showed pneumonia. It is interesting to note that laboratory studies indicated severe dehydration. His field assessment was not indicative of how dehydrated Henry actually was.

CASE 6

Dispatch: 18:00 hrs, 45 y/o female, medical problem, nature unknown

On Arrival: You find 45 y/o Sara, sitting on the kitchen floor awake, looking around, but not focusing. She looks pale.

Initial Assessment Findings

Mental Status—Awake but no verbal response, does not obey command, withdraws to pain
Airway—Open and clear
Breathing—RR 30 with retractions; lung sounds have rales and wheezes all lobes
Circulation—Skin pale, cool, and dry
       Radial pulse regular at 108
       BP 236/126
Chief Complaint—"Isn't acting right" according to husband

Focused History

Events—Husband arrived home from work to find her sitting on the kitchen floor
Previous Illness—Hypertension, urinary tract infection
Current Health Status—Has been complaining of headaches for last several days, was seen by family physician 2 days ago for dysuria, he put her on an antibiotic
Allergies—sulfa and penicillin
Medications—hydrochlorothiazide, nitrofurantoin

Focused Physical

Current VS—P 108, RR 30, BP 236/126
Other Pertinent Findings—pitting edema of ankles noted, pupils equal and reactive, moves all extremities, pulse oximetry 90%
Diagnostic tests—Blood sugar reads "HIGH"

ECG

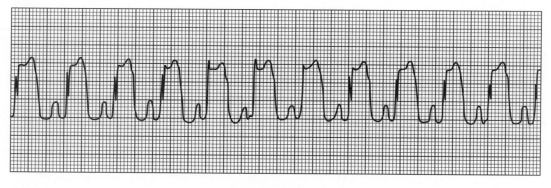

Figure 2-6

QUESTIONS

1. What is significant about Sara's history?

2. Based on the initial assessment, what body systems are affected?

3. What is Sara's Glasgow Coma Score?

4. What is the pathophysiology behind her pale, cool, and dry skin; tachycardia; and hypertension?

5. What is the relationship between Sara's hypertension and pulmonary edema?

6. How would you describe Sara's cardiac rhythm? What is its significance?

7. What is the relationship between Sara's blood pressure and her ECG abnormality?

8. Is there additional information from her history or physical examination that would help you?

9. How serious is Sara's situation?

10. What immediate actions, if any, would you take to treat Sara?

11. What is significant about Sara's pedal edema, pulse oximetry, and blood sugar value?

12. What do you think is causing Sara's current condition?

13. What are the benefits and precautions for using the following pharmacologic agents: sublingual nitroglycerin, furosemide, morphine, nifedipine, diltiazem.

14. How would you treat Sara?

15. Not all patients with hypertensive crises are treated pharmacologically in the field. What are the guidelines for treatment of hypertensive crises in the field?

16. What is Sara at risk for during transport?

17. Is there a relationship between Sara's infection and her present problem?

QUESTIONS AND ANSWERS

1. What is significant about Sara's history?

Her hypertension and current urinary tract infection

2. Based on the initial assessment, what body systems are affected?

CNS—altered mental status

Respiratory—rapid rate of 30, labored, pulmonary edema

Cardiovascular—tachycardia, hypertension

3. What is Sara's Glasgow Coma Score?

GCS 9 (4 spontaneous eye opening, 1 no verbal response, 4 withdraws to pain)

4. What is the pathophysiology behind her pale, cool, and dry skin; tachycardia; and hypertension?

Pale skin is usually due to peripheral vasoconstriction. One of the causes of peripheral vasoconstriction is an epinephrine/norepinephrine release. This would explain her skin color, temperature, and moisture. An epinephrine/norepinephrine response would also explain her tachycardia and hypertension. The question now becomes what stimulated that epinephrine/norepinephrine response?

5. What is the relationship between Sara's pulmonary edema and hypertension?

Hypertension can either cause or be the result of pulmonary edema. When hypertension is the cause, increased hydrostatic pressure in the pulmonary capillary beds exceeds the normal alveolar air pressure. Intravascular fluid is forced across the alveolar membrane and accumulates in the interstitial and alveolar spaces (pulmonary edema).

When hypertension is the result of pulmonary edema, the hypoxemia caused by the pulmonary edema is a stressor that causes a release of epinephrine/norepinephrine. The combined effect of increased preload, increased rate, increased stroke volume, and increased afterload raises cardiac output, thus increasing blood pressure.

6. How would you describe Sara's cardiac rhythm? What is its significance?

Sinus tachycardia with elevated S-T segments. Significantly elevated S-T segments is suggestive of ongoing myocardial injury and ischemia.

7. What is the relationship between Sara's blood pressure and her ECG abnormality?

Sara's significantly elevated S-T segments is one indicator of the insult (acute myocardial injury and ischemia) severe hypertension is causing to her cardiovascular system. The heart's demand for oxygen has outstripped the supply provided to it by its blood flow. Hypoxia causes a lower oxygen content of blood. Hypertension is forcing the heart to work harder (needing even more oxygen than usual) to pump the blood out of the left ventricle and into the aorta against a higher blood pressure.

8. Is there additional information from her history or physical examination that would help you?

Did Sara take all her medication? When was the last time she took her antihypertensive medication? What was she like the last time the husband talked to her?

9. How serious is Sara's situation?

Sara is in a life-threatening situation from acute hypertensive crises. From a field perspective she has signs and symptoms that indicate end organ damage to the heart, lungs, and brain.

10. What immediate actions, if any, would you take to treat Sara?

Oxygen by a non–rebreather mask with a reservoir at 10 to 15 lpm, IV KVO of crystalloid, begin first drug of choice or contact medical control (depending on your protocols).

11. What is significant about Sara's pedal edema, pulse oximetry, and blood sugar value?

Pedal edema takes time to develop. Its presence is consistent with both renal failure and congestive heart failure. Sara's blood sugar value in the absence of a history of diabetes may indicate an extreme epinephrine/norepinephrine response (epinephrine stimulates glycogenolysis and decreases the uptake of glucose by peripheral tissues, together both action increase blood glucose) or undiagnosed diabetes or may be related to her kidney infection.

12. What do you think is causing Sara's current condition?

Sara could be septic because of her history of infection. This would explain her altered mental status and presence of pulmonary edema. However, her hypertension is not consistent with an overwhelming infection. She could be in diabetic ketoacidosis but her edema is not consistent. She may be in kidney failure, which could explain her altered mental status, edema, and extreme elevation in blood pressure. (This is consistent with untreated kidney failure.) It is also possible that Sara has a combination of problems that has caused this presentation.

13. What are the benefits and precautions for the following pharmacologic agents:

Sublingual nitroglycerin—vasodilator, given sublingually

Benefit—short acting, general body vasodilator especially for coronary arteries and pulmonary capillary bed

Precaution—some people have an exaggerated response, either as a result of dose or age, which may lead to a precipitous drop in blood pressure; cerebral vasodilation also occurs

Furosemide—diuretic, given IV

Benefit—almost immediate pulmonary capillary bed vasodilator, takes 15 to 20 minutes to accumulate enough urine to cause diuresis, questionable fall in BP

Precaution—requires constant monitoring, can lead to electrolyte imbalance

Morphine—analgesic, given IV

Benefit—indirectly limits epinephrine/norepinephrine release, general body vasodilator, analgesic

Precaution—depresses respirations, unpredictable fall in BP

Nifedipine—calcium channel blocker, given sublingually or bite and swallow

Benefit—lowers blood pressure steadily, long lasting (approximately 6 hours)

Precaution—may drop BP below desired point, once on board cannot be reversed, has been known to precipitate stroke

Diltiazem—calcium channel blocker, given sublingually

Benefit—lowers blood pressure slowly, can be more controlled, coronary artery vasodilator, effective with pulmonary edema

Precaution—requires close monitoring, may have a cumulative effect when used with other calcium channel blockers

14. How would you treat Sara?

Oxygen, the highest flow she will accept, preferably a non–rebreather mask with a reservoir at 15 lpm; IV normal saline, KVO; sublingual nitroglycerin or furosemide 40 mg IV push or morphine 2 to 3 mg IV push are all appropriate. Nitroglycerin might be used first because of its easy access, ability to vasodilate coronary arteries and pulmonary capillary beds and relatively short half life. Furosemide is more selective in its vasodilation and more specific for pulmonary edema. Morphine may be reserved for a third line medication because of its potential for respiratory depression. Regardless of which medication is used first, frequent reassessment of BP, mental status, and ECG rhythm is necessary. Vital signs should be taken every 2 to 3 minutes.

15. Not all patients with hypertensive crises are treated pharmacologically in the field. What are the guidelines for treatment of hypertensive crises in the field?

Presence of end-organ damage. In the field, important end organs to assess include the heart, lungs, and brain. Pharmacologic treatment is usually determined by the effect on the heart and lungs. In this case, severe pulmonary edema and cardiac ischemia as evidenced by S-T segment elevation were deciding factors in determining treatment. Maintaining cerebral perfusion pressure is a critical point of treatment. If systolic pressure is lowered too fast, cerebral infarct can result. The drug of choice is sodium nitroprusside, which must be closely monitored and the dose precisely delivered to preserve perfusion to the brain. Labetalol is also an excellent drug for hypertensive emergencies, but again, needs to be closely monitored. Necessary monitoring systems for these agents are rarely available in the field.

16. **What is Sara at risk for during transport?**

Stroke, myocardial infarction, and cardiogenic failure with cardiogenic shock.

17. **Is there a relationship between Sara's infection and her present problem?**

Probably. Her peripheral edema may be because of renal failure, which is accompanied by hypertension. Contributing factors to consider also include drug effects. However, this was not the case for Sara.

OUTCOME

Sara was given oxygen by a non–rebreather mask with reservoir at 15 lpm, an IV of normal saline started at KVO, sublingual nitroglycerin administered and furosemide, 40 mg IV push was given. A second set of VS showed P 120, R 30, BP 230/120 and pulse oximetry showed 97%. On arrival at the ED, acute hypertensive crisis was diagnosed and a sodium nitroprusside drip was started. Admission VS: P 116, R 24, BP 220/120. Her S-T segments remained significantly elevated but not to the degree of the initial rhythm strip. After several hours her BP was lowered to 160/80, P 78 and R 18. Her pulmonary edema resolved and S-T segments returned to normal. Sara was eventually diagnosed with early renal failure and diabetes mellitus. Her kidney infection was the stressor that caused her body to decompensate from undiagnosed Type II diabetes mellitus and early kidney failure. Sara eventually became insulin dependent and a dialysis patient.

BIBLIOGRAPHY

American Heart Association. Cummins R. O. (Ed.). (1994). *Advanced cardiac life support textbook.* Dallas, TX: American Heart Association.

Berkow R., & Fletcher A. J. (Eds.). (1992). *Merck manual of diagnosis and therapy.* Rahway, NJ: Merck Research Laboratories.

Bledsoe, B. E., Clayden, D. E., & Papa, F. J. (1996). *Prehospital emergency pharmacology* (4th ed.). Upper Saddle River, NJ: Brady, Prentice Hall.

Bongard F. S., & Sue D. Y. (Eds.). (1994). *Current: Critical care, diagnosis and treatment.* Norwalk, CT: Appleton & Lange.

Calhoun, D. A., & Oparil, S. (1990). Treatment of hypertensive crisis. *New England Journal of Medicine,* (323) 17, 1177-1183.

Camarata P. J., Heros, R. C., & Latchaw, R. E. (1994). "Brain attack": The rationale for treating stroke as a medical emergency. *Neurosurgery,* (34) 1, 144-158.

Chestnut, R. M., et al. (1995). Secondary brain insults after head injuries: Clinical perspectives. *New Horizons,* 3(3): 366-375.

Davis, S. N., & Granner, D. K. (1996). Insulin, oral hypoglycemic agents, and the pharmacology of the endocrine pancreas. In J. G. Hardman & L. E. Limbird (Eds.). *The pharmacological basis of therapeutics* (9th ed., pp. 1487-1518). New York, NY: McGraw-Hill.

Haak S. W., Richardson S. J., Davey S. S., & Parker-Cohen, P. D. (1994). Alterations of cardiovascular function. In K. L. McCance & S. E. Huether (Eds.). *Pathophysiology: The biologic basis for disease in adults and children* (2nd ed., pp. 1000-1081). St Louis, MO: Mosby.

Hart. G. (1990). Strokes causing left vs. right hemiplegia: Different effects and nursing implications. *Geriatric Nursing,* 2, 67-70.

Hobbs W. R., Rall T. W., & Verdoorn, T. A. (1996). Hypnotics and sedatives: Ethanol. In J. G. Hardman & L. E. Limbird (Eds.). *Goodman & Gillman's: The pharmacological basis of therapeutics* (9th ed., pp. 361-392). New York, NY: McGraw-Hill.

Kerr, M. E., & Brucia, J. (1993). Hyperventilation in the head-injured patient: an effective treatment modality? *Heart & Lung,* 22(6), 516-521.

Marion D. W., Firlik A., & McLaughlin M. R. (1995). Hyperventilation therapy for severe traumatic brain injury. *New Horizons,* 3(3), 439-446.

Martini F. H., & Bartholomew E. F. (1997). *Essentials of anatomy and physiology.* Upper Saddle River, NJ: Prentice Hall.

Oates J. A. (1996). Antihypertensive agents and the drug therapy of hypertension. In J. G. Hardman & L. E. Limbird (Eds.). *Goodman & Gillman's: The pharmacological basis of therapeutics* (9th ed., pp. 1383-1410). New York, NY: McGraw-Hill.

Sanders M. J. (1994). *Mosby's paramedic textbook.* St Louis, MO: Mosby.

Tierney L. M., McPhee S. J., & Papadakis M. A. (Eds.). (1994). *Current: Medical diagnosis and treatment.* Norwalk, CT: Appleton & Lange.

Vos J. R. (1993). Making headway with intracranial hypertension. *American Journal of Nursing,* 2, 28-35.

3

Endocrine Emergencies

OVERVIEW

The endocrine system is composed of specialized glands and tissues. This system regulates other glands, organs, and body tissues through substances known as hormones. Some of the functions controlled by the endocrine system through the use of hormones are growth, development, metabolism, reproduction, water reabsorption, mineral distribution, neurotransmitter production, and glucose balance. The major glands in the body include the pituitary and the thyroid.

The pituitary gland, located at the base of the cerebrum, is also known as the master gland. It has two parts, the anterior and the posterior pituitary. The anterior pituitary stores growth hormones and other tropines; the posterior pituitary secretes oxytocin, which stimulates uterine contractions, and antidiuretic hormone or vasopressin, which conserves body water.

The thyroid gland, located on either side of the neck, regulates metabolism, whereas the parathyroid glands, located within the thyroid gland, regulate minerals such as calcium. The adrenal glands, located on top of the kidneys, have two distinct parts. The adrenal cortex produces the multifunctional corticosteroids, whereas the adrenal medulla produces catecholamines such as norepinephrine and epinephrine. The pancreas, located in the upper left quadrant of the abdomen, regulates blood glucose levels through insulin and glucagon. The pineal gland, located in the brain, regulates pigmentation. The ovaries produce female steroids, and the testes produce male steroids.

Endocrine tissue is also found in the liver, thymus, kidneys, heart, stomach, and duodenum, all of which produce hormones unique to the specific organ in which they are found.

Many varieties of endocrine disorders exist. Frequently, the onset and variety of symptoms associated with endocrine disorders are confusing and make identification of the exact problem difficult in the field. Prehospital care is supportive. However, disorders of the adrenal glands, thyroid glands, and pancreas can present severe emergencies that may require immediate interventions.

Adrenal Gland Disorders

The adrenal cortex, located on top of the kidneys, regulates glucocorticoid and mineralocorticoid hormone secretion. Excess adrenocortical hormone secretion presents as Cushing's syndrome. This is characterized by fluid retention observed as a "moon face" and "buffalo hump," along with weakness, hypertension, and fatigue. The weakness and fatigue can predispose to falls.

Hypofunction of the adrenal cortex is Addison's disease. This is rare and is characterized by fatigue, weakness, and weight loss. Hypotension and hypoglycemia are also present. If a patient has a history of Addison's disease and is undergoing treatment, a sudden emergency can be precipitated if medication is abruptly stopped. Weakness and confusion in the presence of hypotension, increased temperature, and abdominal pain can result. This reaction can also happen if someone taking steroids for a long period of time suddenly stops taking the steroid. Field treatment is directed toward supporting perfusion with oxygen therapy and IV fluids.

Thyroid Gland Disorders

The thyroid gland, located on either side of the throat, regulates metabolism. Hypothyroidism is a progressive slowing of all bodily functions. Its most severe result is myxedema coma. Patients present in a coma with edema of the extremities and face, especially the tissues around the eyes. Field treatment is based on correcting the bradycardia and hypotension. An important factor is keeping these patients warm.

Hyperthyroidism is known as thyrotoxicosis or Graves' disease. This results in an increase in body functions. Thyroid storm is an exaggeration of thyrotoxicosis to the level of a life-threatening emergency. Thyrotoxicosis may present as tachycardia or new onset atrial fibrillation without previous cardiac disease. The eyes may appear to bulge and stare; anxiety, tremors, and sweating are also common.

Thyrotoxicosis with fever, cardiac decompensation, and GI symptoms is thyroid storm. The patient will be febrile, often 104° F (40° C) or more. Tachycardia leading to congestive heart failure, confusion and agitation, or even psychotic reactions can occur. GI symptoms include nausea, vomiting, diarrhea, and abdominal pain with dehydration. Treatment includes managing the airway, controlling cardiac dysrhythmias, and supporting perfusion with IV fluids.

Pancreas Disorders

The pancreas, located behind the duodenum and adjacent to the spleen, regulates blood glucose levels with the hormones insulin and glucagon. The islets of Langerhans contains alpha cells that secrete glucagon and beta cells, which secrete insulin. One of the most common endocrine abnormalities encountered in the field is diabetes mellitus, an endocrine disorder caused by insufficient or absent functioning insulin. There are two types of diabetics. A person with type I, or insulin-dependent diabetes mellitus (IDDM), may have very little, if any, functioning insulin. A person with type II, or non–insulin-dependent diabetes mellitus (NIDDM), either has insufficient insulin or has developed insulin resistance.

There are three reactions caused by diabetes mellitus that may be encountered in the field. Hyperglycemia or diabetic ketoacidosis (diabetic coma) develops very slowly, over days to weeks and, in the case of a Type II diabetic, as much as a year. Hypoglycemia (insulin shock) develops very fast, typically within minutes. Another reaction, called hyperglycemic hyperosmolar non-ketotic coma (HHNC) is more typical of the Type II diabetic. In this case there is just enough functioning insulin to prevent ketone formation but not enough to prevent dehydration.

In diabetic ketoacidosis (DKA) the lack of functioning insulin causes a buildup of glucose in the blood stream. The buildup of blood glucose increases the osmotic pull of the blood to the point where body water from the interstitial and intracellular spaces is shifted into the vascular space. The kidneys eventually spill sugar and excess body water (now in the vascular space) in the urine causing polyuria. If the patient can drink enough water to replace what is being lost in the urine, dehydration will be delayed. At the same time, the lack of functioning insulin prevents fat from being deposited and fat stores start to be mobilized. Fat goes to the liver to be metabolized and ketones are formed along with glycerol (which further contributes to the blood glucose level). The ketones are highly acidic and are being formed faster than the muscle cells can use them. Because the acidic ketones have a great potential to change blood pH, the blood buffer system starts working. The pH is also regulated through the respiratory system by the exhalation of carbon dioxide and water vapor and, in this case, ketones. Because of the high acid content of the blood reaching the lungs, respirations are faster and deeper to keep up with the need to exhale CO_2 and ketones. Ketones are volatile and the odor, characterized as acetone or "rotten fruit," is also common. As long as the patient can compensate through the respiratory system to maintain a pH, the body will continue to function.

While acidosis is irritating to the brain, the high osmolality is even less tolerated. Altered mentation, along with confusion, combativeness, seizures, and eventually coma, results.

At the same time fats are being mobilized, protein stores are also being broken with a small amount of glucose, urea and potassium are also created. Urea may cause cess levels of potassium may cause smooth muscle contractions (abdominal pain vomiting) and cardiac dysrhythmias, most frequently tachycardia. High levels of po delay cardiac conduction, causing a wide QRS and tall, peaked T waves.

Common signs and symptoms of DKA include polyuria; thirst (polydip (polyphagia); warm, dry skin; rapid, deep respirations with the odor of acetone (Kussmaul's respirations); tachycardia; altered mentation; and abdominal pain. The blood pressure may be normal or low depending on how well the patient has been able to replace fluid lost through urination. This reaction (ketoacidosis) may be triggered by pregnancy or, in a known diabetic, an infection or a relatively simple illness such as the common cold.

Treatment of DKA is aimed toward correcting the severe dehydration. Normal saline is the solution of choice. It is not uncommon to administer 2 to 4 liters of normal saline to correct the dehydration. While insulin is the treatment immediately started at the hospital, insulin is not given in the field because of the amount of regulation that is necessary.

Hyperosmolar, hyperglycemic, non-ketotic coma is another reaction that occurs, primarily in the Type II diabetic. This reaction may be triggered by a stressful event or an infection. In this reaction, there is just enough functioning insulin that fats are not mobilized and ketones are not present. There is, however, severe dehydration caused by the high levels of glucose causing increased osmotic pull and a corresponding fluid shift. Because many of the patients are older, thirst mechanisms may not be intact, further contributing to dehydration.

Patients frequently present with altered mental status such as confusion and agitation; tachycardia; rapid, shallow respirations; hypotension; and poor skin turgor. Treatment is aimed toward correcting the dehydration. The fluid of choice is normal saline.

Hypoglycemia is caused by not enough food or too much insulin and is a frequent reaction encountered in the field. In a diabetic, hypoglycemia may be triggered by stress, pregnancy, unexpected exercise, an infection, or some medications. Because the brain does not store glucose, its shortage is felt quickly. The brain is particularly sensitive to shortages of glucose (as well as oxygen) and immediate releases of epinephrine and norepinephrine result. These catecholamines stimulate release of stored glucose in the form of glycogen. The effect is short-lived, and signs and symptoms of hypoglycemia occur quickly. Hypoglycemia is a true emergency. If hypoglycemia results in loss of consciousness, brain cells are dying. Immediate treatment is necessary to prevent permanent brain damage and death.

Patients with hypoglycemia have altered mental status; may appear pale, diaphoretic, tachycardic; and have rapid, shallow respirations. Blood pressure may be normal, or in the case of extreme sweating, may be hypotensive. Treatment is glucose, either in the form of food (such as juice or a sandwich), glucose gel, or $D_{50}W$ IV push.

Patients with diabetes are not the only persons who suffer hypoglycemia. Those who are on extreme diets, alcoholics who have been on a binge of drinking, those who have had extreme exercise, and some victims of overdoses are all prone to hypoglycemia. In general, any patient who suffers from an unknown cause of altered mental status or coma should have their blood glucose level assessed and treated accordingly.

CASE 1

Dispatch: 18:45 hrs; 24 y/o unconscious male—manager at apartment will let you in.

On Arrival: You find 24 y/o Tim lying on the couch. He appears to be asleep. You note a rise and fall of his chest. He is in pajamas. From the condition of his clothing and the smell, he has been incontinent of stool and urine.

NOTE: The apartment is not well kept. There are piles of clothing and newspapers in the room. There are dirty dishes and moldy food on the coffee table. The odor is overpowering.

Initial Assessment Findings

Mental Status—Opens his eyes to voice, but no verbal response; localizes pain
Airway—Open and clear
Breathing—RR rapid at 46, no retractions noted; lung sounds clear in all lobes with no difficulty
Circulation—Skin pale, warm, and dry with poor turgor
　　　　　　Radial pulse weak and regular at 110
　　　　　　BP 80/68
　　　　　　Pushes your hands away when abdomen is palpated
Chief Complaint—Unresponsive

Focused History

Events—His sister knew Tim had been ill and became worried when he didn't answer the phone so she called the apartment manager. The apartment manager found Tim in this state and called EMS.
Previous Illness—Insulin-dependent diabetic
Current Health Status—Tim has had the "flu" for the last week, the manager doesn't know anything else.
Allergies—Unknown
Medications—Insulin

Focused Physical

Current Set of VS—P 110, RR 46, BP 80/68
Other Pertinent Findings—"Orange-peel" skin noted on both anterior thighs, pulse oximetry 100%
Diagnostic Tests—BS reads "High"
Other—Refrigerator has one empty bottle of insulin

ECG

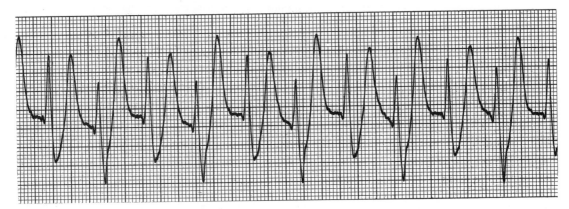

Figure 3-1

1. What is significant about Tim's history?

2. What body systems are affected?

3. What is Tim's Glasgow Coma Score?

4. What is significant about the presence of dirty dishes and moldy food on the coffee table?

5. What is suggested when Tim pushes your hands away when his abdomen is palpated?

6. What is significant about Tim's respirations?

7. What is the relationship between Tim's blood pressure, his skin color, and his tachycardia? What is the relationship between his blood pressure, skin moisture, and turgor?

8. How would you describe Tim's ECG?

9. Would you treat Tim's rhythm pharmacologically? Why or why not?

10. How serious is Tim's situation?

11. What are the possible causes of Tim's present condition?

12. What immediate treatment steps would you take?

13. Is there a recognizable pattern in Tim's signs and symptoms?

14. What is Tim at risk for?

15. Diabetic patients with ketoacidosis often have Kussmaul's respirations. Why wasn't the smell of ketones noticed?

16. Tim pushes your hand away when you palpate his abdomen. Why is this consistent with DKA?

17. What is the most likely reason for Tim's incontinence of urine?

18. What is the relationship between Tim's mental status and his DKA?

19. What is the significance of Tim's "orange-peel" skin on both anterior thighs?

QUESTIONS AND ANSWERS

1. *What is significant about Tim's history?*

   Tim is an insulin-dependent diabetic, and he has been ill for some time.

2. *What body systems are affected?*

   CNS—no verbal response, localizes pain
   Respiratory—rapid rate of 46
   Cardiovascular—tachycardia; pale, dry skin with poor turgor; and hypotension

3. *What is Tim's Glasgow Coma Score?*

   GCS of 9 (3 opens eyes to verbal response, 1 no verbal response, 5 localizes pain)

4. *What is significant about the presence of dirty dishes and moldy food on the coffee table?*

   Eating and the time factor. Tim has probably not been able or aware enough to eat; his current illness has lasted several days at least.

5. *What is suggested when Tim pushes your hands away when his abdomen is palpated?*

   There is the possibility that this is insignificant. However, there is also the possibility that palpating his abdomen is painful and his reaction is to pain.

6. *What is significant about Tim's respirations?*

   At such a rapid rate, you would not expect to get such a good tidal volume. Rapid, deep respirations are typically found with either central neurogenic hyperventilation, which can occur with upper brain stem insult, or with ketoacidosis. In ketoacidosis the rapid, deep respirations are in response to increased acid levels from the ketones. The body is attempting to "blow off" the excess acids in the form of carbon dioxide and vaporized ketones, a characteristic of Kussmaul's respirations. This can occur regardless of the cause of ketoacidosis.

7. *What is the relationship between Tim's blood pressure, his skin color, and his tachycardia? What is the relationship between his blood pressure, skin moisture, and turgor?*

   Tim's tachycardia and pale skin in the presence of hypotension indicate an epinephrine/norepinephrine response with peripheral vasoconstriction, increased heart rate, increased irritability, increased contractility, etc. His skin turgor implies dehydration, explaining the lack of sweating and his blood pressure.

8. *How would you describe Tim's ECG?*

   Wide complex tachycardia, absent P waves, with tall, peaked T waves. This rhythm is an extreme example of the changes seen with hyperkalemia.

9. *Would you treat Tim's rhythm pharmacologically? Why or why not?*

   No, his rhythm is not consistent with ventricular tachycardia. In v-tach the R wave is most often opposite the T and the rate is more frequently around 140 or higher. Tim's BP can be explained by other factors (dehydration). This rhythm is a very distinct example of an electrolyte imbalance for potassium (too much). This might be difficult to tell in the field. In this case, leave his rhythm alone.

10. *How serious is Tim's situation?*

    This is a very serious life threatening condition.

11. *What are the possible causes of Tim's present condition?*

    Diabetic ketoacidosis and/or sepsis. Tim has been ill with the "flu" for several days. Diabetics are at risk for ordinary illnesses becoming more serious because of diabetes. One of the most frequent causes of DKA in adults is intercurrent illness, such as infection, trauma, surgery, or AMI. Since we don't know if the "flu" was an indicator of a diabetic reaction or if it was due to a virus/bacteria, err on the side of the patient and assume both are present until proven otherwise.

12. ***What immediate treatment steps would you take?***

Oxygen, either with a nasal cannula or non–rebreather mask, IV with normal saline and an immediate bolus of 300 to 500 cc, repeated until his BP is up to 90 systolic. The most immediate problem is dehydration from osmotic diuresis. Volume replacement aids in management of acidosis, ketonemia, and hyperglycemia. The amount of fluid replacement frequently exceeds 4 liters in an adult.

13. ***Is there a recognizable pattern in Tim's signs and symptoms?***

Yes, the rapid, deep respirations; warm, dry skin with poor turgor; tachycardia; and low BP in a known diabetic patient indicate diabetic ketoacidosis.

14. ***What is Tim at risk for?***

Further deterioration, possible septic shock, cardiac arrest, permanent brain damage

15. ***Diabetic patients with ketoacidosis often have Kussmaul's respirations. Why wasn't the smell of ketones noticed?***

It may be because a certain percent of the general population can't smell ketones. However, in this case the smell of feces and urine is too strong to differentiate between what is ketones, what is feces, and what is urine. In this situation they are nauseating.

16. ***Tim pushes your hand away when you palpate his abdomen? Why is this consistent with DKA?***

Abdominal pain in patients with DKA is common. Some authors think that the high levels of acid in the blood, particularly the type of acids released in DKA, predispose to pancreatic irritation and irritation of the smooth muscle mass in the small intestine. Both effects can cause abdominal pain. The irritation of the smooth muscle in the small intestine might also have contributed to his incontinence of stool.

17. ***What is the most likely reason for Tim's incontinence of urine?***

DKA results in high levels of blood glucose. This disturbs the osmotic balance of fluid between the intravascular space and the interstitial/intracellular spaces. The osmotic pull of body water into the vascular space from the interstitial and intracellular spaces results in large volumes of blood reaching the kidneys. The kidneys have a threshold for glucose and a sensitivity for amounts of body water (in relation to sodium). When the threshold for glucose is reached and the kidney "spills" sugar, it is diluted (glucose is a large molecule and attracts water) by excess vascular water and excreted as urine. Urine volumes are high and incontinence is common. If body water is not replaced, dehydration can occur rapidly and become severe over a relatively short time period.

18. ***What is the relationship between Tim's mental status and his DKA?***

Diabetic ketoacidosis results in very high glucose and acid levels in the blood. This results in hyperosmolarity and low pH. The brain is very sensitive to both but does not tolerate high osmolarity, as well as it does acidosis. Tim's altered level of consciousness is most closely associated with his hyperosmolarity.

19. ***What is the significance of Tim's "orange-peel" skin on both anterior thighs?***

Repeated injections of insulin in the same place over long period of time may result in atrophy of subcutaneous tissue resulting in skin that is rough and "pebbly" in texture. Its presence in Tim just confirms repeated injections at those sites.

OUTCOME

Tim was admitted to the local hospital with acute diabetic ketoacidosis. Primary treatment was fluid replacement. A second IV of normal saline was started and the second of a total of 8 liters of fluid was begun. His admission BS was 950 mg/dl, Serum K^+ was 8.9. Because the serum K^+ level was so high, a retest was ordered; this time it came back as 9.0. ABGs showed pO_2 120, pCO_2 28, pH 6.9, HCO_3^- 5. Tim was immediately started on an IV drip of regular insulin and was given 1 amp of sodium bicarbonate. A second IV of normal saline was also started in the ED. He was transferred to the ICU. Tim did recover; however, he remained a frequent patient because of the brittle state of his disease.

CASE 2

Dispatch: 10:00 hrs; unconscious child, 8 months old

On Arrival: You find 8-month-old Jeffery lying on his stomach in his crib. He appears to be sleeping and is very pale. You note a slight, rapid, regular movement of his chest wall. He has severe diaper rash and has no diaper on; the odor of urine is overpowering.

Initial Assessment Findings

Mental Status—Unresponsive to voice and pain
Airway—Open and clear
Breathing—RR rapid and shallow at 72; lung sounds clear in all fields
Circulation—Skin very pale, warm, dry, and doughy in texture
      Anterior fontanel sunken
      Brachial pulse very rapid and thready
      BP not taken
Chief Complaint—Unresponsive

Focused History

Events—Mother was unable to wake the baby from his nap.
Previous Illness—Baby has had vomiting and diarrhea for last 3 days. She took the child to the doctor yesterday where the baby was given a shot. She was told to leave the baby's diaper off, give the baby as much Pedialyte as he would take and bring the baby back today to be checked. She went in to take him to the doctor but could not wake him; she then called EMS.
Current Health Status—Vomiting and diarrhea for last 3 days, no fever, severe diaper rash noted yesterday.
Allergies—None known
Medications—Pedialyte

Focused Physical

Current set of VS—P 232, RR 72
Other Physical Findings—Severe diaper rash noted, buttocks excoriated and bleeding but the crib pad is dry, lips cracked, mucous membranes of mouth sticky
Diagnostic Tests—Pulse oximetry reads "ERROR"
Body Weight—20 lbs (9 kg)

ECG

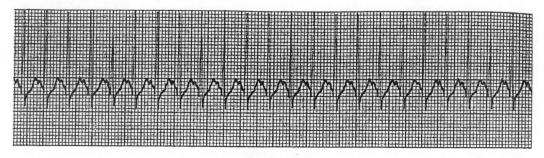

Figure 3-2

QUESTIONS

1. What is significant about Jeffery's history?

2. What body systems is/are affected?

3. What is this baby's Glasgow Coma Score?

4. Are there any additional parts of his history or physical examination you need to know?

5. What is the significance of Jeffery's rapid respiratory rate?

6. What can be determined from the pulse oximetry value?

7. What is the significance of a 3-day history of vomiting and diarrhea in an 8-month-old?

8. What is suggested by Jeffery's sunken fontanel? Could this be confirmed by anything else?

9. What do you think is the cause of Jeffery's current condition?

10. How serious is Jeffery's illness?

11. What would your immediate treatment steps include?

12. What is the most likely reason for Jeffery's pale skin, and why?

13. Jeffery needs an IV. What are appropriate IV fluids for the pediatric patient, and how should they be given?

14. Where would you most likely get an IV started?

15. If you got an IV started, how would you know how much fluid to give?

16. Can Jeffery wait to get an IV until he gets to the hospital?

17. Is there a recognizable pattern to Jeffery's signs and symptoms?

18. What may be causing Jeffery's depressed level of consciousness?

19. How would you describe the baby's rhythm?

20. What is the significance of the rhythm?

21. What is the significance of Jeffery's excoriated, bleeding buttocks?

QUESTIONS AND ANSWERS

1. *What is significant about Jeffery's history?*

   Over 3 days of vomiting and diarrhea, was seen yesterday by physician, has been given Pedialyte

2. *What body systems is/are affected?*

   CNS—Unresponsive to voice and pain
   Respiratory—72 and shallow
   Cardiovascular—Tachycardia of 220, sunken anterior fontanel, skin dry and doughy in texture
   Integumentary—Excoriated, bleeding buttocks

3. *What is this baby's Glasgow Coma Score?*

   GCS of 3 (1 no eye opening, 1 no cry, 1 no motor movement to pain)

4. *Are there any additional parts of his history or physical examination you need to know?*

   How many times yesterday (in an hour) did the mother change Jeffery's diapers? Have the mother describe the color and consistency of Jeffery's diarrhea. How much Pedialyte has Jeffery taken and over what time period? Did she notice a rash at any time?

5. *What is the significance of Jeffery's rapid respiratory rate?*

   At a rate of 72, tidal volume is not adequate. An infant cannot maintain a rate of 60 or over for very long. Jeffery is in respiratory failure and is in danger of impending respiratory arrest.

6. *What can be determined from the pulse oximetry value?*

   Nothing. It is tempting to assume since the RR is 72 that the reading is too low to register. However, there are times that pulse oximetry is inaccurate. This is one of those times.

7. *What is the significance of a 3-day history of vomiting and diarrhea in an 8 month old?*

   The 3 day duration makes dehydration a high risk.

8. *What is suggested by Jeffery's sunken fontanel? Could this be confirmed by anything else?*

   In this case the presence of a sunken fontanel would indicate dehydration. Dehydration could be confirmed by his cracked lips and sticky mucous membranes of his mouth.

9. *What do you think is the cause of Jeffery's current condition?*

   Possibilities include severe dehydration and/or sepsis.

10. *How serious is Jeffery's illness?*

    Very serious. Jeffery is in danger of impending respiratory arrest.

11. *What would your immediate treatment steps include?*

    Ventilate with a BVM with reservoir and O_2 at 15 lpm at a rate of 30 breaths/min. This child needs to be intubated; however, the risks of intubation include a misplaced tube, which may be easily missed. If he can be successfully ventilated using a BVM that may be all that is necessary. The next priority is fluid replacement. Check his blood sugar level. Congenital metabolic defects usually become evident within the first year of life.

12. *What is the most likely reason for Jeffery's pale skin and why?*

    Jeffery probably has extreme vasoconstriction. In infants the epinephrine/norepinephrine response is somewhat different than that of adults; however, vasoconstriction is very active and extremely effective. This response is probably due to his severe dehydration, as well as whatever caused the original vomiting and diarrhea.

13. *Jeffery needs an IV. What are appropriate IV fluids for the pediatric patient, and how should they be given?*

    NS and LR are the best fluids to use because of their physiologic balance of electrolytes. In this case normal saline would be best. Dextrose 5% and water is not recommended for pediatric patients and are inappropriate for dehydration. Fluids are given by bolus to avoid overhydration.

14. Where would you most likely get an IV started?

Jeffery has peripheral vascular shut-down, the only place you will be likely to get an IV started is by the intraosseous route.

15. If you got an IV started, how would you know how much fluid to give?

Administer 20 cc/kg (180 cc) at a time. You would look for a change in mental status, heart rate, or skin color. If Jeffery began to respond by opening his eyes, crying, or moving arms and legs to touch, and you note a decrease in heart rate or improved skin color, then you would know you gave enough.

16. Can Jeffery wait to get an IV until he gets to the hospital?

Only if the transport is extremely short. Jeffery is in shock and needs fluid badly.

17. Is there a recognizable pattern to Jeffery's signs and symptoms?

History of vomiting and diarrhea followed by an altered mental state, tachycardia, rapid respiratory rate, sunken fontanel, and pale skin could indicate dehydration or sepsis.

18. What may be causing Jeffery's depressed level of consciousness?

Hypoxia, acidosis, sepsis, or any combination of these factors.

19. How would you describe the baby's rhythm?

SVT, complexes are narrow and so fast that a clear P wave is not present. However, a P wave can be seen coming off the T wave.

20. What is the significance of the rhythm?

In an infant, to differentiate between a tachycardia resulting from sepsis or hypovolemia and an SVT may be difficult. Generally, in most infants with SVT, the heart rate is greater than 230. In this situation, with these assessment findings, it would be reasonable to assume that the heart rate is in response to acidosis, hypoxia, sepsis, and/or dehydration.

21. What is the significance of Jeffery's excoriated, bleeding buttocks?

Either Jeffery's mom didn't change him often enough and his urine is so strong and concentrated that his skin won't tolerate contact, or he has developed an infection, most likely with candidiasis (yeast), or both.

OUTCOME

Jeffery was ventilated with a BVM at 15 lpm at a rate of 30 to 36 (about every other breath). An IV of normal saline was started by intraosseous and a fluid bolus of 20 cc/kg (180 cc) was administered, with no change, before his arrival at the hospital. On arrival Jeffery was intubated and placed on a ventilator. ABGs showed a PaO_2 of 200%, $PaCO_2$ of 50, pH 7.0, and HCO_3^- of 5. A second intraosseous line of normal saline was started. Initial blood work revealed a blood sugar that was so high it did not register on the machine. A repeat blood sugar was done and a value of 3,000 mg/dl came back. A total of 800 cc of fluid was administered before his transfer to the pediatric ICU. Jeffery was admitted for severe acidosis, severe dehydration, and respiratory failure. His final diagnosis was severe diabetic ketoacidosis. Jeffery was the youngest Type I diabetic patient seen at that institution. He did survive to go home.

CASE 3

Dispatch: 08:30 hrs; unconscious woman, elderly female, possible stroke

On Arrival: On arrival you find 78 y/o Mildred lying in her bed at her home. She appears to be sleeping and looks very pale. Her daughter is present.

Initial Assessment Findings

Mental Status—Unresponsive to voice, withdraws and moans to pain

Airway—Open and clear

Breathing—RR 28 and shallow; lung sounds faint in bases, clear in upper lobes

Circulation—Skin very pale, dry, with tenting noted

> Radial pulse weak and regular at 130
>
> BP 80/54

Chief Complaint—Unresponsive

Focused History

Events—Mildred's daughter last talked to her yesterday afternoon. This morning she called and received no answer so she came to check on Mildred and couldn't wake her, so she called EMS.

Previous Illness—Hypertension

Current Health Status—According to her daughter, Mildred had been complaining of not feeling well, with general body "aching" for the last few days. Her daughter also stated that Mildred hadn't been acting "right;" she had become increasingly lethargic and "especially difficult to deal with."

Allergies—None known

Medications—Minipress (prazosin hydrochloride), which she took regularly

Focused Physical

Current Set of VS—P 136, RR 28, BP 80/54

Other Pertinent Findings—Mucous membranes of mouth dry; during your examination she becomes incontinent of urine; pulse oximetry 98%

Diagnostic Tests—BS reads "HIGH"; 200 cc fluid challenge results in BP 84/60 while LS remain clear

ECG

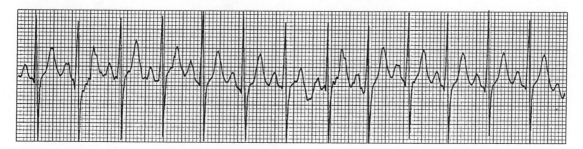

Figure 3-3

QUESTIONS

1. What is significant about Mildred's history?

2. What body systems are affected?

3. What is Mildred's Glasgow Coma Score?

4. What is the relationship between Mildred's tachycardia, hypotension, tenting, and dry mucous membranes?

5. What is the relationship between a high blood sugar and the presence of dry mucous membranes?

6. What is the significance of a high blood sugar in someone who has not eaten in over 8 to 10 hours?

7. How serious is Mildred's condition?

8. What are the possible causes of Mildred's current condition?

9. How important is the history of hypertension when considering the seriousness of her condition?

10. What would your immediate treatment steps include?

11. What is the importance of the initial 200 cc fluid bolus that was given?

12. How would you know when enough fluid had been given?

13. During your treatment and administration of fluid, what assessment signs would indicate respiratory distress?

14. How would you describe Mildred's ECG?

15. Is there any significance to Mildred's incontinence of urine?

16. What are contributing factors to dehydration in the elderly?

17. Of what importance are these contributing factors to prehospital care providers?

18. If the blood sugar is "high" and the patient is dehydrated, <u>why</u> is there no odor of ketones?

QUESTIONS AND ANSWERS

1. What is significant about Mildred's history?

Relatively gradual onset (over last several days) of altered mental state along with vague physical complaints; only known problem was hypertension.

2. What body systems are affected?

CNS—altered mental state
Cardiovascular system—tachycardia, hypotension, dry mucous membranes, tenting
Endocrine—BS reads "high" in presence of dehydration

3. What is Mildred's Glasgow Coma Score?

GCS 7 (1 no eye opening, 2 moaning to pain, 4 withdraws to pain)

4. What is the relationship between Mildred's tachycardia, hypotension, tenting, and dry mucous membranes?

These are all signs of dehydration. Tenting and dry mucous membranes indicate lack of total body water, hypotension reflects loss of blood volume, and tachycardia is a compensatory mechanism to increase cardiac output.

5. What is the relationship between a high blood sugar and the presence of dry mucous membranes?

A high blood sugar indicates a large concentration of glucose within the vascular space. Glucose is a large molecule that causes an osmotic pull. Large concentrations of glucose within the blood will have the osmotic effect of pulling interstitial and intracellular body water into the vascular space. This dehydrates the tissues while maintaining vascular volume. In Mildred's case her dry mucous membranes may be caused by prolonged high blood sugar in the absence of replacement water (in the form of drinking water).

6. What is the significance of a high blood sugar in someone who has not eaten in over 8 to 10 hours?

This is not normal and indicates a problem with metabolism. Lack of sufficient or functioning insulin, high epinephrine/norepinephrine response, or both can result in this condition.

7. How serious is Mildred's condition?

Mildred is severely dehydrated and needs immediate transport.

8. What are the possible causes of Mildred's current condition?

Possibilities include a diabetic reaction such as DKA or hyperosmolar nonketotic coma (HNK), stroke, infection/sepsis, or severe dehydration.

9. How important is the history of hypertension when considering the seriousness of her condition?

It would be nice to know her usual BP; however, that information is not available. Therefore consider that a BP of 80/54 is hypotensive for most people. In the presence of preexisting hypertension, Mildred's blood pressure is even more indicative of a lack of perfusion to vital organs.

10. What would your immediate treatment steps include?

Oxygenation, probably by non–rebreather mask with a reservoir at 10 to 15 lpm. If you choose to ventilate her by a BVM with O_2 at 15 lpm, that is okay, too. (No matter which oxygen delivery system you choose, her respiratory status and oxygenation level must be reassessed and adjusted accordingly.) Mildred needs fluids quickly. Start an IV of normal saline and administer fluid boluses.

11. What is the importance of the initial 200 cc fluid bolus that was given?

In older people especially, the cardiovascular system is usually compromised due to age-related changes. Mildred already has a history of hypertension. Her heart is already working hard to compensate for low volume. Therefore it may not be able to tolerate a sudden influx of a large volume of fluid. Starting with controlled boluses of fluid and reassessing between boluses will give the body a better chance to compensate for the fluid. The fact that her BP gave a marginal increase but her lung sounds remained clear further indicates that more fluid is needed.

12. How would you know that enough fluid had been given?

When there is a change. Look for an increase in level of consciousness, a decrease in heart rate, an increase in BP, or early signs of respiratory distress.

13. During your treatment and administration of fluid, what assessment signs would indicate respiratory distress?

An increase in respiratory rate or effort, a change in skin color, and of course, wheezes or rales. However, in the back of a moving vehicle, lung sounds are very difficult to hear so other signs must be closely observed.

14. How would you describe Mildred's ECG?

Her rhythm is regular and tachycardic with distinct P waves. She has a sinus tachycardia.

15. Is there any significance to Mildred's incontinence of urine?

It certainly doesn't change your treatment; however, it does contribute to the entire picture. If Mildred is indeed dehydrated as a result of high blood sugar levels, then it makes sense that she would have high urine output. (High blood glucose levels would eventually exceed the kidney threshold, causing glucose excretion, which would take high volumes of body water with it—osmotic diuresis.) Unresponsive patients cannot always retain urine (or feces) once their individual capacity is reached.

16. What are contributing factors to dehydration in the elderly?

There are two major factors. The first is the decrease in total body mass. With a loss of muscle mass caused by aging, a major store of body water is lost, and thus a source of compensation. The second is a decrease in the sensation of thirst. As one ages, the thirst sensation becomes less active and predisposes to dehydration. Another related factor is the effect of pharmacologic agents. Many antihypertensive agents have a diuretic effect.

17. Of what importance are these contributing factors to prehospital care providers?

Elderly patients often enter into a state of disease or trauma already dehydrated to some extent. Together, a normal loss of muscle mass in the presence of a preexisting degree of dehydration contributes to an inability to compensate for moderate or even mild insults. The elderly are truly delicate patients to care for.

18. If the blood sugar is "high" and the patient is dehydrated, why is there no odor of ketones?

First, patients with this combination of symptoms are not always diabetic and not all diabetic patients in DKA have a distinctive odor of ketones. Second, there is another type of diabetes, called hyperosmolar hyperglycemic nonketotic coma (HHNK), that is primarily a disorder of older diabetic patients who are non–insulin dependent. They don't have enough insulin to assist in glucose transport across cellular membranes but they have just enough to prevent fat breakdown and ketone production. There is also a relatively limited stress response (probably a result of age-related changes) that also prevents the maximum stimulation of ketogenesis.

OUTCOME

Mildred was oxygenated with a non–rebreather mask and an IV of normal saline started. Repeat boluses of 200 cc were given to a total of 1000 cc. At that point Mildred became verbally responsive but was very confused and did not obey command, GCS 12. VS on arrival were BP 110/76, P 88, R 22. ABGs were within normal limits; however, Mildred's blood sugar was 1149 mg/dl. Mildred was admitted for severe dehydration related to acute HHNK (hyperosmolar, hyperglycemic, nonketotic coma). She was eventually discharged to home with the diagnosis of Type II diabetes and managed with oral hypoglycemic agents.

CASE 4

Dispatch: 10:30 hrs; 34 y/o, unconscious male

On Arrival: You arrive at the scene of a 10 kilometer race. It is a sunny day with a cool breeze and your patient, Robert, is one of the participants. Robert collapsed at the 8 K marker. He is lying supine, appears gray, diaphoretic, and has his eyes closed.

Initial Assessment Findings

Mental Status—Moans and has purposeful response to pain
Airway—Open and clear
Breathing—RR 36 and shallow; lung sounds clear in all lobes
Circulation—Skin cold and wet with a gray tinge and cyanosis around nose and lips
      Radial pulse weak and rapid
      BP 70/42
      Abdomen soft, no response when palpated
Chief Complaint—Collapsed and is unresponsive

Focused History

Events—Robert was maintaining a steady pace for approximately 7 K when he began to fall behind, started weaving between runners, and then collapsed.
Previous Illness—Unknown runner from out-of-town, no identification available other than name, age, and address.
Current Health Status—Unknown
Allergies—Unknown
Medications—Unknown

Focused Physical

Current Set of VS—BP 70/42, P 158, RR 36
Other Physical Findings—Pupils dilated, react sluggishly bilaterally; profusely sweating; pulse oximetry reads "ERROR"
Diagnostic Tests—There is no change after a fluid challenge of 300 cc; blood sugar "Low"

ECG

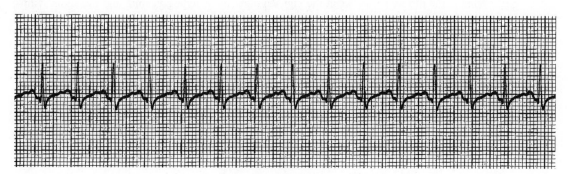

Figure 3-4

QUESTIONS

1. What is significant about Robert's history?

2. What body systems are affected?

3. What is Robert's Glasgow Coma Score?

4. What is the relationship between Robert's hypotension; tachycardia; cold, clammy skin; and cyanosis?

5. Assuming the blood glucose monitor is functioning correctly, what are possible reasons for blood sugar to read "low"?

6. What are possible reasons for the pulse oximetry to give an "ERROR" reading, and do any of these apply to Robert's situation?

7. What could explain Robert's mental status?

8. How serious is Robert's problem?

9. What are possible causes of Robert's current condition?

10. What would your immediate treatment steps include?

11. If you gave D_{50}, would you include thiamine in your treatment?

12. Would you include Narcan (naloxone) in your treatment?

13. How would you describe Robert's ECG? Does it change your approach or treatment?

14. If you suspected Robert was a diabetic, how could you check?

15. If you found no sign of injection sites, and there was no response to D_{50}, what other factors could explain his hypotension; tachycardia; cold, clammy skin; and cyanosis?

16. What are possible reasons for the blood glucose monitor to malfunction or to give an incorrect reading, and do any of these apply to Robert's case?

17. Considering that Robert had no response to the fluid bolus and no response to the D_{50}, now what are your treatment steps?

18. What is the difference between the signs/symptoms of hypoglycemia and the signs/symptoms of heat exhaustion?

19. Can a diabetic patient in hypoglycemia sweat enough to drop the blood pressure as much as Robert's?

20. What would have happened to Robert if an allergic reaction would have been suspected and epinephrine was given?

QUESTIONS AND ANSWERS

1. What is significant about Robert's history?

Extreme exercise before collapse

2. What body systems are affected?

CNS—moans with purposeful response to pain
Cardiovascular—hypotension; tachycardia; cold, clammy skin; cyanosis
Respiratory—rapid, shallow rate

3. What is Robert's Glasgow Coma Score?

GCS 8 (1 no eye opening, 5 purposeful response to pain, 2 moaning)

4. What is the relationship between Robert's hypotension; tachycardia; cold, clammy skin; and cyanosis?

Peripheral vasoconstriction and tachycardia are compensatory mechanisms for hypotension. Clammy skin is an effect resulting from epinephrine and norepinephrine. Cyanosis is a result of either lack of perfusion (resulting from severe vasoconstriction or hypotension) or lack of oxygenation.

5. Assuming the blood glucose monitor is functioning correctly, what are possible reasons for blood sugar to read "low"?

Blood sugar stores can be used up (1) during extreme metabolic demand such as exercise, especially if intake was inadequate before exercise, fever, or environmental extremes; (2) if the pancreas malfunctions producing too much insulin, usually because of a tumor; (3) in the presence of diabetes with too much insulin or exercise; or (4) in the presence of drugs or medication that lower the blood sugar level.

6. What are possible reasons for the pulse oximetry to give an "ERROR" reading, and do any of these apply to Robert's situation?

"ERROR" readings may occur when severe vasoconstriction is present as in hypothermia or shock. Robert is hypotensive and the presence of cold, clammy skin indicates a degree of vasoconstriction is present.

7. What could explain Robert's mental status?

His hypotension, low blood sugar, or a heat-related problem, such as heat exhaustion or heat stroke, could explain his status.

8. How serious is Robert's problem?

This is a true medical emergency. Brain cells without oxygen or glucose die.

9. What are possible causes of Robert's current condition?

Hypoglycemia or a heat-related illness. Both conditions can present in this manner.

10. What would your immediate treatment steps include?

Assist with a BVM and reservoir with oxygen at 15 lpm, start an IV of normal saline, and administer 50 ml of D_{50} slow IV push.

11. If you gave D_{50}, would you include thiamine in your treatment?

Thiamine is necessary for the brain to metabolize glucose. An absence of thiamine in the presence of higher glucose concentrations may cause neurologic damage. Many systems consider thiamine 100 mg IV push as standard care whenever glucose IV is given. Other systems do not. In those systems administration of thiamine is based on the suspicion of alcohol use, appearance of malnourishment, and/or short transport times. There is a window of time such that, if thiamine is required, it can be given after glucose.

12. Would you include Narcan (naloxone) in your treatment?

If you didn't, the reason was probably because hypoglycemia was clearly evident and the circumstances are such that use of a narcotic has a very low probability. The triad of symptoms commonly used to determine naloxone use is: constricted pupils, decreased mental status, and decreased respirations. This triad is not present. It is acceptable not to give naloxone in this situation.

13. *How would you describe Robert's ECG? Does it change your approach or treatment?*

Sinus tachycardia; it does not change approach or treatment.

14. *If you suspected Robert was a diabetic, how could you check?*

Look for a medic-alert tag as a necklace, bracelet, attachment to watch, or ankle bracelet. Look for injection sites. Common sites include the abdomen and both thighs. Insulin-dependent diabetics must give themselves repeated injections over a long time period. Rotating sites helps keep subcutaneous scar tissue at a minimum. However, those sites will develop a particular texture and sometimes a visible change occurs. Those sites feel fibrous and firmer than surrounding tissue.

15. *If you found no sign of injection sites, and there was no response to D_{50}, what other factors could explain his hypotension; tachycardia; cold, clammy skin; and cyanosis?*

Robert has an extreme epinephrine/norepinephrine response. He has just been in extreme exercise that could explain everything *except* his hypotension. Robert is in shock, and the trick is to figure out what type. If it is a hot day, heat exhaustion (fluid loss) could be a possibility. Extreme sweating as a part of a heat-related problem and an allergic reaction are all possibilities. Other possibilities include an internal bleed and a drug-related problem.

16. *What are possible reasons for the blood glucose monitor to malfunction or to give an incorrect reading, and do any of these apply to Robert's case?*

When the machine has not been correctly calibrated or in cases of a broken device. The machine was correctly calibrated and was not broken. These do not apply to Robert.

17. *Considering that Robert had no response to the fluid bolus and no response to the D_{50}, now what are your treatment steps?*

If Robert continues to be cyanotic even with ventilating with the bag-valve-mask, consider intubating. Repeat the fluid bolus and monitor lung sounds and BP. Carefully reassess, listen especially to lung sounds (wheezing, rales), look for wheals, a rash, swollen mucous membranes, anything that would be out of the ordinary. Retest the blood sugar and consider repeating D_{50}.

18. *What is the difference between the signs/symptoms of hypoglycemia and the signs/symptoms of heat exhaustion?*

Both conditions trigger an acute epinephrine/norepinephrine response that then leads to extreme peripheral vasoconstriction, tachycardia, and rapid, shallow respirations. Skin color ranges from extremely pale to ashen in both conditions and can manifest confusion. Both hypoglycemia and heat exhaustion manifest extreme diaphoresis. The history of insulin-dependent diabetes and a low blood sugar may help identify the hypoglycemic diabetic patient, but extreme exercise in hot weather can also lower blood sugar, though usually not as much as a diabetic reaction. The problem in Robert's case was that both were present, so both needed to be treated.

19. *Can a diabetic patient in hypoglycemia sweat enough to drop the blood pressure as much as Robert's?*

It would be unusual for that to happen. However, remember that Robert had two problems compounding one another. A diabetic patient with a hypoglycemic reaction may sweat profusely enough to become dehydrated. Combine that with extreme exercise and you will likely see other "extremes" in symptoms such as cyanotic or ashen, cold skin; extremely high heart rates; and unconsciousness.

20. *What would have happened to Robert if an allergic reaction would have been suspected and epinephrine was given?*

At worst case scenario, the addition of epinephrine might have caused a further increase in heart rate, vasoconstriction, and cardiac contractility thus increasing the oxygen demand and increasing the cardiac workload leading to ischemia of cardiac muscle. At best case scenario, the increase in heart rate, vasoconstriction, and cardiac contractility might have caused a temporary increase in BP without myocardial infarction. In either case, ischemia of cardiac muscle probably would have occurred. Both a myocardial infarction and an epinephrine response have the potential to increase blood glucose levels.

OUTCOME

Paramedics gave Robert a total of 800 cc normal saline in 200 to 400 cc boluses and two amps (total of 100 ml) of D_{50} before arrival at the local hospital. On arrival, Robert was responsive to voice but remained confused, VS: P 100, RR 20, BP 106/72. Hospital lab results showed a blood sugar of 50 mg/dl. That was *after* the two amps of D_{50} in the field. He was given a high-carbohydrate snack in the ED and continued the IV of normal saline at 100 cc/hr. After another 15 to 20 minutes he became fully oriented and was able to tell staff that he was an insulin-dependent diabetic and had taken his medic-alert necklace off for the race because it "bounced around and bothered me." His hypoglycemia was compounded by the fact that he was sweating profusely from the exercise of the race itself and had also suffered sodium and water depletion. He was eventually dismissed from the ED to home.

CASE 5

Dispatch: 07:30 hrs; unconscious 72 y/o female, possible stroke

On Arrival: You find 72 y/o Phyllis, lying in bed with the covers disheveled. She appears to be sleeping, pale, and obese.

Initial Assessment Findings

Mental Status—Unresponsive to voice, withdraws to pain, no verbal response
Airway—Open with blood-tinged saliva
Breathing—RR 8, shallow and labored; lung sounds diminished in bases
Circulation—Skin cool, very dry, and pale, feels doughy
          Radial pulse weak at 50
          BP 90/60
Chief Complaint—Seizure in absence of history of epilepsy

Focused History

Events—Son checks on her regularly and found her having a seizure in bed this morning
Previous Illness—None known, has not seen a physician since children were born
Current Health Status—Seemed to be healthy until husband died 3 months ago. Since then has been quiet and withdrawn with no energy. Son states she gradually stopped all activity since husband died.
Allergies—None known
Medications—None

Focused Physical

Current Set of VS—P 60, RR 8, BP 90/60
Other Pertinent Findings—Skin yellowish but sclera white, face puffy, tongue abraded and seems swollen, she has pitting edema to her knees, abdomen large and distended, pulse oximetry 86% on room air
Diagnostic Tests—Blood sugar 80 mg/dl

ECG

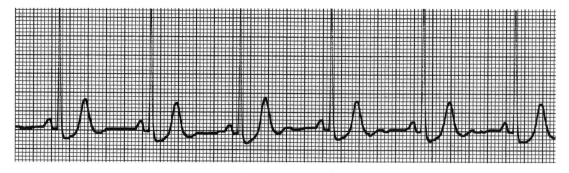

Figure 3-5

1. What is significant about Phyllis' history?

2. What body systems are affected?

3. What is Phyllis' Glasgow Coma Score?

4. What is suggested by Phyllis' slightly bloody saliva?

5. What is the significance of a pulse oximetry reading of 86% on room air?

6. Is her blood sugar low enough to account for her seizure?

7. What is significant about Phyllis' bradycardia?

8. Is Phyllis' heart rate low enough to explain her hypotension?

9. Phyllis is hypotensive but not tachycardic, has pale, cool skin but is not sweating, has pitting edema to her knees and a puffy face but is not tachypneic, has an altered mental status, and has an odd consistency of her skin. What might explain this collection of symptoms, and how should you proceed?

10. How serious is Phyllis' condition?

11. What are your immediate treatment steps?

12. Where would you start the IV and why?

13. Management of Phyllis' airway did not improve her BP. How would you support Phyllis' BP, and what would you need to evaluate to help you decide?

14. Are there any other conservative treatment measures you could do?

15. If Phyllis had a recurrent seizure, what would you do, and why?

16. Phyllis' pulse oximetry was 86%. If she were anemic, what would be the relationship between the two?

17. Phyllis was given a 200 ml fluid bolus, which resulted in bilateral wheezing but her systolic pressure increased to 100. However, even after intubation and ventilation, Phyllis' ABGs were: pH 7.32, $PaCO_2$ 50, PaO_2 80, HCO_3^- 19. What could explain those results?

18. Is there a relationship between anemia and edema?

19. Was there any other part of her history or physical examination that might have been helpful?

QUESTIONS AND ANSWERS

1. What is significant about Phyllis' history?

She hasn't seen a doctor in years, has had a problem for at least 3 months, and sudden onset of a seizure in the absence of a history of seizures.

2. What body systems are affected?

CNS—seizure

Respiratory—RR 8 and labored, pulse ox 86% on room air

Cardiovascular—hypotension; relatively slow heart rate; and doughy, pale, cool skin

Integumentary—excessively dry, doughy skin that is cool

3. What is Phyllis' Glasgow Coma Score?

GCS 6 (1 no eye opening, 1 no verbal response, 4 withdraws to pain)

4. What is suggested by Phyllis' slightly bloody saliva?

She just had a seizure by her son's report; her abraded tongue is suggestive of a grand mal seizure and could explain the bloody saliva.

5. What is the significance of a pulse oximetry reading of 86% on room air?

That isn't a normal value and has to be taken in light of the grand mal seizure she likely had. Sustained skeletal muscle contractions prevent normal respirations and hypoxia is common. Normally, once seizure activity has ceased, normal respiratory function rapidly corrects the hypoxia. The fact that she is not seizing now and has depressed respirations with a pulse oximetry reading of 86% indicates a need for assisted ventilations with high-flow oxygen.

6. Is her blood sugar low enough to account for her seizure?

No, not unless it dropped suddenly and there is no evidence of that.

7. What is significant about Phyllis' heart rate?

The fact that Phyllis has a heart rate of 60 after a grand mal seizure is unusual. Ask how long ago the seizure stopped to better assess the status of her heart rate. If the seizure stopped just before your arrival, a heart rate of 60 is unusual and probably worrisome.

8. Is Phyllis' heart rate low enough to explain her hypotension?

Not usually; however, cardiac ischemia from the seizure may have occurred.

9. Phyllis is hypotensive but not tachycardic, has pale, cool skin but is not sweating, has pitting edema to her knees and a puffy face but is not tachypneic, has an altered mental status and has an odd consistency of her skin. What might explain this collection of symptoms, and how should you proceed?

Her odd collection of symptoms and history of a probable 3-month long problem are indications of a long-term condition field personnel probably can't fix. The normal reaction of the body to hypoxia and hypotension is to have an epinephrine/norepinephrine response, but Phyllis doesn't seem to have one. It is possible, but unlikely, that she has a drug overdose. (There are no empty pill bottles or other indicators.) She doesn't have the collection of signs or symptoms that one might expect when sepsis is present, or when kidney failure is present. Therefore she should be treated by body system, symptomatically, and conservatively.

10. How serious is Phyllis' condition?

She is hypoxic (pulse ox 86%) with an inadequate respiratory rate, hypotensive, relative bradycardia, and has a GCS of 6. She needs to be treated immediately with supportive measures.

11. What are your immediate treatment steps?

Manage her airway, intubate and place an oral airway. If she has another seizure the oral airway will ensure the ET tube will not be kinked closed. Ventilate at 16 to 20/minute and watch her pulse ox for improvement. Start an IV of normal saline.

12. Where would you start the IV and why?

Start the IV midarm if possible and avoid joints. She had one seizure for an unknown reason and may have another. No matter where you start it, to avoid having it pulled out during a seizure, tape it down securely and consider wrapping with gauze or Kerlix.

13. Management of Phyllis' airway did not improve her BP. How would you support Phyllis' BP, and what would you need to evaluate to help you decide?

There are three choices: (1) A 200 cc fluid bolus and reevaluate her lung sounds, (2) give atropine to increase the heart rate, or (3) try a dopamine drip. You would need to take into account the fact that she seems to be "puffy" and has pitting edema (which indicates fluid retention), your transport time to the hospital, and her repeat vital signs and mental status. Of the three treatment choices atropine would be the least invasive. However, since her underlying problem is unknown, it might be best to wait until arrival at the hospital if transport time is short.

14. Are there any other conservative treatment measures you could do?

Keep her warm; her skin is cool to the touch. If you had a thermometer, you could take her temperature.

15. If Phyllis had a recurrent seizure, what would you do and why?

Give her Valium (diazepam) 5 to 10 mg, slow IV push during the seizure activity. Diazepam only works during the seizure activity and is not useful as a preventive measure.

16. Phyllis' pulse oximetry was 86%. If she were anemic, what would be the relationship between the two?

Pulse oximetry cannot distinguish between normal and abnormal amounts of red blood cells (RBCs). If all the available RBCs were saturated, pulse oximetry would indicate a normal saturation level, despite a severe lack of RBCs. Therefore anemia renders pulse oximetry inaccurate, which is why the total picture of the patient needs to be taken into account. In Phyllis' case, however, the determination of hypoxia was correct.

17. Phyllis was given a 200 ml fluid bolus, which resulted in bilateral wheezing but her systolic pressure increased to 100. However, even after intubation and ventilation, Phyllis' ABGs were: pH 7.32, $PaCO_2$ 50, PaO_2 80, HCO_3^- 19. What could explain those results?

Slow, shallow respirations do not allow alveoli to fully expand leading to atelectasis and, over a given time period, pleural effusions occur. This gives rise to inadequate ventilation. Phyllis has a systolic pressure of 90, which was low but ordinarily not low enough to inadequately perfuse the lungs. Phyllis had a ventilation/perfusion problem with inadequate ventilation but perfusion was okay. Usually intubation with positive pressure ventilation (bag-valve-mask) will help open up those alveoli but with pleural effusion present, exchange of oxygen and carbon dioxide is still impaired. The 200 cc bolus of fluid, while a relatively minor amount, was evidently just enough to cause wheezing, which indicated the collection of fluid between the capillaries and the terminal bronchiole of the alveoli was present. Her blood gases were still low, but not as low as they would have been had intubation and ventilation not been done.

18. Is there a relationship between anemia and edema?

Yes, anemia affects blood viscosity. Cardiac output increases to maintain tissue perfusion. The "diluted" blood flows faster and more turbulently than "normal thickness" blood. Increased blood flow within the heart can predispose to congestive heart failure. Because of the lower serum protein levels resulting from some types of anemia, edema might be seen. Relatively minor amounts of fluid can predispose to pulmonary edema in the presence of anemia. However, the degree of pitting edema in Phyllis' case is not explained by anemia alone.

19. Was there any other part of her history or physical examination that might have been helpful?

Did Phyllis have a sudden weight loss/gain? Have a sudden loss/gain of appetite? Have any complaints? Did the family notice a change in her mentation or presence of confusion?

OUTCOME

Phyllis was intubated and ventilated with an IV of normal saline started. A fluid bolus of 200 cc was given with the result of bilateral wheezing but her BP increased to 100 systolic. No further field treatment was given. On arrival at the hospital ABGs showed a pH of 7.32, $PaCO_2/PaO_2$ 50, pO_2 80, HCO_3^- 19. Serum electrolytes showed a sodium level of 108 (135 to 145 mEq/l). A blood count showed anemia with Hgb 9 (12 to 16 gm/dl) and Hct 31% (37% to 45%). Her body temperature was low at 96° F. Her mental status did not improve, and she was placed on a ventilator and admitted to the ICU. Phyllis was diagnosed with myxedema coma, a hypothyroid disorder that results in hypothermia, respiratory depression, bradycardia, delayed reflexes, and dry, rough skin. Dilutional hyponatremia is common, leading to peripheral edema and seizures. (Phyllis' peripheral edema and onset of pulmonary edema after fluid bolus was directly related to her hyponatremia. Her anemia contributed to her CHF, making it more obvious.) This condition is more common in elderly women, especially after a stressor. Phyllis eventually recovered and was dismissed to home.

BIBLIOGRAPHY

American Heart Association. Cummins, R. O. (Ed.). (1994). *Advanced cardiac life support textbook.* Dallas, TX: American Heart Association.

American Heart Association. Chameides, L., & Hazinski, M. F. (Eds.). (1994). *Textbook of pediatric advanced life support.* Dallas, TX: American Heart Association.

Barnwell, M. M., Raskopf, V., Kimball, R., & Tapler, D. (1995). *The Skidmore-Roth outline series: Diabetes.* El Paso, TX: Skidmore-Roth Publishing.

Berkow, R., & Fletcher, A. J. (Eds.). (1992). *Merck manual of diagnosis and therapy.* Rahway, NJ: Merck Research Laboratories.

Beymer, P. L., & Huether, S. E. (1994). Alterations of hormonal regulation. In K. L. McCance & S. E. Huether (Eds.). *Pathophysiology: The biologic basis for disease in adults and children,* (2nd ed., pp. 656-708). St. Louis, MO: Mosby.

Bledsoe, B. E., Clayden, D. E., & Papa, F. J. (1996). *Prehospital emergency pharmacology,* (4th ed.). Upper Saddle, River, NJ: Brady, Prentice Hall.

Bongard, F. S., & Sue, D. Y. (Eds.). (1994). *Current: Critical care, diagnosis, and treatment.* Norwalk, CT: Appleton & Lange.

Davis, S. N., & Granner, D. K. (1996). Insulin, oral hypoglycemic agents, and the pharmacology of the endocrine pancreas. In J. G. Hardman & L. E. Limbird (Eds.). *The pharmacological basis of therapeutics,* (9th ed., pp. 1487-1518). New York, NY: McGraw-Hill.

Farwell, A. P., & Braverman, L. E. (1996). Thyroid and antithyroid drugs. In J. G. Hardman & L. E. Limbird (Eds.). *Goodman & Gilman's: The pharmacological basis of therapeutics,* (9th ed., pp. 1383-1410). New York, NY: McGraw-Hill.

Kelley, S. J. (1994). *Pediatric emergency nursing,* (2nd ed.). Norwalk, CT: Appleton & Lange.

Marcus, R., & Coulston, A. M. (1996). The vitamins. In J. G. Hardman & L. E. Limbird (Eds.). *Goodman & Gilman's: The pharmacological basis of therapeutics,* (9th ed., pp. 1547- 1571). New York, NY: McGraw-Hill.

Martini, F. H., & Bartholomew, E. F. (1997). *Essentials of anatomy and physiology.* Upper Saddle River, NJ: Prentice Hall.

Pons, P. T., & Cason, D. (1997). Conditions by diagnosis. In The American College of Emergency Physicians. *Paramedic field care: A complaint-based approach.* St Louis, MO: Mosby.

Tierney, L. M., McPhee, S. J., & Papadakis, M. A. (Eds.). (1994). *Current: Medical diagnosis, and treatment.* Norwalk, CT: Appleton & Lange.

4

Hematology Emergencies

OVERVIEW

Many disorders of the blood exist, some inherited and some acquired. These disorders are primarily divided into three general types: those that involve the erythrocytes or RBCs, those that involve the leukocytes (WBCs)/lymphoid tissue, and those that involve clotting factors. Specific disorders that may be encountered include conditions such as cancers of the bone marrow or lymph (the various types of leukemia); chronic diseases involving red blood cell production, such as one of the anemias (e.g., pernicious anemia, aplastic anemia, sickle-cell anemia, Cooley's anemia); conditions of too many RBCs, such as polycythemia vera; or diseases of clotting (e.g., hemophilia, von Willebrand's disease).

Patients that present to EMS providers with disorders involving the hematologic system are rare in some areas but are becoming more frequent in others. With technology and current treatment techniques enabling patients with blood disorders to live longer with a better quality of life, EMS providers are more likely to encounter patients with these preexisting problems.

Providers may be called for an emergency directly related to the underlying disease process (as in the case of a sickle-cell anemia patient with acute abdominal pain resulting from a sickle-cell crisis) or to an emergency resulting from a side effect of treatment (as in the case of a leukemia patient on chemotherapy who suddenly starts a profuse nose bleed). It is, however, more common for providers to be called to an emergency where the hematologic disorder is incidental to the call, as in the dispatch to a motor vehicle crash where the injured person also happens to have hemophilia.

In the case of a patient presenting with a chronic disease process involving the blood, there are several characteristics to keep in mind. Airway and breathing may be affected because RBCs exchange oxygen and carbon dioxide at the alveolar level, as well as the cellular level. If a problem exists with the ability of the RBCs to carry oxygen then hypoxemia may result. Other common symptoms involving oxygen transport may include syncope, fatigue, and difficulty walking. Pallor and increased work of breathing are frequently noted.

If a problem exists with the protein content of blood, then peripheral edema may result. Pulmonary edema may occur in some patients with an unrecognized anemia or those undergoing treatment for leukemia.

Circulation may be affected because of perfusion abnormalities. A sickle-cell occlusive crisis may result in ischemia of the joints and capillary beds, causing pain. Disturbance of clotting factors may result in bleeding tendencies as in many of the leukemias. A tendency to form clots along with an increased incidence for angina and bleeding may occur with polycythemia vera, a condition of too many red blood cells. An increased incidence of pulmonary emboli may also be present in these patients.

81

Problems that may be encountered when responding to patients with emergencies directly related to their underlying hematologic diseases include difficulty breathing, bleeding tendencies, pain (usually ischemic in nature), hypoperfusion, and an increased tendency for pulmonary emboli.

Assessment and Treatment

History is very important. If the incident is directly related to the underlying disorder, questions asking when the last incident occurred, how does this incident compare to the last one, and what was done for the last incident, are very helpful. If the disorder is incidental to the nature of the call, questions regarding when the last treatment was received (if appropriate), medications, and medical allergies are pertinent.

EMS providers are trained to recognize the immediate threat to life, the potential threat to life, and the absence of a threat to life. With any patient who presents with an underlying condition that is unfamiliar to the care provider, basic tenets dictate that assessment priorities should be followed and the patient treated symptomatically. It is not necessary that a care provider know exactly what the final diagnosis is to treat. The priorities of airway, breathing, and circulation do not change, no matter what the problem. For those who have chronic conditions and an emergency related to that condition, most patients and their families know more about their own disorder than most medical providers. They may be the best source of information regarding what needs to be done. Contacting medical control should always be an option and should be encouraged in these situations.

CASE 1

Dispatch: 19:45 hrs; 8 y/o male, severe abdominal pain

On Arrival: You find 8 y/o Jarrell, lying in the fetal position on his bed, moaning; he appears pale and is diaphoretic. His mother is present and anxious.

Initial Assessment Findings

Mental Status—Lethargic but oriented and obeys command

Airway—Open and clear

Breathing—RR 32 and shallow; lung sounds faint wheezes in bilateral bases

Circulation—Skin cool, clammy; pale mucous membranes

Radial pulse 130

BP 90/68

Chief Complaint—"My tummy hurts bad."

Focused History

Events—Jarrell was outside sledding (outside temperature 30° F) when he came in complaining of his asthma. After his nebulizer treatment, he went back outside to play. About 30 minutes later he came back in complaining of abdominal and joint pain. He denied any trauma. The abdominal pain has been getting worse over the last hour. His mother was unable to reach the family physician so she called EMS.

Previous Illness—History of sickle-cell anemia, history of exercise-induced asthma

Current Health Status—Frequent episodes of sickle-cell crises, the last one was last month. His last asthma attack that required hospitalization was 2 months ago.

Allergies—None known

Medications—Ventolin (albuterol) inhaler

Focused Physical

Current Set of VS—P 136, RR 32, BP 90/68

Other Pertinent Findings—Mother stated Jarrell was dressed warmly but came in from sledding soaking wet; no sign of trauma; abdomen is tense with pain on palpation; abdominal pain described as steady, sharp, and ranks as an 8 on a 1 to 10 scale, left upper quadrant most painful, denies radiation; hands, feet, elbows appear swollen and are painful to touch; Jarrell denies shortness of breath; pulse oximetry reads "ERROR"; blood sugar 100; weight 80 lbs (36 kg)

Diagnostic Tests—Fluid bolus of 500 ml resulted in no change of VS; however, complaints of joint pain increased

ECG

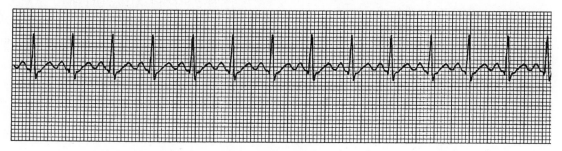

Figure 4-1

QUESTIONS

1. What is significant about Jarrell's history?

2. What body systems are affected?

3. What is Jarrell's Glasgow Coma Score?

4. How would you describe Jarrell's ECG?

5. What are possible reasons for pulse oximetry to read "ERROR"?

6. What is the pathophysiology of sickle cell anemia?

7. What can precipitate a sickle cell crisis?

8. Did Jarrell have any of the precipitating factors present?

9. Is there any other information, from either his history or your physical examination that would be helpful?

10. How does the pathophysiology of sickle-cell anemia relate to Jarrell's present complaint?

11. What is the significance of Jarrell's swollen and painful hands, feet, and joints?

12. Jarrell's vital signs indicate a tachycardia and tachypnea in the presence of a blood pressure of 90 systolic. How could this be explained?

13. The fluid bolus of 500 ml resulted in no change of vital signs but increased complaints of joint pain. What is a likely explanation for the increased complaints of pain?

14. Jarrell describes his pain as being steady and sharp with no radiation and ranks it as an 8 on a 1 to 10 scale. He is lying in the fetal position and points to the left upper quadrant as being most painful. His abdomen is flat and tense and painful to palpation. During the examination, he suddenly complains of a sharp, stabbing pain in his left neck and shoulder. What is the most likely explanation, and of what significance is this?

15. How serious is this situation?

16. How would you initially treat Jarrell?

17. What is Jarrell at risk for?

18. Are there bronchodilators that would be contraindicated in patients with sickle-cell disease?

19. After reviewing the pathophysiology of sickle-cell crisis, what are the main priorities for a patient who has a history of sickle-cell disease?

QUESTIONS AND ANSWERS

1. What is significant about Jarrell's history?

History of sickle-cell anemia and exercise-induced asthma; presence of abdominal pain in absence of trauma; now has joint pain with swollen, painful hands, and feet; on an albuterol inhaler

2. What body systems are affected?

Respiratory—respiratory rate of 32 and bilateral basilar wheezes
Cardiovascular—tachycardia with pale, cool, clammy skin; BP 90 systolic
Other—abdominal pain, specific system unknown; swollen, painful hands and feet with joint pain

3. What is Jarrell's Glasgow Coma Score?

Jarrell's GCS is 15 (4 spontaneous eye opening, 5 oriented, 6 follows command)

4. How would you describe Jarrell's ECG?

Sinus tachycardia without ectopy. Normal P wave, PR interval, narrow QRS <0.10.

5. What are possible reasons for pulse oximetry to read "ERROR"?

His skin is cool and clammy. That suggests that there is peripheral vasoconstriction occurring. That is the most likely reason for the reading of "ERROR".

6. What is the pathophysiology of sickle-cell anemia?

Sickle-cell anemia results from the production of an abnormal form of hemoglobin, called hemoglobin S (Hgb S). It is a genetic molecular defect that is more common in those of African, Mediterranean, Middle Eastern, and East Indian descent. The presence of the abnormal hemoglobin gives the individual the ability to resist the parasitic infections that cause malaria. Hgb S is always present in the blood of a person with sickle-cell anemia; however, it is the deoxygenated form of Hgb S within the RBC, that stretches it into a sickle shape. Sickling usually is not permanent, and intact RBCs can return to normal shape when the Hgb S is reoxygenated. Sickling most frequently occurs in isolated areas (within the body) that have no oxygen content, but can occur anywhere in the body.

Sickled RBCs are stiff and cannot change shape as easily as normal cells when they pass through the microcirculation. As a result, large amounts of sickled RBCs tend to plug the microvasculature, causing vascular occlusion, ischemic pain, and organ infarction. This is the pathophysiology of a vasoocclusive crisis. Sickled RBCs are also more fragile and tend to rupture; thus their lifespan is 10 to 20 days compared to the 120 days for normal RBCs. This hemolysis results in the classic anemia of "sickle-cell anemia."

An exaggerated response may also occur in the spleen causing a sequestration crisis. When undergoing normal hemolysis, a large number of RBCs may become pooled in the spleen, causing a worsening of the anemia and infarction of splenic vessels and hypovolemic shock.

7. What can precipitate a sickle-cell crisis?

Precipitating factors include any circumstance that could lead to increased concentration of Hgb S (dehydration, pregnancy), increased tissue hypoxia (depressed respiratory function as in asthma, pneumonia, high altitude, acidosis), increased oxygen demand (stress, exertion, fatigue), or severe vasoconstriction (exposure to cold). Infections can trigger more rapid hemolysis (hemolytic crisis), an increase in the number of RBCs pooled in the spleen (sequestration crisis), a decrease in the rate of manufacturing new RBCs in the marrow (aplastic crises), or in the case of respiratory infections, interfere with oxygenation of blood.

8. Did Jarrell have any of the precipitating factors present?

Yes, he was outside sled riding, in the wet and cold. It is impossible to tell from the description how cold he might have gotten. His swollen hands and feet might be from the cold or an indicating sign of sickle cell crisis. His condition was complicated by the presence of his exercise-induced asthma. Oxygen demand was increased by exercise in cold weather. Fatigue from the exercise and stress of the asthma and just being outside in the cold are all factors that could play a part.

9. Is there any other information, from either his history or your physical examination, that would be helpful?

This child has two chronic physical conditions, both of which require fairly detailed questions. When was he last seen for his asthma? What happened and what did they do? During his last sickle-cell crisis what treatment was required? Has he had any recent infections such as a sore throat or urinary tract infection?

Sometimes an open-ended question such as "what happened?" will get the most information. For this child it would be important for the receiving hospital to know the type of his last sickle-cell crisis (e.g., vasoocclusive, sequestration, hemolytic, or aplastic). Parents of chronically ill children are frequently very knowledgeable about the disease.

One of the most important questions is "Is this how he usually presents when he has a sickle-cell crisis?" A new pattern (such as abdominal pain) may indicate an emergent problem.

10. How does the pathophysiology of sickle-cell anemia relate to Jarrell's present complaint?

Sickling, which causes sluggish flow and clumping, leads to occlusion of the microvasculature, which initiates tissue hypoxia and ischemia causing pain. Severe abdominal pain often is caused by infarction in abdominal structures. Painful and swollen large joints and surrounding tissues may also be evident because of ischemia and infarction of joints and surrounding tissues.

11. What is the significance of Jarrell's swollen and painful hands, feet, and joints?

There are two possibilities. One possibility is that his swollen extremities are due to frostbite. However, it would be unlikely that his entire arms and shoulders would be affected without having his nose, ears, or other parts of his face also affected. The second possibility is that his swollen, painful extremities and joints are due to the ischemia and hypoxia of a vasoocclusive crisis.

12. Jarrell's vital signs indicate a tachycardia and tachypnea in the presence of a blood pressure of 90 systolic. How could this be explained?

These vital signs in the presence of pale, cool, and clammy skin suggests compensated shock. There is no indication of trauma and no sign of trauma.

13. The fluid bolus of 500 ml resulted in no change of vital signs but increased complaints of joint pain. What is a likely explanation for the increased complaints of pain?

This child has a history of sickle-cell anemia. The process of sickling can be precipitated by cold. If the IV fluids were not warmed, they may have been cold enough to precipitate localized sickling, perceived as joint pain.

14. Jarrell describes his pain as being steady and sharp with no radiation and ranks it as an 8 on a 1 to 10 scale. He is lying in the fetal position and points to the left upper quadrant as being most painful. His abdomen is flat and tense and painful to palpation. During the examination, he suddenly complains of a sharp, stabbing pain in his left neck and shoulder. What is the most likely explanation, and of what significance is this?

Steady, sharp pain is most likely parietal in origin. Pain that arises from the parietal peritoneum is usually sharp, intense, and localized. Lying in the fetal position and having a tense, painful abdomen suggests peritoneal involvement. The sudden sharp, stabbing pain to the left neck and shoulder suggests peritoneal or diaphragmatic irritation with referred pain originating from the spleen. This is consistent with splenomegaly (sequestration) that can occur in sickle-cell crisis, or the rupture of the spleen with its capsule intact and distended as might occur in a trauma patient. In the absence of trauma, this finding suggests peritoneal or diaphragmatic irritation from splenomegaly rather than intraabdominal hemorrhaging.

15. How serious is this situation?

This is a patient whose vital signs and condition could collapse without warning. There are multiple organ system problems to contend with:

Respiratory system—bilateral wheezes interfering with oxygenation (he is at risk for a severe asthma attack)

Circulatory system—abdominal pain with signs of peritoneal irritation and compensated shock consistent with splenic involvement

Musculoskeletal system—swollen, painful hands and feet consistent with vasoocclusive crisis.

16. *How would you initially treat Jarrell?*

Place in position of comfort and keep warm. Administer a bronchodilator such as albuterol by nebulizer to increase air movement and oxygenation. Start an IV with normal saline and warm the fluid. That may mean hanging the IV bag by the heater or coiling the IV tubing inside a warm towel. Infuse by bolus (80 lbs = 36 kg − 20 = 720 ml) with approximately 700 ml of warmed IV fluid. Begin transport immediately. Increase the heat in the back of the ambulance, enough so you can work without your own coat on.

17. *What is Jarrell at risk for?*

He is at risk for severe anemia resulting from sequestering blood in his spleen, complete infarct of an organ, or even a stroke and infection.

18. *Are there bronchodilators that would be contraindicated in patients with sickle-cell disease?*

Bronchodilators in use today have only B_2 activity or both B_1 and B_2 activity, so that they also possess B_2 vasodilation effects. The notable exception is epinephrine, which has B_1, B_2 and A_1 activity. The A_1 vasoconstriction effect of epinephrine may be reason for using with caution in a sickle-cell patient, but there are no contraindications for its use in a life-threatening condition, such as severe asthma, anaphylaxis, symptomatic bradycardia, or cardiac arrest.

19. *After reviewing the pathophysiology of sickle-cell crisis, what are the main priorities for the patient who has a history of sickle-cell disease?*

Oxygenation—Because the process of sickling is dependent on things that lower oxygen tension, oxygenation would be important. However, experts point out that over-oxygenating could cause a rebound effect once it was discontinued. Therefore, unless the patient is hypoxic, use a nasal cannula at 2 to 4 lpm if oxygen is necessary. Since this patient is hypoxic (tachypnea and wheezing) he should be given high-flow oxygen by mask, non–rebreather with a reservoir at 15 lpm.

Hydration—Because sludging and increased blood viscosity further sickling, fluid administration is a critical part of treatment. Administering fluids according to body weight and by bolus is most appropriate.

Preserving body heat—Because hypothermia can precipitate sickling, keeping the patient warm is another priority. This includes removing any remaining wet clothing and covering with blankets, as well as warming IV fluids and increasing the heat in the back of the vehicle.

Prevent further stress—You may not be called for a problem that is directly related to a sickle-cell crisis, but the stress of having to call EMS may cause one. Keeping a calm demeanor and ensuring all questions are answered may go a long way to prevent the onset of a crisis.

Keep in mind that complaints of joint pain, in the absence of trauma, may be an indicator of a vasoocclusive sickle cell crisis. Knowing the priorities of care for these special patients may prevent further complications.

OUTCOME

Jarrell was given high-flow oxygen by a non–rebreather mask with reservoir at 15 lpm and an IV was started with 500 ml of normal saline given by bolus. His complaints of joint pain increased and by arrival at the hospital had begun to vomit and complain of chest pain. Initial VS at the ED showed a P 140, RR 36, and BP 90/76. X-rays and lab work were done, and Jarrell was dehydrated and in shock. He was prepared for an exchange transfusion and admitted with acute sequestration and vasoocclusive sickle-cell crisis. After a rough hospital course, with pneumonia and a cerebral infarction, he was eventually dismissed to home with mild left-sided weakness.

CASE 2

Dispatch: 17:30 hrs; 58 y/o female, difficulty breathing

On Arrival: You find 58 y/o Celia, sitting in a kitchen chair, awake. Her face is flushed and dark red. Her lips are cyanotic. She appears to be gasping for air.

Initial Assessment Findings

Mental Status—Awake, alert, and obeys command
Airway—Open and clear
Breathing—RR 22 and labored with accessory muscle use, talking in 1 to 2 word phrases; lung sounds, rales and wheezes in all lobes
Circulation—Skin flushed, dark red; cyanotic lips and nail beds; cool and clammy to the touch
Radial pulse rapid and irregular at 110
BP 156/92
Chief Complaint—Difficulty breathing

Focused History

Events—Celia was getting dinner prepared when she had sudden, sharp, right-sided chest pain followed by shortness of breath that rapidly got worse. She called for her husband and when he saw her he immediately called EMS.
Previous Illness—Diagnosed with polycythemia vera last year, legally blind in left eye from disease
Current Health Status—Was hospitalized last month for thrombosis in right leg, goes to the ED once a month for phlebotomy to remove a unit of blood
Allergies—Erythromycin
Medications—Tagamet (cimetidine), Zyloprim (allopurinol), and started radioactive phosphate, specific for her polycythemia, yesterday

Focused Physical

Current Set of VS—P 110 and irregular, RR 22 and labored, BP 156/92
Other Pertinent Findings—She denies chest pain now, describes it as "an ache" that gets worse when she takes a deep breath and radiates through to her back. She is also complaining of dizziness, pulse oximetry is 94% on room air, all extremities are dark red with a gray tinge, nail beds are cyanotic, she denies any preexisting cardiac problem, there are no other abnormalities seen. Her husband states she normally looks flushed but not like this.
Diagnostic Tests—None done

ECG

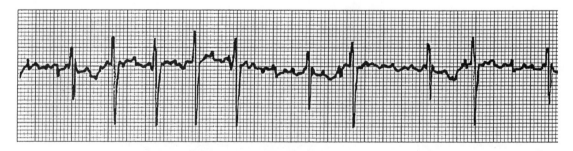

Figure 4-2

QUESTIONS

1. What is significant about Celia's history?

2. What body systems are affected?

3. What is suggested by the pattern of onset of her chest pain and her description of it?

4. Is there an explanation for her pulse oximetry value of 94% on room air?

5. What is your immediate treatment of Celia?

6. How would you describe Celia's ECG?

7. What is the significance of her ECG finding in the presence of her description of onset and type of chest pain and difficulty breathing?

8. What is the significance of Tagamet (cimetidine) and of Zyloprim (allopurinol)?

9. Is there any information, from either her history or physical examination that might be helpful?

10. How serious is Celia's situation?

11. What is Celia at risk for?

12. What do you think is the cause of Celia's current condition?

13. If Celia's VS remained consistent, how would you continue to treat her?

14. What is polycythemia vera?

15. Is a knowledge of this disease process necessary to adequately treat her in the field?

1. What is significant about Celia's history?

Preexisting polycythemia vera indicates a chronic disease, thrombosis last month indicates a potential for problems associated with clots and clot formation, pattern of onset and complaint of pain, on Tagamet (cimetidine) an H_2 blocker commonly given for gastritis, Zyloprim (allopurinol) commonly given for gout, and started radioactive phosphate yesterday.

2. What body systems are affected?

Respiratory—labored breathing, accessory muscle use, talking in 1 to 2 word phrases, presence of rales and wheezes in all lobes, complaint of difficulty breathing

Cardiovascular—dark red face with cyanotic lips, tachycardia with atrial fibrillation; cool and clammy skin

3. What is suggested by the pattern of onset of her chest pain and her description of it?

The onset was sudden and localized (right side) and described as sharp, which then subsided to "an ache." However, when she takes a deep breath her chest pain worsens and radiates through to her back. This seems to point to pleuritic pain with the suggestion of cardiac pain. The sharp pain was immediately followed by shortness of breath that continually worsened. This implies a primary pulmonary problem versus a cardiac problem.

Pulmonary edema with pleuritic chest pain, cyanosis, and acute onset of respiratory failure in a patient with a history of thrombosis strongly suggests a pulmonary embolus (PE). Presence of the chest "ache" radiating to the back may also imply a cardiac component. This suggests the possibility of an ischemic cardiac event either as a result of or in addition to the pulmonary edema and PE.

4. Is there an explanation for her pulse oximetry value of 94% on room air?

A value of 94% isn't low enough to explain Celia's peripheral cyanosis. Her obvious difficulty breathing with wheezes and rales in all lobes suggests that a greater degree of hypoxia is present than what is indicated by her pulse oximetry value. It is possible that the value is not accurate and treatment should be determined by patient findings.

5. What is your immediate treatment of Celia?

Sit her upright if she isn't already, apply oxygen by non–rebreather mask with a reservoir at 15 lpm. Start an IV of NS or LR to run KVO.

6. How would you describe Celia's ECG?

Atrial fibrillation with a rapid ventricular response at a rate of 110.

7. What is the significance of her ECG finding in the presence of her description of onset and type of chest pain and difficulty breathing?

There is no evidence that Celia's atrial fibrillation existed before this time. The new onset of atrial fibrillation in an older patient could be the consequence of an increased demand on the heart or cardiac ischemia unmasking an underlying cardiovascular disease.

In this case, hypoxia, as a result of the pulmonary problem, could precipitate cardiac ischemia, thus creating the dysrhythmia. Another possibility includes the effects of a PE. Cardiac dysrhythmias can occur from a PE as a result of the irritating effect of chemicals of inflammation released by the clotting, lysis, and lung infarction, as well as the hypoxia that can result.

8. What is the significance of Tagamet (cimetidine) and of Zyloprim (allopurinol)?

Tagamet (cimetidine) is an H_2 blocker that is used to prevent or control ulcers and is sometimes used to treat acute or chronic hives. Zyloprim (allopurinol) is used to treat gout by preventing the formation of uric acid crystals. Phlebotomy is the first line treatment for polycythemia vera because it controls complications caused by hypervolemia.

9. Is there any additional information, from either her history or physical examination that might be helpful?

Has this ever happened before? If so how is it the same and/or different? Are there any over-the-counter medications that she is taking? When was her last phlebotomy?

10. How serious is Celia's situation?

This is a potentially life-threatening situation. She is in respiratory failure. Her pattern of signs and symptoms seem to point to a pulmonary embolus. The sudden onset of atrial fibrillation suggests severe stress on the heart and is a possible explanation for the poor peripheral perfusion as evidenced by cyanosis in the presence of a pulse oximetry value greater than 90%.

11. What is Celia at risk for?

Respiratory arrest and cardiac arrest.

12. What do you think is the cause of Celia's current condition?

Her collection of signs and symptoms sound like a pulmonary embolus. Most patients with PE do not have frank pulmonary edema present so soon. This may be caused by the hypervolemia state that occurs in polycythemia vera or it could be the result of a low cardiac output resulting from the dysrhythmia or even an AMI.

13. If Celia's VS remained constant, how would you continue to treat her?

Contacting medical direction might be the best choice. When the paramedic encounters a patient who has a serious illness that is unusual, or happens to be one that the paramedic has little or no familiarity with, then the paramedic should seek medical guidance, if for no other reason than to minimize any risks of treatment. Choices for treatment might include administering a bronchodilator such as Proventil (albuterol) for her wheezing and a vasodilator such as sublingual nitroglycerin. Administering a diuretic such as Lasix (furosemide) 40 mg IV push for her pulmonary edema may be done as a last resort in the field since off-loading body water will further concentrate her blood.

14. What is polycythemia vera?

Polycythemia vera is a condition that causes an overproduction of red blood cells, platelets and white blood cells. Signs and symptoms are usually related to expanded blood volume and increased blood viscosity. Paradoxically anemia and bleeding are common problems. Other medical problems include thrombosis, high incidence of peptic ulcer disease and GI bleeding, epistaxis, and gout (resulting from an overproduction of uric acid). Pruritus and flushed skin are often present. A major part of treatment is regular phlebotomy.

15. Is a knowledge of this disease process necessary to adequately treat her in the field?

Not really. As long as you keep the priorities of care in mind (airway, breathing, and circulation) and how, using treatment modalities and pharmacology, you can help maintain those body systems that control those priorities, you can treat her appropriately.

Keep in mind that there are as many pathophysiologic explanations of medical conditions as there are textbooks. Paramedics are trained to identify actual, potential, and absent life-threats and to treat by supporting key body systems (respiratory, cardiovascular, and central nervous systems). It is not always necessary that we know the exact medical diagnosis, but rather to recognize the significance of what we see in terms of a threat to life and to treat accordingly. A significant part of being competent is recognizing when we need help and contacting medical direction at that time.

OUTCOME

Medics immediately applied oxygen by non–rebreather mask with a reservoir at 15 lpm and started an IV of NS at KVO. A bronchodilator (albuterol) per nebulizer was quickly prepared and administered, as was sublingual nitroglycerin. A second set of VS were: P 90 and irregular, RR 18 and labored, BP 150/86. By the time she reached the ED Celia was talking in complete sentences. Her pulse oximetry did not change significantly. On arrival at the ED, her VS remained stable, her hematocrit was 54% (normal is 37% to 45%), a phlebotomy of 300 ml was begun, and a chest x-ray and ECG were completed. On completion of her phlebotomy she was breathing much more easily with no accessory muscle use. She then was taken to the special procedures room for a V̇Q̇ scan. She was admitted to the ICU with a pulmonary embolus. Her atrial fibrillation eventually converted to a sinus rhythm in the ICU.

One piece of information that was not given to the paramedics was that she missed her last monthly phlebotomy appointment and was 6 weeks behind at the time of this incident. The pulmonary edema was considered an effect of too much blood volume and the PE an effect of blood viscosity.

BIBLIOGRAPHY

Andrews, M. M., & Mooney, L. H. (1994). Alterations in hematologic function in children. In K. L. McCance & S. E. Huether (Eds.). *Pathophysiology: The biologic basis for disease in adults and children,* (2nd ed., pp. 908-939). St Louis, MO: Mosby.

Bachman, D. T., Barkin, R. M., Brennan, S. A., & Recht, M. (1997). Hematologic and oncologic disorders. In R. M. Barkin (Ed.). *Pediatric emergency medicine: Concepts and clinical practice,* (2nd ed., pp. 897-925). St Louis, MO: Mosby.

Berkow, R., & Fletcher, A. J. (Eds.). (1992). *The Merck manual.* Rahway, NJ: Merck Research Laboratories.

Brookoff, D. (1992). A protocol for defusing sickle cell crisis. *Emergency Medicine,* 24: 131-140.

Cohen, A. R. (1983). Hematologic Emergencies. In G. R. Fleisher, & S. Ludwig (Eds.). *Textbook of pediatric emergency medicine,* (3rd ed., pp. 718-744). Philadelphia, PA: Williams & Wilkins.

Dailey, J. F. (1993). *Dailey's notes on blood.* Somerville, MA: Medical Consulting Group.

Guyton, A. C. (1992). Blood cells, immunity, and blood clotting. In *Human physiology and mechanisms of disease,* (pp. 248-279). Philadelphia, PA: W. B. Saunders.

Kelley, S. J. (1994). Hematologic emergencies. In *Pediatric emergency nursing,* (2nd ed., pp. 413-422). Norwalk, CT: Appleton & Lange.

Linker, C. A. (1994). Blood. In L. M. Tierney, S. J. McPhee, & M. A. Papadakis (Eds.). *Current medical diagnosis and treatment: A Lange medical book,* (pp. 415-466). Norwalk, CT: Appleton & Lange.

Mansen, T. J., McCance, K. L., & Parker-Cohen, P. D. (1994). Alterations of erythrocyte function. In K. L. McCance, & S. E. Huether (Eds.). *Pathophysiology: The biologic basis for disease in adults and children,* (2nd ed., pp. 860-877). St. Louis, MO: Mosby.

Martini, F. H., & Bartholomew, E. F. (1997). The cardiovascular system. In *Applications manual: Essentials of anatomy and physiology,* (pp. 89-111). Upper Saddle River, NJ: Prentice Hall.

Reisdorff, E. J. (1993). Sickle cell hemoglobinopathy. In E. J. Reisdorff, M. R. Roberts, & J. G. Wiegenstein (Eds.). *Pediatric emergency medicine,* (pp. 492-499). Philadelphia, PA: W. B. Saunders.

5

Allergy and Anaphylaxis Emergencies

OVERVIEW

Allergies affect approximately 15% of the population. The majority of allergic reactions are minor. The exception is the 1% to 2% of all allergic reactions that result in an anaphylactic reaction that can be life threatening. As emergency care providers, the anaphylactic reaction is the specific allergic reaction most often encountered.

Anatomy, Physiology, and Pathophysiology

Allergic reactions begin with the immune system. Allergens are inappropriate immune responses to antigens. Antigens that cause allergy are termed *allergens*. Common allergens include food, medication, insect venom, pollen, and latex. An anaphylactic reaction is an exaggerated allergic response. Of the four immune mechanisms, type I or the IgE mediated response is the culprit in both atopic (localized allergic reactions) and anaphylactic reactions (generalized reactions producing systemic responses). IgE is produced by B cells in response to a specific allergen and damages the cell membrane of mast cells and basophils. These cells then release histamine, prostaglandins, leukotrienes, and heparin (among other chemicals). Histamine reacts with H_1 and H_2 receptors sites. H_1 receptor sites are in the respiratory system (causing bronchoconstriction) and vascular system (causing vasodilation and increased permeability) and H_2 receptors are also in the vascular system (prolonging vasodilation and permeability) and the GI tract (causing smooth muscle spasms leading to abdominal cramping, vomiting, and diarrhea). Histamine stimulation of H_1 receptors causes the immediate reaction while histamine stimulation of H_2 receptors, along with prostaglandins and leukotrienes, are thought to prolong the reaction.

In some persons, exposure to an allergen causes B cells and basophils to release IgE. Repeated exposure is usually required to produce enough IgE to sensitize a person. Sensitization means enough IgE is produced to damage mast cells or basophils and release their substances. Once sensitized, any further exposure results in an allergic reaction. Anaphylactic shock is an exaggerated, potentially lethal, allergic reaction that primarily involves mast cells. Anaphylactic shock can occur within seconds (as with an injected allergen—bee sting) or take up to as much as an hour to develop (as with an ingested allergen—chocolate). The *speed* of the reaction depends on the degree of sensitivity and the route of exposure. The *type* of reaction depends on the speed of the reaction and the target organ. In general, the more body systems that are involved, the more serious the reaction.

93

Treatment

Treatment options include albuterol, which is a potent bronchodilator; epinephrine, which is a potent inhibitor of mast cell release, as well as having a bronchodilator and vasoconstrictor effect; diphenhydramine, which is a potent H_2 blocker; and dopamine, which is a vasoconstrictor.

Albuterol does not affect any organ system other than the smooth muscles of the bronchioles. It is quick acting and can be repeated. Epinephrine may act within a minute and is rapidly inactivated in the body. It is given subcutaneously (0.3 to 0.5 mg of 1:1,000) or IV (0.1 to 0.3 mg of 1:10,000) in cases of acute cardiovascular collapse. Epinephrine can be repeated every 5 to 20 minutes depending on the problem. Diphenhydramine is primarily an H_2 blocker but also blocks H_1 receptor sites in the blood vessels. Diphenhydramine, 25 to 50 mg, is administered IM or IV and is long acting, up to 4 to 6 hours. Dopamine is a naturally occurring catecholamine that works to increase cardiac contractility and vasoconstriction; the dose is 5 to 20 mcg/kg/min as an IV drip.

Epinephrine remains the drug of choice for anaphylactic reactions, whereas diphenhydramine is very useful (only after epinephrine) for management of anaphylactic reactions during long transports. Dopamine is helpful for maintaining systolic pressure.

CASE 1

Dispatch: 19:00 hrs; 40 y/o male, medical problem, A-1 Restaurant

On Arrival: On arrival you find 40 y/o Mike in the rest room, sitting on the toilet vomiting in the wastepaper container. He is having almost continuous, explosive diarrhea along with his vomiting. He is awake and alert; his color is flushed.

Initial Assessment Findings

Mental Status—Alert and oriented, obeys command
Airway—Open and clear between bouts of vomiting; is able to protect own airway
Breathing—R difficult to determine, approximately 22; lung sounds clear bilaterally
Circulation—Skin flushed, warm, and diaphoretic
        Pulse radial and rapid
        BP 80/52
Chief Complaint—"Terrible abdominal pain"

Focused History

Events—Mike was in the middle of eating his scallops when he suddenly felt like he was going to vomit. When he got to the rest room he realized that he was going to have diarrhea also so he grabbed the wastebasket as he sat on the toilet.
Previous Illness—None
Current Health Status—Good
Allergies—Lobster, artichokes
Medications—None

Focused Physical

Current Set of VS—P 136, R 22, BP 80/52
Other Pertinent Findings—Mike's arms, neck, and torso are all flushed; pulse oximetry 98%
Diagnostic Tests—None performed

ECG

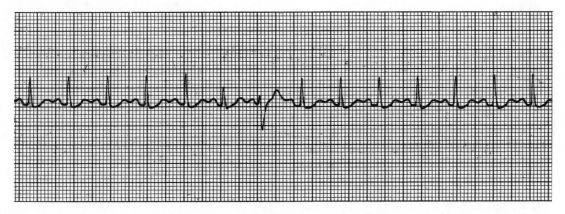

Figure 5-1

QUESTIONS

1. What is significant about Mike's history?

2. What body systems are affected?

3. What are possible causes of Mike's condition?

4. What is the probability of a relationship between Mike's history and his current problem?

5. If an allergic reaction is the problem, why did Mike experience sudden onset of vomiting and diarrhea?

6. How would you describe Mike's ECG?

7. What is Mike at risk for?

8. Are there any other aspects of his history or your assessment that would help you?

9. How serious is Mike's situation and why?

10. What immediate treatment would be appropriate? Why?

11. What would you include in your full treatment?

12. Assuming Mike had an allergic reaction, why didn't wheezing or hives occur?

13. What are the pathophysiologic conditions involving allergic reactions?

14. How does epinephrine work?

15. What other treatment options can be used in acute allergic reactions? How do they work?

16. Why was the epinephrine given SQ and not IV?

17. What is the difference between a non–life-threatening allergic reaction and an anaphylactic reaction?

QUESTIONS AND ANSWERS

1. What is significant about Mike's history?

Allergy to lobster, no other previous history of illness; sudden and acute onset of vomiting and diarrhea when eating scallops.

2. What body systems are affected?

GI tract—vomiting, diarrhea, and abdominal pain
Cardiovascular—tachycardia, hypotension, flushed skin

3. What are possible causes of Mike's condition?

Because most of his physical signs and symptoms involve the GI system, and this episode seems to be associated with eating, possibilities include food poisoning, gastroenteritis, or an allergic reaction.

4. What is the probability of a relationship between Mike's history and his current problem?

Mike's history of allergy to lobster and his current sudden and acute onset of symptoms while eating another variety of shellfish have a very high probability of being related. This is further supported by the presence of flushed skin and hypotension, other signs of allergic reaction.

5. If an allergic reaction is the problem, why did Mike experience sudden onset of vomiting and diarrhea?

The type of reaction depends on the target organ. In Mike's case one target organ seems to be his GI tract. Acute mucosal edema of his GI tract together with smooth muscle spasm is causing crampy abdominal pain, vomiting, and diarrhea.

6. How would you describe Mike's ECG?

Sinus tachycardia with a single PVC.

7. What is Mike at risk for?

Acute dehydration, respiratory system involvement, cardiovascular collapse, losing consciousness.

8. Are there any other aspects of his history or your assessment that would help you?

What usually happens when he eats lobster? Did he feel okay this morning? Did he have any nausea, vomiting, or diarrhea earlier today? Does he itch? How soon after eating did the signs and symptoms start?

9. How serious is Mike's situation? Why?

Mike is already hypotensive and losing body fluid rapidly. He is also at risk for respiratory involvement. He needs immediate treatment.

10. What immediate treatment would be appropriate? Why?

Normally the answer would be to give oxygen; however, in Mike's case administering oxygen would be extremely difficult. Oxygen by blow-by or O_2 cannula could be tried. In this case, the next choice is to stop the reaction and that calls for epinephrine. Mike will not lie down because of his explosive diarrhea. It will be difficult to get him off the toilet until his diarrhea is under control. Mike is awake, and most people are acutely embarrassed to be incontinent in public, regardless of their situation. Epinephrine will help to reverse the reaction and, although diarrhea won't be eliminated, delivery of epinephrine will help to bring it under control. The choice is to give it either SQ or IV. In some systems the choice is based on whether severe cardiovascular collapse is present (such as a systolic BP less than 70). In other systems the paramedic makes the choice based on the situation. The dose of epinephrine would be 0.3 to 0.5 mg 1:1,000 SQ or 0.1 to 0.3 mg 1:10,000 IV, if profoundly hypotensive.

11. What would you include in your full treatment?

After oxygen by mask non–rebreather with reservoir at 15 lpm, IV access of normal saline with fluid bolus, and initial epinephrine (either 0.3 to 0.5 mg 1:1,000 SQ or 0.1 to 0.3 mg IV push), reassessment of mental status and vital signs will dictate further treatment. If hypotension continues, continuing fluid boluses, repeating epinephrine, and/or starting a vasopressor such as dopamine, 5 to 20 mcg/kg/min is appropriate. If the patient stabilizes, diphenhydramine 10 to 25 mg slow IV push may also be recommended.

12. *Assuming Mike had an allergic reaction, why didn't wheezing or hives occur?*

Allergic reactions vary according to the allergen, method of contact, and where a particular patient's concentration of mast cells and histamine receptors exist. Most people have mast cells concentrated in the skin and vessels. Histamine receptors are throughout the respiratory tract and GI tract. In Mike's case the GI tract had the immediate contact and thus the immediate reaction of vomiting and diarrhea. His reaction also affected the vascular system, causing widespread vasodilation. This resulted in his flushed skin and hypotension. His tachycardia is probably related to both the reaction to the allergen and his hypotension. Even though not all body systems are necessarily involved in anaphylactic reactions, there is no way of telling if Mike will not have respiratory involvement or if it just hasn't happened yet.

13. *What are the pathophysiologic conditions involving allergic reactions?*

Environmental antigens, known as allergens (the substance one is allergic to), react with certain antibodies, IgE, formed as a result of prior exposure to the same or similar allergen. These antigen specific antibodies are already attached to mast cells (in the tissue) or basophils (in the blood). The trigger to release histamine, heparin, and other vasoactive chemicals from these cells is the specific binding of an allergen to the cell-bound IgE. Histamine causes most of the effects seen in allergic reactions. Vasodilation, increased permeability of blood vessels, bronchoconstriction, increased gastric acid secretion, and increased intestinal motility are all effects of histamine.

14. *How does epinephrine work?*

Epinephrine is a catecholamine that stimulates both alpha-receptors (which cause vasoconstriction) and beta-receptors (B_1 increases cardiac contractility, automaticity; B_2 stimulates bronchodilation). But perhaps of critical importance in anaphylaxis is the ability of epinephrine to stabilize the cell membranes of mast cells and basophils, thus limiting the further release of histamine.

15. *What other treatment options can be used in acute allergic reactions? How do they work?*

Treatment options include bronchodilators to counteract the bronchoconstriction effect of histamine; diphenhydramine to block the histamine receptor sites, thus limiting the effect of additional histamine release; normal saline or lactated Ringer's solution to replace fluid that has shifted into the interstitial spaces; dopamine to help increase cardiac contractility and cardiac output and to stimulate peripheral vasoconstriction; and methylprednisolone as a long-acting antiinflammatory to provide extended suppression of the allergen/antibody reaction.

16. *Why was the epinephrine given SQ and not IV?*

Some references (such as the Bledsoe text, Mosby's Paramedic Text, and the Merck Manual) suggest that the IV route for epinephrine may be used when cardiovascular collapse is present. Some systems define cardiovascular collapse as a systolic pressure of 70 or below. The rationale is that at pressures above 70 systolic, epinephrine can still be absorbed very quickly from the subcutaneous route and, since epinephrine is relatively hard on the body, there will be less negative effect while still obtaining the maximum positive effect. In this case if epinephrine had been given IV, the dose and dilution would be 0.1 to 0.3 mg of a 1:10,000 dilution.

17. *What is the difference between a non–life-threatening allergic reaction and an anaphylactic reaction?*

A non–life-threatening allergic reaction most frequently involves only one body system (e.g., urticaria by itself). However, if that one body system is a critical one, for example, the respiratory system, it may become life threatening. An anaphylactic reaction is usually sudden, occurring within seconds or minutes of exposure (there are some exceptions of up to an hour after exposure), involves the cardiovascular and/or respiratory systems, and is profound. In the majority of cases, the presence of skin flushing, hypotension, and tachycardia signal the presence of an anaphylactic reaction.

OUTCOME

Mike was admitted with a diagnosis of acute allergic reaction with anaphylaxis. In the field he was treated with epinephrine 0.3 mg, 1:1,000 SQ. An IV of normal saline was started and a total of 700 ml was infused before arrival at the hospital. On arrival his admission vital signs were: P 120, R 20, BP 100/72. He still was vomiting and had diarrhea but the frequency was considerably less for both. Mike was admitted to the ICU after both diphenhydramine (Benadryl) 50 mg slow IV push and methylprednisolone (Solu-Medrol) 100 mg IM were started in the ED, and a total of 1700 ml of normal saline infused. He was discharged 2 days later.

CASE 2

Dispatch: 13:30 hrs; 3 y/o male, possible allergic reaction

On Arrival: When you enter the home the first thing you hear is a fussy cry. You find 3 y/o Jimmy squirming on his mother's lap. He is covered with hives.

Initial Assessment Findings

Mental Status—Awake, oriented according to mother, moving all extremities as he tries to scratch all places at once, obeys command, GCS 15

Airway—Open and appears to be clear

Breathing—R 40 and labored with faint, audible wheezes; lung sounds have wheezes in all lobes

Circulation—Skin covered with urticaria

Radial pulse rapid at 188

BP unable to assess because of wrong cuff size

Chief Complaint— "It itches all over."

Focused History

Events—Jimmy first began complaining of itching about an hour ago. Approximately 30 minutes ago his mother first noticed red marks appearing so she called his physician. In the short time it took for the physician to call her back, Jimmy had hives all over. The physician directed her to call EMS.

Previous Illness—Several bouts with ear infections

Current Health Status—Current ear infection

Allergies—None known

Medications—On ampicillin for current ear infection

Focused Physical

Current Set of VS—P 188, R 40, unable to assess BP (wrong cuff size)

Other Pertinent Findings—Wt. 30 lbs, hives over entire body

Diagnostic Tests—None performed

ECG

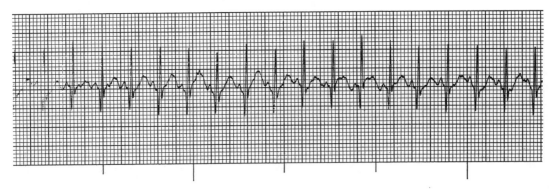

Figure 5-2

QUESTIONS

1. What is significant about Jimmy's history?

2. What body systems are affected?

3. What is Jimmy's Glasgow Coma Score?

4. What is the significance of the presence of urticaria?

5. What is the significance of the presence of wheezing?

6. How would you describe the ECG?

7. What are the possible causes of Jimmy's condition?

8. Is Jimmy's rhythm unusual for this situation?

9. How serious is Jimmy's situation?

10. Are there any other aspects of his history or your assessment that would help you?

11. What immediate treatment is appropriate? How would you deliver it?

12. What additional treatment would you choose?

13. Does it matter which treatment, epinephrine or a bronchodilator, is given to Jimmy first?

14. How does epinephrine work in an allergic reaction?

15. Jimmy had no known allergies and had taken ampicillin before this incident. Why did he suddenly develop an allergy to ampicillin?

16. What is the pathophysiology of angioedema and urticaria?

QUESTIONS AND ANSWERS

1. **What is significant about Jimmy's history?**

    On an antibiotic (ampicillin), current ear infection, no previous history of allergy

2. **What body systems are affected?**

    Integumentary—presence of urticaria
    Cardiovascular—rapid heart rate
    Respiratory—rapid rate and generalized wheezes

3. **What is Jimmy's Glasgow Coma Score?**

    GCS 15 (4 eye opening, 5 verbal response, 6 motor response)

4. **What is the significance of the presence of urticaria?**

    Urticaria is local wheals and erythema in the dermis characterized by severe itching. Urticaria typically occurs when there is an exaggerated inflammatory reaction. Generalized urticaria usually only occurs during allergic reactions.

5. **What is the significance of the presence of wheezing?**

    Wheezing in the presence of urticaria *strongly* suggests an allergic reaction. The wheezing is extensive, involving all lung fields, and is becoming audible. Wheezing is a lower airway problem, while stridor is an indication of an upper airway problem. In this case, there is no way of knowing if wheezing will remain the full extent of the reaction or if the reaction will continue to stridor and fully obstruct Jimmy's airway.

6. **How would you describe the ECG?**

    Sinus tachycardia. In children, SVT (P wave buried in preceding T, narrow QRS) is usually not apparent until rates are 200 or higher.

7. **What are the possible causes of Jimmy's condition?**

    Allergic reaction, most probably a result of ampicillin.

8. **Is Jimmy's rhythm unusual for this situation?**

    It is fast, even for a 3 year old. However, in this situation, a rate that fast (in the presence of an allergic reaction) would not be considered unusual.

9. **How serious is Jimmy's situation?**

    There is a direct threat to Jimmy's airway. Obstruction of the upper airway from angioedema (swelling caused by exudate), pulmonary edema, and bronchoconstriction of the lower airways are all potential life threats. Another indicator of the seriousness of this situation is the presence of multiple body systems affected. There is a higher probability of anaphylaxis the more body systems that are involved.

10. **Are there any other aspects of his history or your assessment that would help you?**

    Has Jimmy taken ampicillin for previous ear infection? How long ago did he take his last dose? Is there any over-the-counter medication he is also taking? When did he last eat? How long after he ate did the reaction begin?

11. **What immediate treatment is appropriate? How would you deliver it?**

    Oxygen can be administered by having Jimmy's mother hold a mask non–rebreather, at 10 to 15 lpm, close to Jimmy's face. A bronchodilator, such as albuterol (Proventil) 1 unit dose, can be prepared and then administered by nebulizer mask at 5 to 7 lpm O_2.

12. **What additional treatment would you choose?**

    A dose of epinephrine, 0.01 mg/kg of 1:1,000 for subcutaneous injection. If long transport times are involved, administration of diphenhydramine 5 to 15 mg IM may also be considered.

13. Does it matter which treatment, epinephrine or a bronchodilator, is given to Jimmy first?

All things being equal, probably not. However, this decision will be based on which one is the easiest, and therefore the quickest, to do. Since the airway is the immediate problem and preparation of a bronchodilator is relatively quick and easy to do, the bronchodilator might be administered first. Bronchodilators will not treat urticaria. In Jimmy's case, epinephrine would treat both the bronchoconstriction and urticaria. However, in cases of long transport, a long-acting medication such as diphenhydramine may be very useful to continue to treat the urticaria and to prevent any late phase or slow onset of additional symptoms.

14. How does epinephrine work in an allergic reaction?

In addition to the alpha (vasoconstriction) and beta (B1 increases cardiac contractility, automaticity; B2 stimulates bronchodilation) effects of epinephrine, this catecholamine stabilizes the cell membranes of mast cells and basophils, thus limiting the further release of histamine and other chemicals of anaphylaxis.

15. Jimmy had no known allergies and had taken ampicillin before this incident. Why did he suddenly develop an allergy to ampicillin?

To develop an allergic reaction, a person needs to be sensitized to that substance. In other words, he needs to come into contact with that substance before the incident that results in the allergic response. For many people the allergic reaction comes after repeated contact with the allergen. It is impossible to predict when an allergic response will occur, if ever.

16. What is the pathophysiology of angioedema and urticaria?

Urticaria is a manifestation of the fluid shift that occurs when blood vessels dilate and become permeable. Fluid leaks out of the capillaries into the interstitial and intracellular spaces. As the subcutaneous and dermal layers swell, nerve endings are stretched and irritated causing the sensation of itching. Scratching, however, often causes a burning feeling because of the stretched and irritated nerve endings. A similar effect in the lungs causes fluid to leak into the alveoli and may produce pulmonary edema.

The process of urticaria is generally limited to the epidermis and dermis. If the process extends to the subcutaneous layer, some sources then term the process angioedema. Many textbooks use the terms, *urticaria* and *angioedema,* interchangeably. Antihistamines, (especially H_1 receptor blockers), such as diphenhydramine, are especially useful for management of angioedema, urticaria, and their associated itching.

OUTCOME

Jimmy was given epinephrine 0.15 mg of 1:1,000 SQ and transported. En route he was also given albuterol (Proventil), 1 unit dose, by nebulizer mask at 6 lpm O_2. On arrival at the local hospital he no longer had audible wheezes and his urticaria was fading. He was given Sus-Phrine (a long acting, oil-based epinephrine preparation) and sent home with an oral diphenhydramine (Benadryl) prescription. He was diagnosed with an allergic reaction to penicillin.

CASE 3

Dispatch: 10:00 hrs; 23 y/o female, medical problem, nature unknown

On Arrival: You find 23 y/o Karen lying on her stomach on the couch in her pajamas. She is awake and appears anxious. Her husband is with her.

Initial Assessment Findings

Mental Status—Alert and oriented, anxious, obeys command

Airway—Open and clear

Breathing—R 22, talking in complete sentences; lung sounds are clear but faint, even with deep breaths

Circulation—Skin slightly pale, warm, and dry

Pulse radial and regular at 108

BP 110/72

Chief Complaint—Just doesn't feel well

Focused History

Events—She woke up this morning and felt fine, had breakfast and lay down to watch TV and became restless, felt anxious, and didn't know why, then realized that she just didn't feel well. Her husband thought she was pale and didn't know what to do so he called EMS.

Previous Illness—Chronic back problems with a slipped disc in the lumbar area

Current Health Status—Had surgery 5 days ago for a disc removal, came home yesterday

Allergies—None known

Medications—Advil (ibuprofen) for pain

Focused Physical

Current Set of VS—P 108, R 22, BP 110/72

Other Pertinent Findings—Pulse oximetry shows 95% (Karen is a nonsmoker). There are no other obvious signs of abnormality. The dressings on her back appear intact with no sign of infection. She moves all extremities with equal sensation.

Diagnostic Tests—None performed

ECG

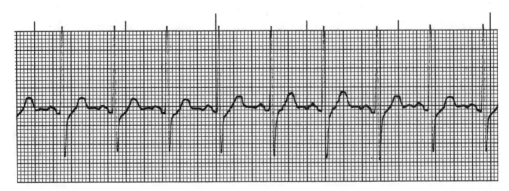

Figure 5-3

QUESTIONS

1. What is significant about Karen's history?

2. What body systems are affected?

3. What is Karen at risk for?

4. Of the conditions Karen is at risk for, which ones can present with anxiety and tachycardia?

5. How serious is Karen's situation? Why?

6. Are there any other aspects of her history or your assessment that would help you?

7. How would you describe Karen's ECG?

8. What are possible causes of Karen's condition?

9. Of the possible causes of Karen's condition, which ones have a low probability? Which causes have a high probability?

10. What immediate treatment would be appropriate?

11. En route to the hospital Karen starts scratching her back and complains of itching. On inspection of her back, you see a fine rash that looks like measles beginning at midscapular level. Her chest and abdomen are clear. How does your impression of her problem change?

12. What would you also need to reassess?

13. How would your treatment change?

14. Would you consider this a life-threatening problem?

QUESTIONS AND ANSWERS

1. *What is significant about Karen's history?*

   Previously healthy with the exception of disc problem, recent surgery for disc removal, on medication, no known allergies.

2. *What body systems are affected?*

   CNS—anxious
   Respiratory—faint lung sounds, pulse ox at 95% on room air
   Cardiovascular—tachycardia

3. *What is Karen at risk for?*

   Pulmonary emboli, because of her history of recent surgery, and infection. She is relatively stable physically, but her anxiety and tachycardia are signs of another problem not readily identifiable.

4. *Of the conditions Karen is at risk for, which ones can present with anxiety and tachycardia?*

   Any condition that can cause an epinephrine/norepinephrine response. In Karen's case both the problems she is at risk for can produce an epi/norepi response.

5. *How serious is Karen's situation. Why?*

   Karen is currently stable with a high potential for becoming unstable. Her presentation is difficult because there is no clear sign or symptom of a specific problem. Her sudden onset of anxiety is worrisome, particularly because she is at risk for pulmonary emboli. Faint lung sounds even with a deep breath seem to indicate pulmonary involvement. But it is difficult to tell exactly what the involvement is. The pulse ox at 95%, even though within normal limits, is relatively low for a 23 y/o who is a nonsmoker with no previous pulmonary problem. There is cause to suspect a more serious problem.

6. *Are there any other aspects of her history or your assessment that would help you?*

   Has Karen taken Advil before? Did she feel well yesterday? Any additional activity? Any pain or discomfort? Have bowel and bladder function been normal? What do her stools look like? Any nausea, vomiting, and/or diarrhea?

7. *How would you describe Karen's ECG?*

   Sinus tachycardia

8. *What are possible causes of Karen's condition?*

   Pulmonary emboli, infection, delayed reaction to anesthesia, reaction to medication, internal bleeding, spinal cord injury, and hyperventilation syndrome.

9. *Of the possible causes of Karen's condition, which ones have a low probability? Which causes have a high probability?*

   There is low probability for cord damage. Karen has good movement and sensation. Hyperventilation syndrome is a low probability because her respiratory rate isn't fast enough, although an increased tidal volume can occur with a normal respiratory rate. A reaction to anesthesia is also a low probability because the time frame is too long. High probability conditions include pulmonary emboli because of the history of recent surgery and immobility; a reaction to medication is possible (ibuprofen); internal bleeding is also possible. Karen might have developed a "silent" GI bleed secondary to ibuprofen.

10. *What immediate treatment would be appropriate?*

    Oxygen with a nasal cannula or non–rebreather mask to raise pulse ox levels to 98% or 99%. Think about starting an IV just in case a line is needed. Normal saline or lactated Ringer's at KVO or with a saline lock is appropriate.

11. *En route to the hospital Karen starts scratching her back and complains of itching. On inspection of her back, you see a fine rash that looks like measles beginning at midscapular level. Her chest and abdomen are clear. How does your impression of her problem change?*

    With the appearance of a rash that itches, an allergic reaction is strongly suggested.

12. What would you also need to reassess?

Recheck vital signs and reassess respiratory status. Listening to lung sounds in the back of a moving vehicle is practically impossible. Reassessment of respiratory status would include her ability to talk in complete sentences, skin vitals (color, temperature, moisture), respiratory rate, depth and presence of retractions, or accessory muscle use.

13. How would your treatment change?

To a great extent it would depend on the reassessment findings. If wheezing were audible, she complained of wheezing, or other respiratory involvement were noted, then a bronchodilator, such as albuterol, 1 unit dose per nebulizer at 5 to 7 lpm O_2 would be appropriate. If wheezing would become more extensive or her blood pressure would start to fall, consider epinephrine SQ, 0.3 to 0.5 mg 1:1,000. If cardiovascular collapse with a systolic pressure <70 were evident, then epinephrine IV, 0.1 to 0.3 mg 1:10,000 could be considered. If no appreciable change were noted in respiratory status and vitals remained stable, then diphenhydramine 10 to 25 mg IV or IM would be appropriate to treat hives and prevent progression of the allergic reaction.

14. Would you consider this a life-threatening problem?

With just the information that was given, this is not a life threat. However, if symptoms extended to hypotension or obstruction of the airway, a potential for life threat would be present.

15. In your situation, what part of Karen's assessment would most likely be missed?

OUTCOME

Karen was given oxygen by mask, non–rebreather at 15 lpm and an IV of normal saline started at KVO. Her pulse oximetry improved to 98%. En route, she began to itch. Her entire back was covered with a fine, measleslike rash. Her vital signs remained stable. By the time she arrived at the hospital, Karen's trunk, legs, and arms were covered with the same measleslike rash. She was given diphenhydramine (Benadryl) 25 mg IM and subsequently dismissed to home. Her diagnosis was allergic reaction to ibuprofen.

CASE 4

Dispatch: 14:00 hrs. An unconscious male, possible heart attack

On Arrival: You find 50 y/o Bob lying on his side in the back yard approximately 5 feet from a running lawn mower. Bob is wearing a T-shirt, shorts, and tennis shoes. He appears sunburned and is unresponsive. A neighbor is present.

Initial Assessment Findings

Mental Status—Unresponsive to voice and pain
Airway—Open and clear
Breathing—R weak and shallow at 4; lung sounds none on L, very faint wheezes on R
Circulation—Skin red, warm, and diaphoretic
      Radial pulse not present, carotid weak and rapid
      BP unable to determine
Chief Complaint—Unresponsive

Focused History

Events—Bob was apparently mowing his lawn when his neighbor happened to glance out his window, saw Bob on the ground, and called EMS
Previous Illness—Hypertension
Current Health Status—Good
Allergies—Unknown
Medications—"Something for his blood pressure"

Focused Physical

Current Set of VS—P weak and rapid, unable to count, R agonal, BP unable to determine
Other Pertinent Findings—There are no tan lines, Bob is red all over; two blanched wheals on back of Bob's R lower leg, pulse oximetry reads 70%
Diagnostic Tests—None performed

ECG

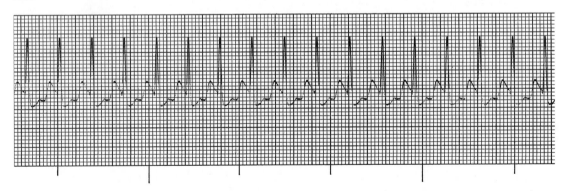

Figure 5-4

QUESTIONS

1. What are your priorities?

2. What is your immediate response?

3. What body systems are affected?

4. What is most significant about Bob's physical findings and his current problem? Why?

5. Assuming Bob is now intubated, being ventilated, and on the cardiac monitor, what would you do next?

6. What effect do you want epinephrine to have?

7. How would you describe Bob's ECG?

8. Would it be appropriate to give adenosine or verapamil, or would it be appropriate to cardiovert this rhythm?

9. What effect will the epinephrine have on his rhythm?

10. If the epinephrine had little effect, what would your options include?

11. How long would you wait to repeat the dose of epinephrine?

12. With Bob's history of hypertension and age, should epinephrine be used?

13. What effect does dopamine have? Should dopamine be used?

QUESTIONS AND ANSWERS

1. What are your priorities?
Shut off the lawn mower; establish airway, breathing, and circulation.

2. What is your immediate response?
Bob needs to be intubated and ventilated.

3. What body systems are affected?
CNS—unresponsive
Respiratory—agonal rate, limited lung sounds
Cardiovascular—weak rapid pulse, no obtainable BP, widespread vasodilation

4. What is most significant about Bob's physical findings and his current problem? Why?
Bob is flushed all over with respiratory compromise and hypotension in the presence of two blanched wheals. These are significant findings that strongly suggest a profound allergic reaction to an insect sting or bite.

5. Assuming Bob is now intubated, being ventilated, and on the cardiac monitor, what would you do next?
Start an IV of normal saline or lactated Ringer's, give epinephrine 0.3 to 0.5 mg of 1:10,000 IV push, follow with a 500 cc bolus of fluid and begin transport as soon as possible.

6. What effect do you want epinephrine to have?
Peripheral vasoconstriction, bronchodilation, strengthen cardiac muscle contractility for an end result of increase in blood pressure, ease of ventilation, and increased perfusion.

7. How would you describe Bob's ECG?
SVT, at a rate of 168. Close inspection shows regular R-R intervals and a QRS <0.10. SVT is consistent with reflex tachycardia from anaphylaxis.

8. Would it be appropriate to give adenosine or verapamil, or would it be appropriate to cardiovert this rhythm?
No to all the above. The underlying cause of the dysrhythmia should be treated.

9. What effect will the epinephrine have on his rhythm?
The SVT is secondary to hypotension and hypoxemia from an allergic reaction.
With an increase in blood pressure and perfusion and increased supply of oxygen to the pulmonary capillaries (from bronchodilation), the heart rate should slow down.

10. If the epinephrine had little effect, what would your options include?
Options include repeating the epinephrine once and repeating the fluid bolus. Dopamine is another pharmacologic option. You can use premix or mix as 400 mg or 800 mg in 500 cc (200 to 400 mg in 250 cc) and start at 5 mcg/kg/min or as directed in your local protocols.

11. How long would you wait to repeat the dose of epinephrine?
There should be a 3 to 5 minute delay between doses to give the drug time to circulate. The time frame between doses is relatively short because you administered the medication intravenously.

12. With Bob's history of hypertension and age, should epinephrine be used?
Yes. Even with his history, Bob's situation is life threatening. Epinephrine is the drug of choice. There are no contraindications for epinephrine in cardiac arrest or anaphylaxis. Bob may die if measures are not taken immediately.

13. What effect does dopamine have? Should dopamine be used?

Dopamine has both alpha and beta effects depending on the dose. At low doses (1 to 2 mcg/kg/min) renal and mesenteric artery vasodilation occurs; at 5 to 10 mcg/kg/min increased cardiac contractility occurs; at 10 mcg/kg/min increased rate and some increased peripheral vasoconstriction can be noted; at 15 to 20 mcg/kg/min primarily alpha effects of peripheral vasoconstriction are present. Increased cardiac contractibility and increased peripheral vasoconstriction are the desired effects. Individual responses are varied, so close monitoring of patient response is warranted.

If Bob doesn't respond with an increase in BP, dopamine is a reasonable choice.

OUTCOME

Bob was admitted to the local hospital with an acute allergic reaction with anaphylaxis. He was intubated and ventilated in the field, an IV of normal saline was started and a total of 1200 cc was given. He was also given 0.5 mg epinephrine, 1:10,000 IV that was repeated twice. On arrival, he was responding to command, was breathing on his own, had a BP of 86 systolic, and pulse ox was up to 87%. He received dopamine by drip and methylprednisolone in the ED. He was admitted to the ICU where there was some concern regarding the effect of the epinephrine on his heart. However, there seemed to be no deleterious effects, and Bob was dismissed to home 2 days later with instructions on how to use his new EpiPen.

BIBLIOGRAPHY

American Heart Association. Cummins, R. O. (Ed.). (1994). *Advanced cardiac life support textbook.* Dallas, TX: American Heart Association.

American Heart Association. Chameides L., & Hazinski M. F. (Eds.). (1994). *Textbook of pediatric advanced life support.* Dallas, TX: American Heart Association.

Berkow R., & Fletcher, A. J. (Eds.). (1992). *Merck manual of diagnosis and therapy.* Rahway, NJ: Merck Research Laboratories.

Bledsoe, B. E., Clayden, D. E., & Papa, F. J. (1996). *Prehospital emergency pharmacology,* (4th ed.). Upper Saddle, River, NJ: Brady, Prentice Hall.

Bongard, F. S., & Sue D.Y. (Eds.). (1994). *Current: Critical care, diagnosis and treatment.* Norwalk, CT: Appleton & Lange.

Gyetvan, M. C. (Ed.). (1994). *Nursing timesavers: Respiratory disorders.* Springhouse, PA: Springhouse Corporation.

Kelley, S. J. (1994). *Pediatric emergency nursing,* (2nd ed.). Norwalk, CT: Appleton & Lange.

Martini, F. H., & Bartholomew, E. F. (1997). *Essentials of anatomy and physiology.* Upper Saddle River, NJ: Prentice Hall.

Rote, N. S. (1994). Alterations in immunity and inflammation. In K. L. McCance, & S. E. Huether (Eds.). *Pathophysiology: The biologic basis for disease in adults and children,* (2nd ed., pp. 268-298). St Louis, MO: Mosby.

Rote, N. S. (1994). Immunity. In K. L. McCance, & S. E. Huether (Eds.). *Pathophysiology: The biologic basis for disease in adults and children,* (2nd ed., pp. 205-233). St Louis, MO: Mosby.

Tierney, L. M., McPhee, S. J., & Papadakis, M. A. (Eds.). (1994). *Current: Medical diagnosis and treatment.* Norwalk, CT: Appleton & Lange.

6

Toxicology Emergencies

OVERVIEW

The incidence of poisonings and overdoses are fairly common. However, patients suffering from an overdose or poisoning can be among the most confusing cases to work with in the pre-hospital arena. Patient situations may also involve a very strong emotional or psychiatric component, especially if the event was purposeful. This may require use of additional patient care skills and a concentration on scene safety.

There is also a significant number of events that are accidental or unintentional. Whether the event is accidental or purposeful may not be readily apparent, and a strong index of suspicion should be maintained.

Anatomy, Physiology, and Pathophysiology

Methods of exposure include ingestion, injection, absorption, and inhalation. The method of patient exposure may not be the only method of exposure. Therefore the care provider must be especially vigilant regarding personal safety.

Because of the wide variety of poisons and substances that can be overdosed, there is an equally wide potential for a variety of body systems affected. There is very little that can be universally stated about signs and symptoms of the overdose or poisoning patient. The critical body systems involved are the central nervous system, the respiratory system, and the cardiovascular system. Other common body systems often affected include the digestive system, along with the liver, pancreas, and the renal system.

Effects on the central nervous system may include irritation or suppression manifesting as altered mental status (anxiety and confusion to paranoia to drowsiness to coma), ocular effects (blurred or double vision or photophobia), tinnitus, and/or seizures. Effects may extend to the peripheral nervous system causing tremors or deficits such as numbness, tingling, or varying degrees of paralysis. Paralysis of the respiratory muscles is particularly ominous.

Respiratory effects may include respiratory depression perceived as a sensation of shortness of breath or difficulty breathing. Physical effects may include alterations in respiratory rate and/or effort along with sudden onset of bronchoconstriction and/or pulmonary edema. Central nervous system effects may extend to the respiratory centers of the brain. Respiratory depression is particularly dangerous.

Cardiovascular effects may include widespread vasodilation or constriction, myocardial muscle failure, or myocardial irritation. Physical effects may be hypotension, hypertension, pulmonary edema, or cardiac dysrhythmias.

Common GI effects include nausea and vomiting. Gastric irritation leading to abdominal pain, bleeding, and diarrhea are also frequent. The effects on the liver are frequently not immediately apparent. Approximately 80% of the liver is destroyed before alterations in liver function tests are evident. Similarly, kidney failure usually takes hours before signs and symptoms manifest themselves. The liver and kidney are particularly vulnerable in cases of toxicity because all substances that enter body fluids pass through the liver to be detoxified and almost all pass through the kidney to be excreted.

The onset of signs and symptoms may be dependent on the dose (low doses of fluoride are considered nontoxic and healthful, whereas high doses are very toxic), the body system affected (acetaminophen affects the liver and immediate signs and symptoms are nonexistent), and patient age (organophosphates are particularly toxic to children). They may be immediate or delayed.

Having a working knowledge of all poisons or a knowledge of the effects of all substances taken in large amounts is unreasonable. Several sources are available to help with the volume of information needed. One of the most common sources of information is the regional poison control centers that are located throughout the country. In addition, there are poisondex listings available on computer or microfiche. The American Association of Poison Control Centers (AAPCC) coordinates a data collection system of poison exposures that occur in the United States. The centers serve as the main source of information for poisonings and overdoses.

Assessment

Because of the sheer number of substances encountered in poisoning and overdose calls, the variety of signs and symptoms are enough to frustrate the most experienced provider. History often provides the keys for suspecting the cause of the problem. However, it should never be assumed that the patient's signs and symptoms are related solely to an overdose or toxic ingestion. All other reasonable causes, supported by history, environment, gender, age, and/or previous illness that may explain the assessment findings must also be considered.

Priorities of assessment do not vary. Airway, breathing, circulation, and mental status continue to be the focus of any primary assessment. During the primary survey immediate life-threatening problems are identified. Appropriate resuscitative measures are performed as each problem is encountered. Further assessment should concentrate on those body systems affected. A detailed physical examination should pay special attention to the skin for clues to the method of exposure. Areas that appear reddened, blistered, or discolored should be noted and the care provider should avoid direct contact with these areas. Any unknown substance on the patient's clothing or skin should be suspect and decontamination procedures followed.

Repeated physical assessment is very important to note trends. A high index of suspicion should be maintained and treatment needs anticipated.

Treatment

The primary survey and resuscitative measures are essentially accomplished simultaneously. A few immediately life-threatening poisonings are specifically treated (amyl nitrite or sodium nitrite for cyanide, oxygen for carbon monoxide, naloxone for narcotics) during this phase before undertaking a full detailed physical assessment.

Oxygen should be administered to all patients with an altered mental status. The only exception is definite paraquat poisoning. An ECG monitor should be placed on the patient and cardiac dysrhythmias treated according to ACLS guidelines for specific dysrhythmias. IV access should be established and a blood glucose level obtained in all patients with altered mental status. Dextrose 50% and thiamine should be administered if hypoglycemia is confirmed.

Specific antidote treatment for certain specific symptomatic toxic exposures/overdoses should be administered if toxins are known and/or confirmed. Several common antidotes include the following:

Poison	Antidote
Acetaminophen	N-acetyl-cysteine (Mucomyst)
Atropine	Physostigmine (anticholinergics)
Calcium channel blockers	Calcium chloride
Carbon monoxide	Oxygen
Carbamates	Atropine
Clonidine	Naloxone
Cyanide	Amyl nitrite, sodium nitrite, or sodium thiosulfate
Diazepam	Flumazenil (Romazicon)
Ethylene glycol	Ethyl alcohol
Fluoride	Calcium gluconate
Iron	Deferoxamine
Methanol	Ethyl alcohol
Narcotics	Naloxone (Narcan)
Organophosphates	Atropine or pralidoxime
Phenothiazines	Diphenhydramine (Benadryl)
Propranolol	Glucagon
Tricyclic antidepressants	Sodium bicarbonate

CASE 1

Dispatch: 12:30 hrs; unconscious child, 13 y/o, medical problem, nature unknown

On Arrival: You find a 13 y/o old female, Tonya, lying on her bedroom floor. She appears very pale; there is minimal chest wall movement. Her mother is present and is extremely upset.

Initial Assessment Findings
> **Mental Status**—Unresponsive to voice and finger pinch
> **Airway**—Open and clear
> **Breathing**—RR agonal at 4-6/min; lung sounds clear bilaterally
> **Circulation**—Skin pale, cool, and dry; mucous membranes very pale
>> No palpable radial or carotid pulses
>> BP cannot be auscultated or palpated
> **Chief Complaint**—Unresponsive

Focused History
> **Events**—Mother stated Tonya passed out in gym class today; the teacher called her to take Tonya home. Mother made arrangements to take Tonya to the doctor at 2:00 PM, then came to call her to lunch and found her unresponsive on her bedroom floor. She immediately called 911.
> **Previous Illness**—No illness, but has attention deficit disorder, diagnosed at the age of 3, also has chronic bed-wetting for which she started medication 5 days ago.
> **Current Health Status**—Complained of not feeling "good" this AM. Mother thought she was just trying to get out of going to school and made her go anyway.
> **Allergies**—None known
> **Medications**—Takes Ritalin (methylphenidate) and Trofanil (imipramine) regularly; pill count corresponds with dosing schedule

Focused Physical
> **Current Set of VS**—P 0, RR 4 to 6, BP 0
> **Other Significant Findings**—When she is ventilated and chest compression are started, Tonya weakly moves her arms, the action appears purposeful (to push rescuer off chest). Her abdomen is soft with no distention. She weighs approximately 105 lbs.
> **Diagnostic Tests**—Fluid challenge 500 ml, no change in VS or LS

ECG

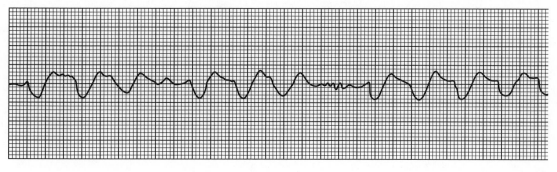

Figure 6-1

QUESTIONS

1. What is significant about Tonya's history?

2. What body systems are affected?

3. How would you describe Tonya's ECG?

4. What is the relationship between Tonya's cardiac rhythm and her cardiovascular, respiratory, and central nervous systems?

5. What would be the initial treatment?

6. When chest compressions are started, she exhibits weak arm movement that seems purposeful (to push the rescuer off her chest). What is the most likely explanation for this?

7. Because there is a response to chest compressions, should they be stopped?

8. What is her Glasgow Coma Score (GCS), and how would you report it?

9. Previously healthy children rarely code, and to exhibit an ECG such as this one is even more unusual. What are the possible causes for Tonya's condition?

10. What additional questions could be asked that might help narrow down the causes for Tonya's condition?

11. Paramedics at the scene gave a fluid bolus. Is that acceptable treatment? If so, how much fluid should they have given?

12. What is the worst possible outcome of a fluid bolus for Tonya?

13. Would you cardiovert, or would you defibrillate?

14. How would you treat Tonya?

15. When defibrillating a child, how are the joules calculated?

16. In this situation, what considerations would need to be made for defibrillating Tonya?

17. What is Trofanil (imipramine) and its possible effects?

18. What is Ritalin (methylphenidate) and its possible effects?

19. Does the information regarding imipramine and methylphenidate relate in any way to Tonya's condition?

20. Given the information on imipramine and methylphenidate, are there any additional treatment alternatives?

QUESTIONS AND ANSWERS

1. What is significant about Tonya's history?

Syncope during exercise, which implies a problem with cardiac output, either volume, rate and/or rhythm, or strength of contraction may be involved; recent new medication, because of the possibility of allergy or drug reaction; and no known recreational drug use.

2. What body systems are affected?

CNS—only responds to pain of chest compression, GCS 7
Respiratory—agonal respirations
Cardiovascular—hypotension, lack of perfusion, bizarre rhythm

3. How would you describe Tonya's ECG?

Assuming that the complexes seen are ventricular, the QRS is wide, bizarre, and occurs in groups but is indistinct, making a rate determination difficult. As far as giving the rhythm a name, the paramedics in the field described it as "something between V-fib and V-tach."

4. What is the relationship between Tonya's cardiac rhythm and her cardiovascular, respiratory, and central nervous systems?

Tonya's rhythm is not a rhythm that generates an adequate cardiac output, thus the lack of a detectable pulse and blood pressure. The presence of agonal respirations suggests at least some perfusion to the brain stem is occurring.

5. What would be the initial treatment?

Tonya is in cardiorespiratory arrest. Her airway is clear but respirations are inadequate. She needs to be ventilated with a bag-valve-mask and oxygen, chest compressions started, and then intubated with an IV of crystalloid begun.

6. When chest compressions are started, she exhibits weak arm movement that seems purposeful (to push the rescuer off her chest). What is the most likely explanation for this?

Ventilations with the bag-valve-mask and chest compressions are improving perfusion to the brain, at least enough to cause a perception of pain, ability to localize, it and an attempt to react to it.

7. Because there is a response to chest compressions, should they be stopped?

Check for the return of a pulse. A pulse may have returned as a result of oxygenation and ventilation. If there is no pulse, continue chest compressions.

8. What is her Glasgow Coma Score (GCS), and how would you report it?

Her GCS is 7 (1 eye opening; 1 verbal response; 5 motor response). Report it in relation to treatment; initially GCS 3, during ventilations and chest compressions, a weak, purposeful motor response noted.

9. Previously healthy children rarely code, and to exhibit an ECG such as this one is even more unusual. What are the possible causes for Tonya's condition?

If a child has a cardiac arrest, the most frequent cause is respiratory arrest. Tonya has no respiratory history and she had agonal respirations on arrival. There was no obstruction noted. Her ECG (wide, bizarre QRS with no distinct P wave) is not typical of someone who has a respiratory related problem. In this case, respiratory arrest is not a likely primary cause.

Although a congenital cardiac anomaly might explain her ECG, it is not probable that this condition would go undetected for 13 years. This possibility is unlikely. Additional possibilities include severe anemia that could be caused by extended menses, a spontaneous or induced abortion, or a perforated ulcer. Anemia is a possibility due to the extreme pallor of her mucous membranes. However, her rhythm is not typical of someone who has a severe internal bleed.

Tonya could be having a drug-related problem, either from recreational use or a reaction between the medications she is already taking. This is more likely since a new medication was added only 5 days ago. A drug-related problem is a strong possibility and might be a likely explanation for her ECG.

It is also possible that Tonya could have been exposed to a poison of some sort. If the yard has been sprayed recently or if there were chemicals around that she could have been exposed to, such as fertilizers, insecticides, and so on, this might explain her condition. This is another strong possibility and could explain her ECG.

Her history and findings (with the exception of her ECG) do not seem to indicate that a severe electrolyte imbalance has occurred, though this does remain a possibility and might help explain her ECG. If an electrolyte imbalance is present it is most likely a secondary effect to a primary cause.

An anaphylactic reaction is also possible but not likely because of the prolonged time since exposure. Also her ECG is not typical of an anaphylactic reaction.

10. What additional questions could be asked that might help narrow down the causes for Tonya's condition?

Ask if she has started her menses; if so, how long has it lasted? Ask about the possibility of vaginal bleeding (asking about pregnancy is touchy, the information you need may be given more readily if phrased in terms of bleeding rather than pregnancy). Ask about exposure to chemicals, if the lawn has been sprayed or if she has been around chemicals. Ask about drug use, and if her friends use drugs. Ask what she did yesterday, if her behavior was different and if it was, how did it differ? What was her behavior this morning? What did she act like? What did she do? She complained of not feeling well, was she more descriptive? Is there the appearance or possibility of anorexia or bulimia?

11. Paramedics at the scene gave a fluid bolus. Is that acceptable treatment? If so, how much fluid should they have given?

At first glance, a fluid bolus is acceptable because hypotensive children are usually hypotensive because of dehydration, bleeding, sepsis, or vasodilation, rather than pump failure. In fact, PALS recommends a 10 to 20 ml/kg bolus delivered twice in an arrest of unknown or suspicious cause. Hypovolemic shock may require a third bolus of 20 ml/kg. Tonya weighed 105 lbs, which is 47.7 kg or 48 kg, at 20 ml/kg equals a 960 ml bolus. A 10 to 20 ml/kg bolus would be 480 to 960 ml bolus.

12. What is the worst possible outcome of a fluid bolus for Tonya?

Pulmonary edema. An important consideration is the fact that her rhythm is unusual, which might suggest a conduction defect and is not one that can support cardiac output. With such a rhythm, think of the possibility of inducing pulmonary edema.

13. Would you cardiovert or would you defibrillate?

She is pulseless and unresponsive without CPR, thus she meets the criteria for defibrillating, regardless of how you interpret this rhythm (coarse V-fib or VT). This rhythm does not have enough of an R wave to cardiovert.

14. How would you treat Tonya?

Intubate, ventilate at 20/minute, chest compressions, IV access of crystalloid (Ringer's lactate or normal saline), and bolus with fluid (480-960 ml). Reassess lung sounds carefully. Cardioversion is not an option, there is not enough of an "R" wave to be detected. Defibrillation is a possibility and, since Tonya can feel (purposeful movement during CPR), the issue of sedation may be considered. However, whether or not she can feel once CPR has ceased is also a consideration. In any case this rhythm is not one that supports perfusion. Defibrillation times 3 is reasonable. Because of her responsiveness during CPR, pharmacologic therapy may be done first. Epinephrine, 0.01 mg/kg IV push and, if this rhythm is interpreted as ventricular tachycardia, lidocaine, 1 mg/kg are also logical treatments. If drug ingestion is suspected, naloxone 0.4 to 2 mg is also a logical treatment.

15. When defibrillating a child, how are the joules calculated?

Although the optimal energy dose for defibrillation in infants and children has not been established, the AHA recommends an initial shock of 2 J/kg, with the second and third increased to 4 J/kg. For a 105 lb child, or 48 kg, the initial defibrillation would be 96 joules. 100 joules is the logical setting, with the second and third shock at 200 joules.

16. *In this situation, what considerations would need to be made for defibrillating Tonya?*

The first consideration is to decide if this rhythm is one that will respond to defibrillation, the second important consideration, is the evidence that she can feel pain. Electrotherapy without sedation, in any patient that can feel, should be avoided. Sedation itself has considerations depending on the agent used. In most systems, prehospital sedation is accomplished with IV Valium (diazepam) slow IV push. The pediatric dose is 0.1 to 0.4 mg/kg (a common dose is 0.25 mg/kg) to a total of 5 mg. Respiratory depression is always a possibility when administering diazepam. Tonya has already been intubated and her respirations are being controlled. To help your decision, ask these questions: If diazepam was *not* used, what is the worst that could happen? In this case she would feel the discharge. If diazepam *was* used, what is the worst that could happen? The worst is a respiratory arrest. However, she already presented with agonal respirations that needed to be assisted. How could it be controlled? You would ventilate, as you already are. Would the time it would take to sedate, delay treatment enough to make a difference in the outcome? That would depend on whether the drug was with you or if you needed to send someone after it.

17. *What is Trofanil (imipramine) and its possible effects?*

Imipramine is a tricyclic antidepressant (TCA) that, in small doses, is used to treat persistent bedwetting in older children. TCAs are known for their cardiac dysrhythmias, hypotension, seizures, and pulmonary edema. Sinus tachycardia, QRS $\geq$ 100 msec, ventricular tachycardia, and fibrillation are common results of overdoses of TCAs.

18. *What is Ritalin (methylphenidate) and its possible effects?*

Methylphenidate is a prescription amphetamine currently recommended for treatment of pediatric attention deficit disorders. Toxicity is due to sympathetic overdrive with hypertension, tachycardia, supraventricular, and ventricular dysrhythmias as common side effects.

19. *Does the information regarding imipramine and methylphenidate relate in any way to Tonya's condition?*

The information on imipramine suggests that Tonya has suffered an overdose. Her signs and symptoms (wide, bizarre rhythm and hypotension) fit the clinical picture of a TCA overdose. The cardiac effects of methylphenidate are similar to imipramine (tachycardia, PVCs, and vasoconstriction), but hypotension and conduction defects are not common side effects.

20. *Given the information on imipramine and methylphenidate, are there any additional treatment alternatives?*

Sodium bicarbonate is the treatment of choice for serious TCA overdoses. Alkalinizing the blood increases the protein binding of the drug. Binding reduces the amount of free drug, thus decreasing its activity and promoting its excretion.

The AHA recommends 1 mEq/kg of sodium bicarbonate given IV push, over 1 to 2 minutes. Another method is to start a sodium bicarbonate drip of 0.5 mEq/kg/hr. The rate is adjusted according to the width of the QRS or to maintain a blood pH of 7.5 to 7.55.

OUTCOME

After intubation and hyperventilation at 24 to 30/minutes, chest compressions were started. Tonya's reaction was startling to the rescuers but when compressions were stopped, she returned to a GCS of 3 with no pulse so CPR was continued. An IV was started and a 500 cc fluid bolus was given with no results. Two doses of epinephrine at 0.5 mg (0.01 mg/kg) IV push and 50 mg lidocaine (1 mg/kg) IV push were equally unsuccessful. On arrival at the hospital her reaction to CPR was equally startling to the ED staff. After confirming pulselessness and absence of pressure without CPR, she was sedated and immediately defibrillated with no change in the rhythm. Sodium bicarbonate, 50 mEq IV push was administered along with an additional 600 ml bolus of normal saline. Her rhythm started showing a narrowing of the QRS and her BP was obtained at 40 systolic by Doppler. An IV of norepinephrine was started and her BP increased to 70 systolic. At this point, wheezing was detected bilaterally, an IV of dopamine was also started, and she was admitted to the ICU. Two hours later she was diagnosed with pulmonary edema. This was managed with diuretics and fluid restriction. She was dismissed 1 week later with no neurological deficit.

The cause of the overdose was never really determined. A pharmacist present on Tonya's arrival theorized that she may have had an idiosyncratic reaction between her medications where the methylphenidate somehow interfered with the excretion of the imipramine. However, this was never confirmed, and she was immediately taken off the imipramine.

CASE 2

Dispatch: 09:30 hrs; 31 y/o unconscious man

On Arrival: You find a 31 y/o male, Terrel, lying prone on the floor of a living room. He appears to be sleeping, looks pale, and there is no chest wall movement. His friend is there.

Initial Assessment Findings

Mental Status—Unresponsive to voice and pain
Airway—Open and clear
Breathing—RR 4-6/minute and shallow, lung sounds bilateral diffuse rales and wheezes
Circulation—Skin pale, cool, and dry
        No palpable radial or carotid pulses
        Unable to palpate or auscultate
Chief Complaint—Unconscious, unresponsive

Focused History

Events—The friend states that Terrel fell asleep after a party last night. EMS was called because the friend could not wake Terrel up this morning. There was some cocaine, marijuana, pills, and beer. The friend does not know what or how much Terrel might have taken.
Previous Illness—Unknown
Current Health Status—Known recreational drug user
Allergies—Unknown
Medications—Unknown

Focused Physical

Current Set of VS—P 0, RR 4-6, BP 0, pulse oximetry ERROR
Other Pertinent Findings—When Terrel is rolled over, greenish mucoid drainage is noted around and in his nostrils; there are track marks on both arms in various stages of healing; pupils are dilated, equal, and slow to react
Diagnostic Tests—Blood sugar 22

ECG

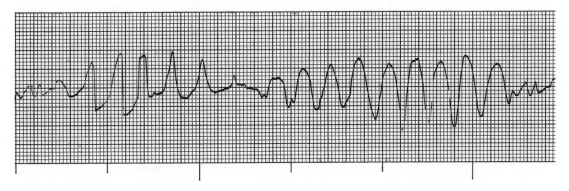

Figure 6-2

QUESTIONS

1. What is significant about Terrel's history?

2. What body systems are affected?

3. What is his Glasgow Coma Score?

4. How would you describe Terrel's ECG?

5. Terrel's ECG is unusual. What is it, and what could be the cause?

6. What is the relationship between Terrel's ECG and his current cardiovascular, respiratory, and CNS status?

7. What are the possible causes of Terrel's current condition?

8. What are possible reasons for the pulse oximeter to read ERROR?

9. What are possible causes of Terrel's pulmonary edema?

10. What would be the initial treatment?

11. If the rhythm stayed the same, would your treatment differ from that of any other code?

12. How would you continue treatment?

13. If this patient were treated as any other code patient in V-fib or pulseless V-tach, would the patient be harmed?

14. If Terrel was successfully resuscitated, what additional actions should be taken?

15. What are the indications for Narcan (naloxone)?

16. How does magnesium sulfate work?

17. What might be likely causes of Terrel's hypoglycemia?

18. If Terrel were an insulin-dependent diabetic, what sign might you check for?

19. What is the significance of the greenish, mucoid nasal drainage?

20. If resuscitation were successful, what is this patient at risk for?

QUESTIONS AND ANSWERS

1. *What is significant about Terrel's history?*

He was present at a party where drugs were being used and he is a known drug user, both of which increase the suspicion that recreational drugs are involved; he has been unconscious for some time, which increases the seriousness of the problem.

2. *What body systems are affected?*

CNS—Unconscious, unresponsive, GCS 3

Respirations—Agonal, 4 to 6; pulmonary edema

Cardiovascular—No pulse, no BP, nonperfusing rhythm

3. *What is his Glasgow Coma Score?*

GCS 3 (eye opening 1; verbal response 1; motor response 1)

4. *How would you describe Terrel's ECG?*

Wide, bizarre QRS complexes; ventricular tachycardia of multiple morphology, specifically torsades de pointes.

5. *Terrel's ECG is unusual. What is it, and what could be the cause?*

Torsades de pointes ("twisting of the points") is a ventricular tachydysrhythmia characterized by a continuously changing QRS vector. There are two main causes. The most frequent cause is drug induced. Agents include tricyclic antidepressants, disopyramide, or antidysrhythmics such as quinidine, procainamide, lidocaine, amiodarone, nifedipine, and digitalis. The second cause is the group of rare, congenital long Q-T syndromes. (Hypokalemia has also been known to cause torsades.)

6. *What is the relationship between Terrel's ECG and his current cardiovascular, respiratory, and CNS status?*

Ventricular tachycardia, including torsadess, is considered potentially lethal and an unstable rhythm. In this case the rhythm doesn't generate adequate cardiac output. There is no pulse, no blood pressure, and an inadequate circulation to the brain. Agonal respirations are seen when the brain stem is inadequately perfused. Presence of pulmonary edema could, in part, be caused by inadequate left ventricular function.

7. *What are the possible causes of Terrel's current condition?*

The most obvious one is a drug overdose. Lidocaine, procainamide, mannitol, and furosemide are all substances commonly used to "cut" street drugs. Lidocaine and procainamide are both known to precipitate torsades. Mannitol and furosemide are diuretics known to be potassium "wasters" and hypokalemia is another cause of torsadess. It is equally possible that TCAs or another recreational drug or even a particular combination of drugs triggered this event. Hypoglycemia is not a known cause of torsades, but in this situation it could be a factor. It is also possible that Terrel is a diabetic.

8. *What are possible reasons for the pulse oximeter to read ERROR?*

There are several reasons for pulse oximetry to read ERROR. Tissue perfusion may be so low that a capillary pulse cannot be detected. This may be caused by peripheral vasoconstriction, lack of volume, or both. Other reasons include a reading so low that the machine cannot read it, hypothermia, too much light in the room, inadequate contact with the capillary bed, or too much extremity movement.

9. *What are possible causes of Terrel's pulmonary edema?*

It is most likely due to several reasons, of which inadequate left ventricular function (as a result of drugs or inadequate oxygenation or both) is only one. Lack of motion for a prolonged period will cause pulmonary secretions to settle. Both conditions predispose to fluid collection.

Narcotics are known to cause pulmonary edema independent of route of administration. This is probably due to pulmonary capillary damage. In polydrug overdoses, a neurogenic factor may also be involved.

10. *What would be the initial treatment?*

Clear the airway, hyperventilate then intubate, begin chest compressions while preparing to defibrillate, defibrillate times 3, IV access

11. *If the rhythm stayed the same, would your treatment differ from that of any other code?*

Yes. Because the patient is hypoglycemic, you would need to administer 50% dextrose. Magnesium sulfate is the drug of choice for treating torsades. Electrical pacing can be useful for overdrive pacing, but because capture rates are variable, many physicians prefer magnesium sulfate. The dose of magnesium sulfate is 1 to 2 g, slow IV push over 1 to 2 minutes.

12. *How would you continue treatment?*

After the first three shocks, if the rhythm stayed the same, it would be acceptable to administer magnesium sulfate, 1 to 2 g, slow IV push over 1 to 2 minutes. Magnesium is the treatment of choice for torsades. Twenty-five grams of 50% dextrose is appropriate for hypoglycemia and should be given either just before or just after the magnesium sulfate (flush the line with 20 cc of normal saline after each medication administration). The exact order will be determined by which medication is more accessible and ready to give. In some systems 2 mg Narcan (naloxone), slow IV push would also be given as standard overdose treatment.

13. *If this patient were treated as any other code patient in V-fib or pulseless V-tach, would the patient be harmed?*

It is difficult to say that one could "harm" a clinically dead patient. However, the point is that epinephrine and lidocaine do not have any effect on torsades. The harm comes in delay of correct treatment, not in inducing further harm. Torsades should be suspected whenever ventricular tachycardia is refractory to lidocaine, procainamide, and bretylium. However, treatment of any dysrhythmia may not last or even work if hypoglycemia is not corrected.

14. *If Terrel was successfully resuscitated, what additional actions should be taken?*

Torsades is suppressed by magnesium sulfate but will recur if the precipitating mechanisms are not removed or corrected. Therefore a drip of 1 to 2 g of magnesium sulfate should be initiated and administered over an hour. The blood sugar level should be reassessed on the way to the hospital, especially if transport time is longer than 15 minutes. Repeat assessment of tidal volume and pulmonary edema.

15. *What are the indications for Narcan (naloxone)?*

Indications include known or suspected narcotic overdose, presence of respiratory depression, and constricted pupils. In this situation, pupils were dilated and reacted equally. Remember that the effects of hypoxia (causing pupil dilation) can override the effect of the narcotic (causing pin-point pupils). The decision to administer naloxone would be based on local protocols.

16. *How does magnesium sulfate work?*

Magnesium is an intracellular action that functions as a cofactor in many enzyme reactions. For example, it is essential for the function of the sodium-potassium ATPase pump and it acts as a physiological calcium channel blocker and blocks neuromuscular transmission. Therefore lack of magnesium can hinder replenishment of intracellular potassium, prolong calcium influx, and neuromuscular transmission. It is known that magnesium stores can be depleted in acute myocardial infarction. It is thought that these mechanisms play a part in precipitating refractory V-fib. Exactly how it breaks v-fib and torsadess is thought to be a result of its action at the Na^+-K^+ ATPase pump to stabilize the cell membrane. Magnesium will treat torsades even with normal magnesium levels.

17. *What might be likely causes of Terrel's hypoglycemia?*

Diabetes is one likely cause, but not the only one. Many drugs are also known to lower blood sugar levels. It is equally possible that Terrel had not eaten before his recreational drug use and, in combination with the drugs (some drugs interfere with the release or utilization of glycogen and/or glucagon), his blood sugar could have dropped.

18. **If Terrel were an insulin-dependent diabetic, what sign might you check for?**

    Check areas commonly used for injection sites and look for the typical skin changes associated with chronic irritation. The skin acquires a lumpy feel resulting from the accumulation of scar tissue in the subcutaneous layer. Absence of such findings do *not* negate the possibility of diabetes, it just confirms a site of repeated subcutaneous injection, which may be insulin. If a drug alert necklace, wallet card, or watch tag is present then diabetes can be confirmed.

19. **What is the significance of the greenish, mucoid nasal drainage?**

    Infection. Snorting as a route of recreational drug use commonly results in chronic sinus infections or localized infections of necrotic mucous membranes. The worst infection possibility would be erosion of the posterior sinus wall causing a brain abscess and/or meningitis or encephalitis.

20. **If resuscitation were successful, what is this patient at risk for?**

    Recurrence of torsadess, recurrence of hypoglycemia and seizures.

OUTCOME

After clearing his airway, intubating and ventilating, three successive shocks were delivered with no change in his rhythm. An IV was established and 2 g magnesium sulfate given slow IV push. The rhythm converted to a bradycardic sinus rhythm that increased to a rate of 72 to 80 with administration of 25 g of dextrose 50%. VS: P 72 and regular, BP 80/Systolic, RR no spontaneous respirations, pulse oximetry 80%. Narcan 2 mg was given with no noticeable effect and transport begun. On arrival at the hospital, VS had not changed, an IV of dopamine at 5 mcg/kg/minute was begun with a resulting rise in BP to 100 systolic. An infusion of magnesium sulfate at 10 mg/minute was also begun. Admission blood work including CBC, electrolytes, enzymes, and toxicology screen was drawn. Admission blood alcohol was 0.25 mg/dl. The pulmonary edema improved but spontaneous respirations did not. Terrel was placed on a ventilator and admitted to the ICU. Shortly after arrival in the ICU the patient suffered grand mal seizures which were initially managed by Valium (diazepam) then, as the seizures continued, Ativan (lorazepam). A brain scan showed extensive cerebral edema. He was diagnosed with hypoxic brain syndrome. Two days later he suffered another seizure, developed intractable V-fib and died. His drug scan showed large amounts of strychnine, procainamide, and alcohol with smaller amounts of cocaine, heroin, cannabis, and mannitol.

CASE 3

Dispatch: 12:30 hrs; 30 y/o unconscious male

On Arrival: You find 30 y/o Harold, sitting at the kitchen table, face forward in a plate of scrambled eggs. His breathing is audible; he is snoring and seems to be sleeping. His wife is present.

Initial Assessment Findings

Mental Status—Unresponsive to voice and pain

Airway—Full of scrambled eggs and saliva, snoring loudly

Breathing—RR 12, shallow and regular; lung sounds clear on left with localized wheezes, mid-axillary area on right

Circulation—Skin pale, cool, and dry
        Radial pulse intact at 76
        BP 100/56

Chief Complaint—Unresponsive

Focused History

Events—Wife states he got home from working the night shift, was talking to her while he ate breakfast and suddenly put his face in his food and started to snore. When asked why she didn't call then, she stated she thought he was "just real tired" so let him sleep. She didn't get worried until she couldn't wake him up.

Previous Illness—None known

Current Health Status—Suffered broken ribs about 5 days ago but was unable to take off work so has been working (lifting boxes at local factory) ever since.

Allergies—None known

Medications—Tylox (oxycodone)

Focused Physical

Current Set of VS—P 76, RR 12, BP 100/56

Other Pertinent Findings—Old bruise noted on lower right chest wall, midaxillary area, slight crepitus when palpated; pupils constricted; no other significant findings noted.

Diagnostic Tests—Pulse oximetry 90%; blood sugar 80 mg/dl

ECG

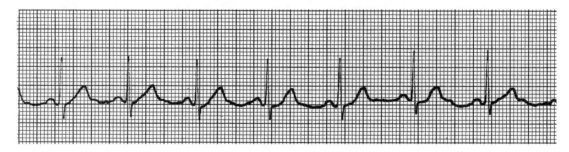

Figure 6-3

QUESTIONS

1. What is significant about Harold's history?

2. What body systems are affected?

3. What is his Glasgow Coma Score?

4. What immediate treatment steps would you take?

5. How would you describe Harold's ECG?

6. Which cranial nerve affects pupil size, and where does it come from?

7. What is the significance and possible causes of bilaterally constricted pupils?

8. What are the possible explanations for a pulse oximetry value of 90%?

9. What are the possible explanations for the localized wheezing in the posterior midchest area?

10. Is there a relationship between Harold's vital signs, oxygenation, and mental status?

11. What other history or physical findings might help with determining what might be wrong?

12. What type of medication is Tylox (oxycodone), and how does it work?

13. What are the possible causes of Harold's current condition?

14. How would you continue treatment?

15. If resuscitation is successful, what is Harold at risk for?

16. Harold's blood sugar was tested. Was this necessary?

17. How does Narcan (naloxone) work, and what is the dose?

18. What precautions should be observed when giving Narcan (naloxone)?

19. When a patient has overdosed on an unknown substance are there any guidelines to observe for administration of naloxone?

QUESTIONS AND ANSWERS

1. **What is significant about Harold's history?**

   Sudden onset of altered mental status, history of broken rib, and now taking medication

2. **What body systems are affected?**

   CNS—with altered mental status, bilateral constricted pupils
   Respiratory—rate of 12, shallow, pulse oximetry 90%

3. **What is his Glasgow Coma Score?**

   GCS = 3 (1 eye opening, 1 verbal response, 1 motor response)

4. **What immediate treatment steps would you take?**

   Remove his face from the eggs and clear his airway.

5. **How would you describe Harold's ECG?**

   Sinus rhythm, regular rate, normal PR interval, normal width QRS, no ectopy.

6. **Which cranial nerve affects pupil size, and where does it come from?**

   The third cranial nerve—oculomotor nerve—arises from the top of the brain stem (specifically the midbrain) and controls 4 of the 6 muscles that move the eyeball, as well as the size of the pupil and the shape of the lens.

7. **What is the significance and possible causes of bilaterally constricted pupils?**

   Usually indicates a brain stem effect. This may be a result of drugs or irritation of the brain stem from infection or stroke.

8. **What are the possible explanations for a pulse oximetry value of 90%?**

   Harold has a history of fractured ribs on the right, visible presence of a bruise, and localized wheezing on the right. It is logical to also assume that the right lung may not be ventilating as well as the left. A respiratory rate of 12 with a decreased tidal volume is an additional factor. The threat of possible aspiration must also be included. Together these factors could explain a pulse oximetry value of 90%.

9. **What are the possible explanations for the localized wheezing in the posterior midchest area?**

   Since it is located in the approximate area of the bruise and fractured rib, it is possible that there is a small lung contusion. It is equally possible and highly probable that Harold aspirated. Even though a narcotic is involved and narcotics (especially heroin, Darvon [propoxyphene] and methadone) are known to cause pulmonary edema, Harold's wheezing is focal rather than bilateral, which makes a narcotic cause unlikely.

10. **Is there a relationship between Harold's vital signs, oxygenation, and mental status?**

    Harold's blood pressure is adequate to perfuse his brain and the pulse oximetry value, while somewhat low, is not enough to explain his altered mental status. There is no direct or obvious relationship.

11. **What other history or physical findings might help with determining what might be wrong?**

    Ask if you can see his prescription bottle and determine the number of pills he has taken since the prescription was filled. Ask his wife if she knows how often he takes his medication. Ask if he has access to other drugs, uses drugs recreationally, or if this has happened before. Does he have any environmental exposure at work? Ask for more information about how he broke his ribs. What happened? How long ago? When did he see the doctor?

12. **What type of medication is Tylox (oxycodone), and how does it work?**

    It is a synthetic narcotic also known as Percodan. Narcotics are CNS depressants that bind with pain receptor sites in the brain (thalamus, reticular formation, lower brain stem, and spinal cord) producing analgesia, decreased anxiety, and sedation. Because the site of action is usually the midbrain and brain stem, the cough reflex, and respiratory centers are also depressed. As little as 15 mg has been known to cause respiratory depression in adults. The oculomotor nerve (CN III), whose origin is in the midbrain, is also affected resulting in bilateral pupil constriction. Nausea, vomiting, and seizures can also occur. Cardiac effects include peripheral vasodilation and orthostatic hypotension.

13. ***What are the possible causes of Harold's current condition?***

    The most likely cause is an overdose of his medication. It is also possible that another injury was incurred when he broke his ribs. However, he has been working ever since his accident so a bleed or associated head injury, while possible, is unlikely.

14. ***How would you continue treatment?***

    Administer high-flow oxygen, assist ventilations with a bag-valve-mask, and start an IV of crystalloid, normal saline or Ringer's lactate. A saline lock would also be acceptable. Give Narcan (naloxone) 2 mg, slow IV push and transport.

15. ***If resuscitation is successful, what is Harold at risk for?***

    Extreme anxiety and confusion with a return of mental status; pneumonia, most likely from aspiration.

16. ***Harold's blood sugar was tested. Was this necessary?***

    Yes. Many drugs affect blood sugar metabolism, either by dropping or raising the blood level. Designer drugs are particular offenders. Hypoglycemia can potentiate a drug-induced coma and render any specific treatment ineffective.

17. ***How does Narcan (naloxone) work and what is the dose?***

    Naloxone, or Narcan, is a narcotic antagonist that competes for binding sites in the brain. It also displaces narcotic molecules from opiate receptors and thus can reverse respiratory depression associated with narcotic overdose. The standard dose is 0.4 to 2 mg IV, which can be repeated. Higher doses (up to 10 mg) may be needed for propoxyphene (Darvon) overdoses. Suspect another disease process or overdose on nonopioid drugs if no results are seen.

18. ***What precautions should be observed when giving Narcan (naloxone)?***

    Naloxone will immediately precipitate withdrawal-like symptoms when given to a person physically addicted to a narcotic. Extreme combativeness in known addicts has occurred with such regularity that often providers are cautioned to restrain the patient and then only give enough to reverse respiratory depression rather than risk injury in the back of a moving vehicle.

    Naloxone has a half-life of 12 to 20 minutes. Most narcotics have a longer half-life and signs/symptoms of narcotic overdose may recur, requiring repeated doses of naloxone. An IV drip of naloxone may be necessary for narcotics such as methadone, Darvon (propoxyphene), Tylox (oxycodone) and Lomotil (diphenoxylate).

19. ***When a patient has overdosed on an unknown substance, are there any guidelines to observe for administration of naloxone?***

    Generally, most protocols call for the administration of naloxone for unconsciousness and/or respiratory depression when any drug overdose is suspected. In some patients rebound increases in sympathetic nervous system activity have resulted in ventricular dysrhythmias and pulmonary edema after administration of naloxone for polydrug use. However, this is an uncommon reaction and is rarely seen in the field. Some systems advocate use of naloxone only when narcotics are suspected and bilateral pupil constriction is noted or respiratory depression is present.

OUTCOME

Harold's airway was immediately cleared, and he was ventilated with a bag-valve-mask. A check of his empty prescription bottle showed that 8 pills should be present. An IV was started and 2 mg naloxone was given IV push with no result. He was loaded into the ambulance and transport begun. As the unit pulled away from the curb, Harold woke up and was extremely confused and anxious. Explanations were given and he was reassured only to lose consciousness on arrival at the ED. Another 2 mg of naloxone was quickly administered in the ED. After a few minutes he again awoke suddenly and was extremely anxious and confused, expressing the belief that he must be crazy. After a naloxone drip was started, his mental status remained constant. Harold admitted to taking an oxycodone almost every hour to manage his pain when he worked. His total dose was calculated at 40 mg over an 8 hour period. Harold was observed for 23 hours and dismissed.

The brand of oxycodone, Tylox, also contains acetaminophen. This was also a concern although, in this case, the dose was only 4 grams, taken over an 8 hour period. A toxic dose of acetaminophen is 10 g as a single ingestion in an adult.

CASE 4

Dispatch: 14:40 hrs; Unconscious 2 y/o, possible overdose

On Arrival: A woman in her sixties runs out of the house carrying a flaccid, unresponsive 2 y/o child. The child appears pale with cyanotic/gray face.

Initial Assessment Findings

Mental Status—Unresponsive to voice and pain
Airway—Open and clear
Breathing—RR agonal at 3-4/minute, shallow; lung sounds clear, all lobes
Circulation—Skin cool, dry, pale with cyanotic/gray color to face
        Pulse not detectable
        BP may be 30 systolic, difficult to hear
Chief Complaint—Unresponsive

Focused History

Events—Grandmother put Sammy down for a nap at 2:00 PM, at 2:30 PM she checked on him and found him on the floor, unresponsive with an open bottle of her heart pills beside him. She then called EMS. The prescription bottle is for Isoptin (verapamil) 120 mg. There are 10 to 12 pills on the floor. The bottle of 60 is empty.
Previous Illness—None
Current Health Status—Good
Allergies—None known
Medications—None

Focused Physical

Current Set of VS—P 0, RR 4, BP 30 systolic
Other Pertinent Findings—No muscle tone; pupils are equal, dilated, and very slow to react; the child appears to weigh 25 lbs.
Diagnostic Tests—Blood sugar 226 mg/dl, pulse oximetry reads ERROR

ECG

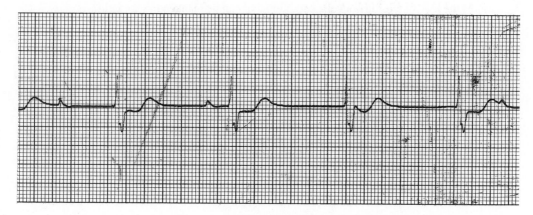

Figure 6-4

1. What is significant about Sammy's history?

2. What body systems are affected?

3. What are accurate ways to assess perfusion in a child?

4. How serious is Sammy's condition?

5. What is verapamil, and what does it do?

6. What additional information is critical for determining specific hospital treatment?

7. How would you describe Sammy's cardiac rhythm?

8. Is Sammy's rhythm consistent with a verapamil overdose?

9. Sammy's rate and rhythm do not seem to justify the profound shock evident. Why?

10. What are possible explanations for the pulse oximetry reading of ERROR?

11. What is Sammy in danger of?

12. What is your immediate priority?

13. What is the proper size bag-valve-mask (BVM) for Sammy?

14. What are the risks of using a bag-valve-mask (BVM) without intubation and how can the risks be minimized or prevented?

15. What are the guidelines to follow for determining when to begin CPR on a child?

16. What is Sammy's weight in kg?

17. Where would sites for rapid vascular access most likely be found in this patient?

18. What are all the possible treatment modalities for this situation and why?

19. How would you continue treatment for Sammy?

20. If resuscitation is successful, what is Sammy at risk for?

21. Is the high blood sugar level a condition that can be managed in the field?

QUESTIONS AND ANSWERS

1. *What is significant about Sammy's history?*

Found at the scene with an empty pill bottle of verapamil, which the child is believed to have ingested; found flaccid and unresponsive, which increases the seriousness of the situation.

2. *What body systems are affected?*

CNS—unresponsive

Respiratory—agonal respirations (hypoxia)

Cardiovascular—peripheral vascular collapse, inadequate perfusion, bradycardia, hypotension, altered cardiac conduction

Endocrine—high blood sugar level

3. *What are accurate ways to assess perfusion in a child?*

First look at degree of activity and mental status. In general, the sicker the child, the quieter the child. When hypoperfusion to the brain is sudden, there are few warning signs before unconsciousness. When hypoperfusion is gradual, confusion, agitation and lethargy may alternate. Failure to recognize parents and failure to respond to a painful stimulus are ominous signs in a previously normal child.

Skin color and temperature are also valuable indicators of perfusion. Presence of central cyanosis in a child indicates hypoxemia. Sammy has a gray color to his face that indicates not only hypoxemia but also stasis of blood. Skin temperature must be taken into account with the ambient temperature.

Pulse rate and location are also valuable indicators of perfusion. As peripheral vasoconstriction occurs, pulses are more difficult to feel; thus the location of a pulse is a gross indicator of the extent of peripheral shut-down. The presence of bradycardia is an ominous sign in a child with shock.

4. *How serious is Sammy's condition?*

Sammy is in critical condition with profound shock and hypoxia.

5. *What is verapamil, and what does it do?*

Verapamil is a calcium channel blocker. Calcium channel blockers interfere with transport of calcium and other ions through the Ca^{++}-dependent slow channels in cardiac muscle, SA and AV nodes, and vascular smooth muscle, resulting in relaxation of arterial smooth muscle (lowering peripheral resistance) and a negative inotropic effect on the heart (decreased strength of contraction). The degree to which this occurs depends on which calcium channel blocker is involved. For instance, verapamil causes peripheral vasodilation but has a greater tendency to result in bradycardia, AV block, and decreased contractility than Procardia (nifedipine), which primarily causes peripheral vasodilation, or Cardizem (diltiazem), which is more moderate in its effects of vasodilation and decreased contractility.

Toxic doses of verapamil can result in AV dissociation, sinus arrest, bradycardia, and asystole. Reflex compensating mechanisms may be insufficient at toxic levels. The combination of decreased contractility, bradycardia, and vasodilation can result in profound shock. At toxic levels, calcium channel blockers also inhibit the release of insulin.

6. *What additional information is critical for determining specific hospital treatment?*

How many pills were originally in the bottle? When was the prescription filled? How many pills were gone before Sammy took them? Were there any other pills that Sammy could have taken?

7. *How would you describe Sammy's cardiac rhythm?*

This is a third degree block. If you look closely, however, the P wave is intermittent, not constant. This suggests a degree of severity of the conduction interference induced by the verapamil. The existing QRS complexes are narrow and regular at a rate of 40 to 60, suggesting that a junctional escape pacemaker is initiating ventricular depolarization.

8. Is Sammy's rhythm consistent with a verapamil overdose?

Yes, toxic doses of calcium channel blockers can result in sinus arrest and any of the dysrhythmias belonging to the syndrome of AV dissociation. If there is no association between the P waves that are present and the QRS complexes then the dysrhythmia of third degree block is present. The rate is slow enough that there is time for a P wave to generate a QRS if not blocked. The existing QRS complexes are narrow, regular, and between a rate of 40 to 60, suggesting that they are junctional in origin and escape beats rather than irritable in nature.

9. Sammy's rate and rhythm do not seem to justify the profound shock evident. Why?

Calcium channel blockers affect more than cardiac conduction. Inotropic action is severely compromised and, in the presence of extreme arterial vasodilation, profound hypoperfusion has resulted. Sammy is also hypoxic, further compounding the problem.

10. What are possible explanations for the pulse oximetry reading of ERROR?

Pulse oximetry is inaccurate in states of peripheral collapse or hypotension.

11. What is Sammy in danger of?

Aspiration and cardiac arrest.

12. What is your immediate priority?

Establish an airway and ventilate this child. Intubate, if possible, otherwise continue to ventilate with a bag-valve-mask, applying slow, *gentle* pressure just until chest rise is seen. Reassess the pulse.

13. What is the proper size bag-valve-mask (BVM) for Sammy?

The infant/toddler/preschool age size (app. 750 ml bag). However, larger bags can be used effectively as long as proper techniques are used. Most children will not need the entire volume of the bag to be ventilated adequately. Applying gentle pressure only until chest rise is seen will ensure an adequate tidal volume without overinflating the lungs.

14. What are the risks of using a bag-valve-mask (BVM) without intubation, and how can the risks be minimized or prevented?

The risks include gastric inflation with associated passive regurgitation leading to aspiration. Gastric inflation also contributes to inadequate tidal volume resulting from distention of the stomach against the diaphragm. These risks can be minimized by proper positioning of the airway, avoiding forceful inflations and releasing pressure on the bag when chest rise begins. Applying cricoid pressure during assisted ventilation is useful in adults, older children, and adolescents. Its use in infants, toddlers, preschool age, and young school age children is questionable.

When the stomach is distended and hard, passing a nasogastric (NG) tube will help relieve pressure and prevent aspiration.

15. What are the guidelines to follow for determining when to begin CPR on a child?

According to the American Heart Association (AHA) subcommittee on Pediatric Resuscitation and the American Academy of Pediatrics, "if a pulse is not palpable or the heart rate is less than 60 and signs of poor systemic perfusion are present, chest compressions should be started."

16. What is Sammy's weight in kg?

One kg equals 2.2 lbs. At 25 lbs, Sammy weighs approximately 11 kg (25 lb ÷ 2.2 = 11.36 kg)

17. Where would sites for rapid vascular access most likely be found in this patient?

In cases of profound hypotension, an intraosseous route would probably be the most likely place for successful cannulation. However, the antecubital spaces, external jugular veins and the dorsum of the foot are all places where veins may be readily accessible.

18. What are all the possible treatment modalities for this situation and why?

Options include: transcutaneous pacing, epinephrine, atropine, dopamine, norepinephrine and calcium chloride.

Transcutaneous pacing, though unusual in children, is indicated here because of the profound symptoms. Pacing to increase the heart rate, thus increasing cardiac output, would be the goal. Pacing could be done quickly if the appropriate size electrodes were available. Children that weigh 15 kg or more usually accommodate adult size pads. Sammy weighs 11 kg, the medium-

or child-size pads would be more appropriate with anterior/posterior placement of electrodes. If pacing were started and cardiac output resulted in an increase in level of consciousness, sedation would also be appropriate.

Epinephrine (endogenous catecholamine), 0.01 mg/kg of a 1:10,000 solution for the first dose. The second and all subsequent doses should be 0.1 mg/kg of a 1:1,000 solution. Epinephrine can also be given down the ET tube. In that case the dose would be 10 times the IV dose or 0.1 mg/kg of a 1:1,000 solution, diluted in 3 to 5 ml of normal saline. In a code situation, epinephrine would stimulate beta effects of increased heart rate and increased cardiac contractility and alpha effects of peripheral vasoconstriction. The effect on contractility is dependent on the child's development. All three effects raise cardiac output. Epinephrine can also be repeated.

Atropine (parasympathetic blocker), 0.02 mg/kg (minimum dose 0.1 mg) given IV or ET, may be effective for a sinus bradycardia but is not known for effective treatment of third degree block in adults. In a child, atropine enhances AV conduction and can be effective in bradycardias with AV block. However, atropine should be used to treat bradycardia only after adequate ventilation and oxygenation have been ensured. When clinical evidence of shock is present in a child, epinephrine may be more effective.

Dopamine (endogenous catecholamine), produces both a direct and indirect stimulation of cardiac receptors. Infants and toddlers may have limited response because of incomplete sympathetic innervation. Infusion rates of 5 to 10 mcg/kg/minute increase cardiac contractility while rate of 10 to 20 mcg/kg/minute cause vasoconstriction and increased heart rate. Because of the immature development of a 2 year old, the effect on contractility may be limited. The corresponding increase in oxygen demand, as well as tachycardia, may be problematic. An infusion of 10 mcg/kg/minute is a reasonable starting dose for a child in shock with an adequate volume. However, effective response of dopamine also depends on a stable rhythm. Children may not respond predictably because of variability in the patient's own endogenous catecholamine response, pharmacokinetics, organ system function and available stores of norepinephrine.

Norepinephrine (endogenous catecholamine) 0.05 mcg/kg/minute, is a potent peripheral vasoconstrictor. Because of its tendency to cause tachycardia, increase the myocardial work load and increase oxygen consumption, norepinephrine is used as a last resort in shock states where the volume is normal. Epinephrine infusions have replaced use of norepinephrine in some systems.

Calcium chloride (extracellular electrolyte) therapy is indicated for treatment of suspected calcium channel blocker overdose. The dose is 10 to 25 mg/kg for calcium channel blocker overdose. Calcium gluconate is not recommended for calcium channel blocker overdoses.

19. How would you continue treatment for Sammy?

After ventilating and confirming absence of a pulse, begin CPR. Start an IV of crystalloid, normal saline (NS), or lactated Ringer's (LR) and give a fluid bolus of 20 ml/kg (20 ml/kg × 11 kg = 220 ml NS or LR). Reassess VS. During this time period, and if access is available, call your local poison control. However, treatment should not delay transport. If perfusion has not improved and/or pulse not palpable after ventilation and fluid bolus, poison control will direct you to give the treatment of choice, which is calcium chloride 10%, 10 to 25 mg/kg (10 mg × 11 kg to 25 mg × 11 kg) or 110 to 275 mg diluted in 50 cc normal saline and infused over 5 minutes. If calcium chloride is not available, the next best treatment is epinephrine, 0.01 mg/kg (0.01 mg × 11 kg) or 0.11 mg of 1:10,000 slow IV push. Epinephrine will not only help increase the heart rate, it will also minimize the effect of the AV block, increase contractility as the child's development allows, and increase peripheral vasoconstriction. The IV dose can be repeated and an infusion begun.

Although dopamine is often the drug of choice for adult post-resuscitations, epinephrine is the drug of choice for pediatrics. Like dopamine, epinephrine has dose-related actions. Low-dose infusions (<0.3 mcg/kg/minute) are associated with alpha effects (vasoconstriction).

A transcutaneous pacer may be considered if an epinephrine infusion is not possible or practical. Care must be given to manage the discomfort that may result from its use. IV Valium (diazepam) is a common drug of choice for field sedation. Neither atropine, norepinephrine, nor dopamine are likely drugs of choice.

20. If resuscitation is successful, what is Sammy at risk for?

Aspiration pneumonia, pulmonary edema, and tachycardia. Aspiration pneumonia is a common result of depressed mental status, especially in pediatric overdoses. Pulmonary edema, as a result of fluid overload, is easily handled by furosemide (Lasix) and positive pressure ventilation. Tachycardia from use of epinephrine requires monitoring and high-flow oxygen to assist with the increased oxygen demand by the myocardium. The heart rate will slow as the epinephrine is metabolized by the body.

21. *Is the high blood sugar level a condition that can be managed in the field?*

No. Once adequate perfusion is restored and normal liver and pancreatic function resumes, blood sugar values will return to normal. It is, however, an indicator that a significant overdose has occurred.

OUTCOME

Sammy was immediately suctioned and ventilated with minimal improvement in skin color and no change in heart rate, intubation was attempted with no success. Ventilations with a BVM continued, CPR was begun and an intraosseous line (IO) was started with normal saline while poison control was notified. The drug of choice, calcium chloride was not available. A fluid challenge of 200 ml was given and 0.1 mg epinephrine, 1:10,000, was given IO and repeated. On arrival at the hospital, Sammy's junctional rhythm had increased to a rate of 100 and a carotid pulse was present. Sammy was immediately given 200 mg of calcium chloride 10%, another bolus of fluid; an epinephrine infusion was started, x-rays and lab tests were done and he was admitted to the pediatric ICU. The total dose of verapamil taken was calculated at 4.8 g. After a bout of respiratory failure (resulting from aspiration pneumonia) and liver failure (secondary to verapamil), Sammy was eventually dismissed to home, neurologically intact.

CASE 5

Dispatch: 17:30 hrs; Persons ill, nature unknown.

On Arrival: You find two patients; one is a 48 y/o female in bed, and she has been vomiting and has been incontinent of stool, with diarrhea. She appears to be sleeping; her color appears normal. The second patient is her 16 y/o son, who also is in bed and appears to be sleeping; his color also appears normal.

Initial Assessment Findings:

	Mother	Son
Mental Status—	When awakened, alert and oriented	When awakened, alert and oriented
Airway—	Open and clear	Open and clear
Breathing—	RR 20, normal effort	RR 24, normal effort
	Lung sounds clear	Lung sounds clear
Circulation—	Skin normal	Skin normal
	Radial pulse regular at 108	Radial pulse 110
	BP 164/86	BP146/90

Chief Complaint—Headache and abdominal pain (mother and son)

Focused History

Events—The husband came home from work and found his wife and son sick in bed, so he called EMS. He tells you the thinks they "got some bad food"; all three family members had turkey and dressing for Thanksgiving the day before.

Previous Illness—Neither patient has a previous illness

Current Health Status—Both were previously healthy

Allergies—No allergies for either patient

Medications—No medication for either patient

Focused Physical

Current Set of VS for Mother—P 108 and regular, R 20, BP 164/86

Current Set of VS for Son—P 110 and regular, R 24, BP 146/90

Other Pertinent Findings—Pulse oximetry 99% for mother, 100% for son

Diagnostic Tests—None performed

ECG—Mother's

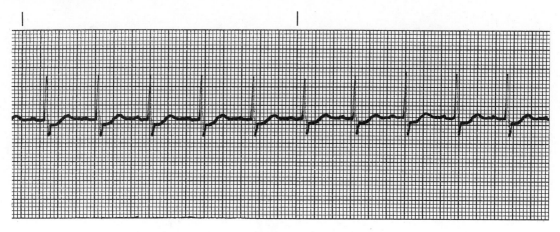

Figure 6-5

QUESTIONS

1. What is significant about the history?

2. What body systems are affected?

3. What is the Glasgow Coma Score for the patients?

4. How would you describe the mother's ECG?

5. Is there a relationship between the mother's abdominal pain and fecal incontinence?

6. What is significant about the husband not being ill?

7. What is significant about the combination of headache, abdominal pain, vomiting, and diarrhea?

8. Is there any other information, either from the history or your physical examination that might be helpful?

9. What are possible causes of the mother and son's present condition?

10. How would you begin treatment?

11. Even though tidal volumes seem to be adequate, what is the value of placing patients in this situation on a non–rebreather mask?

12. Are there other actions that should be taken not related to immediate patient treatment?

13. Under what circumstances are pulse oximetry devices inaccurate?

14. If this is a problem of an inhaled toxin, what are the types of toxic mechanisms common to inhaled toxins?

15. Is the mother's ECG consistent with hypoxia and an inhaled toxin?

16. Outside of warning placards on transport vehicles, are there any detectable signs of the presence of an inhaled toxin at a scene?

17. Is there a difference in the signs and symptoms of CO poisoning and common food poisoning (salmonella or staph)?

QUESTIONS AND ANSWERS

1. *What is significant about the history?*

   More than one person in a single dwelling is ill with similar signs and symptoms, which implies a contagious disease or an environmental toxin; one person who ate the same food is not ill, which implies that there may be another problem.

2. *What body systems are affected?*

   CNS—headache is nonspecific

   Cardiovascular—tachycardia, BP relatively high for persons at rest with no previous history

   GI/GU—abdominal pain, mother has been incontinent

3. *What is the Glasgow Coma Score for the patients?*

   Mother GCS 15; Son GCS 15

4. *How would you describe the mother's ECG?*

   Sinus tachycardia.

5. *Is there a relationship between the mother's abdominal pain and fecal incontinence?*

   Probably. Diarrhea in a person with normal bowel function and tone is usually due to hyperperistalsis. Increased peristalsis is often perceived as abdominal cramping or "gas pains" and can be painful. If is comes fast enough the patient may not have time to make it to the bathroom.

6. *What is significant about the husband not being ill?*

   If the husband also ate the turkey and dressing, food poisoning is unlikely. The husband also spent the day away from the house. This implies that there may a factor about the household environment that may be significant.

7. *What is significant about the combination of headache, abdominal pain, vomiting, and diarrhea?*

   This combination of symptoms is fairly nonspecific. However, what is significant is that they occur at the same time in the same house with family members who have been together for an extended period. The remaining family member, who hasn't been with them, is well.

8. *Is there any other information, either from the history or your physical examination that might be helpful?*

   Is there anyone else in the household? If so, are they ill? Did the husband feel well this morning when he got up? When did the mother and son first feel ill? Are there any pets? Where are they and are they ill? Where is the food? Have they eaten anything after the husband left for work? Has there been any painting, stripping, or cause for any other chemicals to be used in the house lately?

9. *What are the possible causes of the mother and son's present condition?*

   It is possible that food poisoning is the culprit if they ate something different from the husband. It is more likely that there is something in the house causing their illness. Toxic fumes are a possibility. The most common toxic inhalant, especially during cold weather, is carbon monoxide.

10. *How would you begin treatment?*

    Oxygen by non–rebreather mask with reservoir at 15 lpm and move to vehicle. Initiate an IV of normal saline KVO or by saline lock.

11. *Even though tidal volumes seem to be adequate, what is the value of placing patients in this situation on a non–rebreather mask?*

    When a toxic substance is suspected, a mask non–rebreather may deliver over a 90% concentration of oxygen. Using a mask non–rebreather will also decrease the amount of substance that is inhaled.

12. *Are there any other actions that should be taken that are not related to immediate patient treatment?*

    If available, contact the local utilities district or a local engine company with a carbon monoxide detector to evaluate the premises. If a toxic substance is suspected, evacuate ill parties and family members to the vehicle to complete your assessment and care.

13. *Under what circumstances are pulse oximetry devices inaccurate?*

Pulse oximetry is inaccurate when vasoconstriction or hypothermia are present. It is also inaccurate in certain cases of poisoning, especially carbon monoxide and cyanide poisoning. This is because pulse oximetry detects the percentage of bound hemoglobin, but it cannot tell to what the hemoglobin is bound. In cases of carbon monoxide, where CO displaces oxygen on the hemoglobin molecule, or in cases of cyanide poisoning, where oxygen stays bound to the hemoglobin because it cannot be utilized by the cells, pulse oximetry values will be misleading and inaccurate.

14. *If this is a problem of an inhaled toxin, what are the types of toxic mechanisms common to inhaled toxins?*

(1) Simple asphyxiants, which displace oxygen from the air, such as carbon dioxide or methane; (2) chemical asphyxiants, which inhibit oxygen delivery or use by the cell, such as carbon monoxide or cyanide; (3) irritants, which cause mucosal damage in the respiratory tract, such as ammonia, chlorine, or phosgene; (4) chemical asphyxia and irritation, which inhibit oxygen delivery or use combined with mucosal damage, such as hydrogen sulfide or ozone; and (5) direct organotoxicity, such as vinyl chloride causing liver cancer; or (6) any combination of the above, such as certain hydrocarbons that are toxic inhalants, interfering with diffusion of oxygen, as well as sensitizing the myocardium to endogenous catecholamines.

15. *Is the mother's ECG consistent with hypoxia and an inhaled toxin?*

Yes, the presence of tachycardia indicate a degree of hypoxia and irritability.

16. *Outside of warning placards on transport vehicles, are there any detectable signs of the presence of an inhaled toxin at a scene?*

Most inhaled toxins are not detectable. If they are detectable, it is usually too late by the time it is realized. The most reliable sign at a scene is a pet that is ill. In the absence of a pet, there are only two others, odors or irritant signs such as burning eyes or cough. Several inhaled toxins have very distinct odors, such as the rotten egg smell of mercaptons or hydrogen sulfide and the bitter almond odor of hydrogen cyanide. However, what is most dangerous about inhaled toxins is that most can not be detected.

17. *Is there a difference in the signs and symptoms of CO poisoning and common food poisoning (salmonella or staph)?*

Carbon monoxide poisoning signs and symptoms include headache, tachycardia, tachypnea, nausea, and vomiting, with long-term exposure resulting in intestinal damage. Signs and symptoms of common food poisoning include nausea, vomiting, diarrhea, headache, dehydration, and tachycardia. The biggest difference is not in the signs and symptoms as much as it is in the history.

OUTCOME

This is a disturbing case because neither patient was transported. It was easily determined that the husband ate the same food and a check of the family dog determined that the dog spent the day outside and was not ill. When the husband discovered that the medics would not help him clean up his wife's diarrhea, the husband preferred to call the family physician, which he did, in their presence. The family physician thought the family had a touch of the flu and instructed the husband to force fluids and if they were not improved by the next day to bring them to the office. The medics assumed that the physician knew more than they did so they left. By the next day, the husband awoke with chest pain. When ABGs were done, high levels of carboxyhemoglobin were discovered. The family was notified and treated by hyperbaric chamber. The wife suffered long-term sequela of arthritis and frequent thrombophlebitis. Neither the wife nor the son had any recollection of EMS ever being present.

The significance of multiple family members exhibiting the same signs and symptoms was missed. If a disease was not the cause, then something in the environment (an ingested or inhaled toxin) was. The implication here is that if it is toxic to the residents, then it is also toxic to the responders. Ill persons and family members should have been removed to the transport vehicle. It would not have taken long to ask an engine company with a CO detector to come and assess the environment. Even if CO was not suspected, these people were obviously ill and needed to be checked. Another more costly error was the assumption that an off-site physician's assessment of the situation was more accurate than the on-site medic's assessment.

BIBLIOGRAPHY

Allicson, E. J. (1989). Tricyclic antidepressants. In E. K. Noji & G. D. Kelen (Eds.). *Manual of toxicologic emergencies.* St Louis, MO: Mosby.

American Heart Association. Cummins, R. O. (Ed.). (1994). *Advanced cardiac life support textbook.* Dallas, TX: American Heart Association.

American Heart Association. Chameides, L. & Hazinski, M. F. (Eds.). (1994). *Textbook of pediatric advanced life support.* Dallas, TX: American Heart Association.

Baird, M. S. (1995). Torsades de pointes: Success equals recognition. *Journal of Emergency Nursing* (21)2: 142-143.

Baldessarini, R. J. (1996). Drugs and the treatment of psychiatric disorders: Depression and mania. In J. G. Hardman, L. E. Limbird, P. B. Molinoff, R. W. Ruddon, & A. G. Gilman (Eds.). *Goodman & Gilman's pharmacologic basis of therapeutics,* (9th ed., pp. 431-460). New York, NY: McGraw-Hill.

Berkow, R. & Fletcher, A. J. (Eds.). (1992). *Merck manual of diagnosis and therapy.* Rahway, NJ: Merck Research Laboratories.

Bledsoe, B. E., Clayden, D. E., & Papa, F. J. (1996). *Prehospital emergency pharmacology,* (4th ed.). Upper Saddle, River, NJ: Brady, Prentice Hall.

Dickinson, E. T. (1992). Magnesium comes of age. *Journal of Emergency Medical Services* (5) 60-61.

Eichelberger, M. R., Ball, J. W., Pratsch, G. L., & Clark, J. R. (1998). Pediatric cardiopulmonary resuscitation. In *Pediatric emergencies,* (2nd ed.) Upper Saddle River, NJ: Brady, Prentice Hall.

Kelley, S. J. (1994). *Pediatric emergency nursing,* (2nd ed.). Norwalk, CT: Appleton & Lange.

Madden, C. (1989). Narcotics/opioids. In E. K. Noji & G. D. Kelen (Eds.). *Manual of toxicologic emergencies.* St Louis, MO: Mosby.

Martini, F. H., & Bartholomew, E. F. (1997). *Essentials of anatomy and physiology.* Upper Saddle River, NJ: Prentice Hall.

Merigian, K. S. (1989). Cocaine. In E. K. Noji & G. D. Kelen, (Eds.). *Manual of toxicologic emergencies.* St Louis, MO: Mosby.

Reisine, T. & Pasternak, G. (1996). Opioid analgesics and antagonists. In J. G. Hardman, L. E. Limbird, P. B. Molinoff, R. W. Ruddon, & A. G. Gilman (Eds.). *Goodman & Gilman's pharmacologic basis of therapeutics,* (9th ed., pp. 521-555). New York, NY: McGraw-Hill.

Sanchez, R. L. (1989). Carbon monoxide. In E. K. Noji & G. D. Kelen, (Eds.). *Manual of toxicologic emergencies.* St Louis, MO: Mosby.

Spicer, S. S. (1989). Calcium-channel blockers. In E. K. Noji and G. D. Kelen, (Eds.). *Manual of toxicologic emergencies.* St Louis, MO: Mosby.

Tobey, R. C., Birnbaum, G. A., Allegra, J. R., Horowitz, M. S., & Plosay, J. J. (1992). Successful resuscitation and neurologic recovery from refractory ventricular fibrillation after magnesium sulfate administration. *Annals of Emergency Medicine* (21) 92-96.

7

Neonatal Emergencies

OVERVIEW

Caring for infants can be as stressful as caring for the pregnant patient. Neonates are both amazingly delicate but also surprisingly resilient. Normal, uncomplicated childbirth is a process whereby the care provider monitors and aids in the birth of an infant, an event that can be the highlight of a provider's career. When complications arise, rapid identification of the problem and efficient management using basic procedures will often contribute to a positive outcome. Of the complications that can occur, hypothermia is the most frequent, followed by hypoxia. Premature infants have a higher rate of hypoxia and are more susceptible to hypothermia. Meconium staining also presents an emergency but is not common in the field.

The most frequent response by the newborn to hypothermia or hypoxia is bradycardia. Bradycardia in the infant responds quickly to stimulation, oxygen, and ventilation.

Resuscitation of the newborn follows the inverted pyramid with the basic assessment principles of airway, breathing, and circulation still present. There is, however, an important difference. Resuscitation of the newborn includes temperature as a first priority. Warming and drying (temperature) the newborn, followed by positioning and suctioning (airway), stimulation (breathing), and assessment of heart rate and color (circulation) will effectively resuscitate the majority of infants born in the field. Although skin color is an important parameter in all patients, there is a difference with an infant. An infant may have peripheral cyanosis despite an adequate respiratory rate and a heart rate greater than 100. Peripheral cyanosis is an indication of the sympathetic response that occurs during the process of birth and is considered normal. However, if *central cyanosis* is present, administer 100% oxygen until the cause is determined. Ideally, oxygen should be warmed and humidified. However, this is not always possible in the field.

If respirations do not begin within 5 to 10 seconds after stimulation, begin ventilation with a bag-valve-mask. If respirations begin but the heart rate is not adequate (greater than 120), oxygen should be administered by the blow-by technique. If this does not improve the infant's color and increase the heart rate, or the heart rate is 100 or less, then ventilating with a bag-valve-mask at a rate of 40 to 60 is recommended. If the heart rate drops below 80, chest compressions are indicated. Care should be taken not to ventilate so vigorously that a pneumothorax results or gastric over-inflation compromises respiratory tidal volume. If the above measures are unsuccessful, IV access through the IO route is then recommended. Using the umbilical vein for IV infusions is not a usual practice by field personnel. Pharmacologic intervention is limited to epinephrine, 1:10,000 dilution at 0.01 mg/kg.

If meconium staining is noted, treatment differs. The trachea should be suctioned before other resuscitative steps are taken. Suction the mouth before the nose.

Stable newborns should be given to the mother as soon as possible. The bonding process will be enhanced, and the heat radiating from the mother's body will help keep the infant warm. Do not forget about the father. If the father is present, and the child is stable, include the father in the bonding process with the mother.

CASE 1

Dispatch: 19:30 hrs; 30 y/o female, possible delivery in progress

On Arrival: You are greeted at the door by a 9 y/o girl who tells you her mother is having her baby brother. You find 30 y/o Sharmane standing, bracing herself on the kitchen table. She is alert, and her color is good. She tells you she thinks the baby is coming.

Initial Assessment Findings

Mental Status—Alert, oriented, and obeys command

Airway—Open and clear

Breathing—RR 20; lung sounds are not assessed

Circulation—Skin color is good; she is warm and dry

> Pulse regular at 100
>
> BP 132/76

Chief Complaint—Regular contractions

Focused History

Events—She wasn't feeling well today and was experiencing low back pain. Her water broke about 30 minutes ago, and about that same time her contractions started. She called her husband, but he was on a service call so she left a message to come take her to the hospital. When she felt the urge to push she called EMS.

Previous Illness—Asthma

Current Health Status—Good, pregnancy normal; due date in 6 days

Allergies—None known

Medications—Brethine (terbutaline sulfate), prenatal vitamins

Focused Physical

Current Set of VS—P 100, RR 20, BP 132/76

Other Pertinent Findings—This is Sharmane's fifth child; all four other children (the oldest is 9) are standing around watching; Sharmane is having contractions about 30 seconds apart for 45 seconds; she appears to be straining to push

Diagnostic Tests—None done

1. What is significant about Sharmane's history?

2. What is important about a pregnant woman, in labor, who has had four previous pregnancies?

3. What is significant about your observations?

4. What is your first priority?

5. You check Sharmane and the baby is crowning. How would you proceed?

6. How could you manage the children?

7. When the baby's head is born, there are two things that should be done, one is to suction the baby's nose and mouth. What is the other?

8. If you would discover the cord around the baby's neck, what would you do?

9. Should you suction the baby's nose or mouth first, or does it matter?

10. After the head is delivered, the shoulders will rotate to an anteroposterior position (relative to the mother's anatomy). What do you need to do to assist delivery of the rest of the baby's body?

11. Once the baby's body has exited the vaginal canal, what are appropriate actions to take?

12. How long should you wait to clamp the umbilical cord, and where should you clamp it?

13. How can you stimulate the newborn to ensure good respiratory effort?

14. What parts of a newborn assessment should be completed before giving the baby to mom?

15. The baby boy you just delivered initially cried, then quieted and is looking around. He has a pink trunk with cyanotic feet and hands, is actively moving his arms and legs, and has an apical pulse of 146 and an irregular repiratory rate of 42. Is this normal or does this baby need resuscitation?

16. What is the medical term for cyanotic feet and hands, or peripheral cyanosis, in the presence of a pink or reddish trunk in a newborn?

17. During the immediate time period after exiting the vaginal canal, what is the newborn at risk for developing, and how do you prevent it?

18. After giving the baby to Sharmane, you note that blood continues to ooze from the vaginal canal. What actions are appropriate?

19. There are important issues of documentation when a baby is born. What specifics must be documented?

20. If Sharmane continues to bleed profusely en route to the hospital, what could you do to slow down or control the bleeding?

21. If, on the way to the hospital, you inspected for the amount of vaginal bleeding and discovered that the umbilical cord seemed to lengthen, what does that indicate?

QUESTIONS AND ANSWERS

1. What is significant about Sharmane's history?

Due date for pregnancy in 6 days; four previous pregnancies; water has already broken about 30 minutes ago and now has urge to push; uncomplicated pregnancy; history of asthma and the bronchodilator terbutaline

2. What is important about a pregnant woman, in labor, who has had four previous pregnancies?

The process of childbirth is usually rapid in the multiparous patient.

3. What is significant about your observations?

Contractions started and membranes ruptured 30 minutes ago; contraction about 30 seconds apart that last for 45 seconds; she is straining to push. These indicate that the patient is in active labor. The urge to push indicates that the fetus' presenting part has descended into the pelvis.

4. What is your first priority?

To check for crowning.

5. You check Sharmane and the baby is crowning. How would you proceed?

Delivery is imminent, so transport is not recommended at this time. Get her to a place where she can lie down, or at least get her into a comfortable position. With a gloved hand on the baby's head, exerting gentle pressure to control the birth, have your partner open the OB kit and hand you the suction bulb. Your partner should open the drapes and get them placed, if possible. Then proceed to deliver the baby. If time permits, obtain IV access in the hand or forearm with a large-bore catheter using NS or LR KVO.

6. How could you manage the children?

Have them get some clean towels or stand by their mother's head.

7. When the baby's head is born, there are two things that should be done, one is to suction the baby's mouth and nose. What is the other?

Check for the cord around the baby's neck. This occurs about 10% of the time.

8. If you discover the cord around the baby's neck, what would you do?

Try and ease the cord over the baby's head or around the baby's shoulders. If these attempts are not successful, then use the clamps to clamp the cord and cut the cord between the clamps.

9. Should you suction the baby's nose or mouth first, or does it matter?

Most prehospital textbooks advocate suctioning the mouth first, then the nose as does the American Heart Association's Pediatric Advanced Life Support course. Earlier editions of prehospital texts advocated the opposite, nose first then the mouth. This has probably led to much of the confusion regarding which to suction first. Theoretically, the mouth can hold more foreign material than the nose, so suctioning the mouth first would control a major source of aspiration. As long as both the mouth and nose are suctioned rapidly in sequence, the current standard of care is met and the potential for aspiration is minimized.

10. After the head is delivered, the shoulders will rotate to an anteroposterior position (relative to the mother's anatomy). What do you need to do to assist delivery of the rest of the baby's body?

Apply *gentle* downward pressure on the upper side of the head to deliver the upper (anterior) shoulder under the symphysis pubis. Then gently lift the head with both hands to slide the lower (posterior) shoulder over the perineum. The rest of the body should follow easily. Keep the baby at the level of the mother's uterus while the cord is pulsating.

11. Once the baby's body has exited the vaginal canal, what are appropriate actions to take?

The baby should be suctioned again if necessary and immediately dried. During this period the baby should be observed and assessed. The cord should be clamped and cut.

12. How long should you wait to clamp the umbilical cord, and where should you clamp it?

The recommended time period is a minute or two after complete delivery. If you are busy taking care of the baby or mother, four or five minutes won't be detrimental. Keeping the baby at the level of the mother's vagina, repeat suctioning if necessary and apply the first clamp about 6 to 12 inches away from the infant, with the next clamp 1 to 2 inches distal to the first. Then the cord can be cut between the two clamps.

13. How can you stimulate the newborn to ensure good respiratory effort?

Usually the process of suctioning is enough to stimulate good breaths, but drying the infant with a soft towel is another method of stimulation that is often used.

14. What parts of a newborn assessment should be completed before giving the baby to mom?

The newborn should be assessed for appearance or color, pulse, grimace (irritability reflex response to suctioning), activity (muscle tone), and respiratory effort. These are known as the APGAR score.

15. The baby boy you just delivered initially cried, then quieted and is looking around. He has a pink trunk with cyanotic feet and hands, is actively moving his arms and legs, and has an apical pulse of 146 and an irregular respiratory rate of 42. Is this normal or does this baby need resuscitation?

This baby is grossly normal. A normal newborn heart rate is greater than 100, with most around 140. A normal respiratory rate is between 30 and 60 with most at 40. It is normal for a newborn to have an irregular respiratory rate. Cyanotic extremities are considered normal in a newborn.

16. What is the medical term for cyanotic feet and hands, or peripheral cyanosis, in the presence of a pink or reddish trunk in a newborn?

Acrocyanosis. This is due to the massive sympathetic response at birth causing severe peripheral vasoconstriction, leaving hands and feet poorly perfused. The tongue and mucous membranes are the best sites in a newborn to assess color as an indication of cardiovascular efficiency.

17. During the immediate time period after exiting the vaginal canal, what is the newborn at risk for developing, and how do you prevent it?

Hypothermia. Make sure the infant is dried and wrapped in dry towels, cover the head with a knit cap or towel, then give the baby to mom. Mom is radiating body heat from the delivery process, and her body can keep the baby warm.

18. After giving the baby to Sharmane, you note that blood continues to ooze from the vaginal canal. What actions are appropriate?

Sharmane will continue to ooze blood until the placenta delivers. However, it is important to observe and inspect the immediate entrance to the vaginal canal for any tears. Vaginal tears tend to be a source of bleeding that can be controlled by direct pressure.

19. There are important issues of documentation when a baby is born. What specifics must be documented?

Time of birth, initial infant assessment and time (1 minute), and second infant assessment and time (5 minutes). Document appearance of amniotic fluid (meconium stained or not), presenting part, and any difficulties during delivery (cord around the baby's neck, aspiration). Document your neonate assessment in terms of your findings (vital signs, skin color, and general activity) rather than a specific APGAR score.

20. If Sharmane continues to bleed profusely en route to the hospital, what could you do to slow down or control the bleeding?

Massage the uterus or put the baby to breast. Massaging the uterus stimulates uterine contractions that help constrict open vessels from the site of separation of the placenta. Putting the baby to breast stimulates production of oxytocin, from the posterior pituitary. This hormone also causes contractions of uterine smooth muscles. If a vaginal tear is the source of vaginal bleeding, uterine massage and administration of oxytocin will be ineffective, direct pressure usually controls that type of bleeding effectively. Since most complications of childbirth occur within the first hour after labor, frequently monitor the mother's general well-being, BP, and hemorrhaging.

21. *If, on the way to the hospital, you inspected for the amount of vaginal bleeding and discovered that the umbilical cord seemed to lengthen, what would that indicate?*

The lengthening of the umbilical cord suggests that the placenta has separated. Generally the placenta is delivered without assistance and should be taken to the hospital with Sharmane in the plastic bag provided in most OB kits. If not fully expelled, gentle traction on the cord should deliver the placenta. However, when the placenta is not completely separated and too much tension is placed on it, there is the risk of incomplete separation of the placenta or uterine inversion. Both of these have the potential to cause massive bleeding and are to be avoided.

OUTCOME

Sharmane delivered a healthy 7-pound baby boy at home. Initial APGAR 9, five minutes later his APGAR was 10. Sharmane had minimal vaginal bleeding, there were no tears noted. During transport she began breast-feeding the baby. Shortly after arrival at the hospital she delivered the placenta. Sharmane and her new son were dismissed to home later that evening.

CASE 2

Dispatch: 02:00 hrs; 36 y/o female, possible delivery in progress

On Arrival: You are greeted at the door by a man who appears stunned. He repeatedly states, "But she was taking birth control pills." He leads you to his wife in the bedroom. Thirty-six y/o Holly is sitting in bed, looking at a male infant who is lying between her legs. Holly appears equally stunned. The umbilical cord is still attached to the infant who appears very small. The infant is gray, has a chest rise and fall, but is not moving.

Initial Assessment Findings of the Infant

Appearance—Face and trunk gray in color, extremities very pale and mottled
Pulse—Apical pulse is 110
Grimace—No facial expression, eyes closed
Activity—No spontaneous movement
Respiratory Effort—Airway open with some mucus present, respiratory rate 10 and irregular

Focused History of Mother

Events—Holly started having severe abdominal pain shortly after dinner this evening. She went to bed early. Her abdominal pains continued and worsened in severity until finally she woke her husband. Shortly thereafter her water broke and she realized she was having a baby. Her husband then called EMS. The baby was born just before the medics arrived.
Previous Illness—None
Current Health Status—Holly stated she began gaining weight and "lost my waist" so she started dieting and exercising. She has been taking oral birth control pills for about 5 years. She has no idea when she could have gotten pregnant. Both Holly and her husband are cooperative but extremely surprised.
Allergies—None known
Medications—Ortho-Novum (oral contraceptive)

Focused Physical of Infant

Current Set of VS—Apical pulse 110, RR 10 and irregular
Other Pertinent Findings—There is no meconium staining noted, the cord stopped pulsating as you approached the newborn, at your best guess the baby appears to weigh about 4 pounds.

QUESTIONS

1. What are the implications of Holly's history of an unknown pregnancy?

2. How does the heart and respiratory rate for this baby differ from what is normal?

3. This baby weighs about 4 pounds; what are low–birth-weight newborns at risk for?

4. What effect does hypothermia have on a newborn?

5. How could you manage hypothermia in this baby?

6. What are your immediate priorities for this baby?

7. What would be your first action?

8. When suctioning this infant, how long should suction continue?

9. You have dried and warmed the baby, started suctioning, and rubbed the baby's back. You noticed weak extremity movement and the respirations are up to 16/min, but the apical pulse is now 100. How would you continue resuscitation?

10. What are the side effects associated with the use of a BVM, and how could they be avoided?

11. An infant BVM is too big for a preemie, but it is all you have to use. What would be your best indicator of adequate tidal volume and appropriate inflation pressure for this baby?

12. If you had to intubate this baby, what size ET tube would you start with?

13. At what point would you start chest compressions?

14. What is the best way to increase this baby's heart rate?

15. If you had to start an IV, where would you start it?

16. If pharmacologic agents would be necessary, which one(s) would be your choice, and what dose would you use?

17. You have oxygenated with warmed oxygen by wrapping the oxygen tubing around a very warm towel and wrapped it again with a dry towel. You started gentle bagging at 30/min and closely observed the newborn's heart rate. After dropping to a low of 90, the baby's heart rate is now 146. His extremities remain pale but there is good muscle tone, and the baby is beginning to cry and move around. What are your current priorities for this newborn?

18. Whenever we have a child as a patient, we also have the parents as patients. Assuming that Holly has no physical problem post delivery, how could Holly and her husband best be cared for while their baby is being treated?

19. You noted in your initial assessment that no meconium staining was noted. If it were present, what would it look like?

20. In your current situation, what part of this infant's assessment would most likely be missed?

QUESTIONS AND ANSWERS

1. What are the implications of Holly's history of an unknown pregnancy?

No prenatal care is a risk factor associated with the need for neonatal resuscitation; unsure of gestational age of newborn.

2. How does the heart and respiratory rate for this baby differ from what is normal?

Normal newborn heart rate is around 140 (100 to 180) with a normal respiratory rate around 40 (30 to 60). This baby has a heart rate of 110 with a respiratory rate of 10.

3. This baby weighs about 4 pounds, what are low–birth-weight newborns at risk for?

A major risk is hypothermia due to two factors: a large surface-to-mass ratio and cardiorespiratory distress.

4. What effect does hypothermia have on a newborn?

Surfactant can break down, acidosis is exacerbated, and recovery is delayed due to hypothermia. The effect of hypothermia on this premature baby is profoundly greater than the effect on a full-term newborn. Premature newborns are more likely to suffer hypothermia because of the absence of brown fat. This newborn baby is severly acidotic due to hypoxia (hypoventilation and inadequate perfusion).

5. How could you manage hypothermia in this baby?

Options include: quickly drying the amniotic fluid covering the infant, removing wet linens from contact with the baby, wrapping the dried infant with a warm towel or blanket, or placing towel-wrapped latex gloves filled with warm water around the infant. Because of the infant's depressed state, and probable need for resuscitation, you may not be able to place the infant directly with the mother. In a normal situation, the mother's body radiates heat, so placing the baby with the mother will keep the infant warm.

6. What are your immediate priorities for this baby?

Your priorities follow the inverted pyramid for neonatal resuscitation. The first priority is to prevent heat loss by drying and keeping the baby warm. Second, open the airway by proper positioning (place the baby on his back with the neck in a neutral position with a 1-inch roll under the shoulders) and suction the mouth and nose. Third, assess breathing and respiratory effort; stimulate (rubbing bare back or flicking soles of feet), and administer supplementary oxygen (blow-by, PPV, or intubation) as needed. Reassess heart rate and color, and finally begin chest compressions if needed.

7. What would be your first action?

Immediately begin to dry and warm this newborn. Cutting the cord can wait.

8. When suctioning this infant, how long should suction continue?

No longer than 3 to 5 seconds.

9. You have dried and warmed the baby; started suctioning, and rubbed the baby's back. You noticed weak extremity movement and the respirations are up to 16/min but the apical pulse is now 100. How would you continue resuscitation?

Oxygenate with warmed and humidified oxygen if possible. Oxygen from the tank is very cold but can be warmed by wrapping the oxygen tubing around a very warm towel. Use the blow-by technique by blowing oxygen across the nose of the newborn with the end of the tubing within a half-inch of the nares. If blow-by oxygenation does not improve the respiratory effort and rate, then use a small bag-valve-mask (750 ml or less) with reservoir and 100% oxygen to assist ventilations at a rate of 40 to 60 per minute. If pressure-monitoring devices are present, the infant may require up to 35 to 40 cm H_2O pressure for the first breath or two to overcome resistance. From that point on, 15 to 20 cm H_2O pressure should be sufficient.

10. **What are the side effects associated with the use of a BVM, and how could they be avoided?**

    Gastric distention and a pneumothorax are the main side effects. They can be avoided by neutral positioning of the head and neck and delivering the proper tidal volume (6 to 8 ml/kg) with only shallow depression of the BVM. Close observation of the gastric area for distention is also helpful.

11. **An infant BVM is too big for a preemie, but it is all you have to use. What would be your best indicator of adequate tidal volume and appropriate inflation pressure for this newborn?**

    Observation of adequate chest wall movement is the best indicator of appropriate inflation pressure.

12. **If you had to intubate this baby, what size ET tube would you start with?**

    Remember, this child is most likely a preemie (low birth weight of 4 pounds and inaccurate estimate of gestational age) so start with a 2.5 ET. A size 3 will probably be too big.

13. **At what point would you start chest compressions?**

    Begin chest compressions if the neonate's heart rate falls below 80, or is between 80 and 100 and not rising with continued assisted ventilations at 100% FiO_2.

14. **What is the best way to increase this baby's heart rate?**

    Oxygenate and control the respiratory rate.

15. **If you had to start an IV, where would you start it?**

    The most likely place is an intraosseous line. Umbilical access is also available and is an easy access. It is not, however, always recommended. Placing a catheter too deeply may inject fluid or medication toward or into the hepatic duct. A dose of epinephrine directly into the liver would be fatal for an infant who otherwise may have a chance to live.

16. **If pharmacologic agents would be necessary, which one(s) would be your choice, and what dose would you use?**

    Epinephrine is the drug of choice at the same dose for both IV and ETT routes, at 0.01 to 0.03 mg/kg (0.1 to 0.3 mg/kg of a 1:10,000 solution).

17. **You have oxygenated with warmed oxygen by wrapping the oxygen tubing around a very warm towel and wrapped it again with a dry towel. You gently assist ventilations at 40/min and closely observed the baby's heart rate. After dropping to a low of 90, the baby's heart rate is now 146. His extremities remain pale but there is good muscle tone and the baby is beginning to cry and move around. What are your current priorities for this newborn?**

    Keep this baby warm and, if the situation warrants, give the baby to his mother while you continue to oxygenate and closely monitor the newborn's respiratory rate and effort, color, heart rate, and activity. The process of bonding with mother is very important and, if at all possible, needs to be started as soon as possible.

18. **Whenever we have a child as a patient, we also have the parents as patients. Assuming that Holly has no physical problem post delivery, how could Holly and her husband best be cared for while their baby is being treated?**

    They need to be told what is happening in clear and simple terms. They are very surprised and may be asking many questions that you cannot answer. Women have been known to get pregnant while taking birth control pills. More of a history could be obtained. Holly needs to be asked if she has taken any over-the-counter medications for her abdominal pain before the birth. Decide with the parents to what hospital you will be taking them. Your policies regarding transport of infant, mother, and father need to be followed. Ask if there is someone who needs to be notified and offer to call, either before leaving or at the hospital.

19. *You noted in your initial assessment that no meconium staining was noted. If it were present, what would it look like?*

Meconium is the first bowel movement of the infant that normally occurs after birth. It is so dark green that it usually looks black. If it happens before birth, it is a sign of fetal distress. When mixed with amniotic fluid, it may look like pea-green soup, leaving a greenish tinge to the baby, hence the name "meconium staining." Meconium is thick and sticky. If it is aspirated by the infant, it causes pneumonia and sepsis. Therefore, if meconium staining is seen or suspected, the infant is prevented from taking the first breath by avoiding any stimulation that would provoke the start of spontaneous respirations, until after repeated endotracheal suctioning to remove meconium from the lower airway. After this is done an endotracheal tube is left in place, and ventilations are assisted by a BVM with O_2. Now the mouth and nose can be suctioned clear of fluid and meconium.

OUTCOME

The infant was severely depressed on initial assessment (1 minute APGAR 3). The infant was rapidly dried and wrapped in a clean, dry towel. A warm pad was made with hot towels, placed in plastic sacks, and wrapped in more towels. The infant was laid on this "warming pad," suctioned, and ventilated with 100% O_2 at 30/min with a BVM. Transport was initiated. After several minutes of ventilation, the infant pinked up, began moving, and started crying. On arrival at the hospital, the infant had an APGAR of 9 (because of extremity cyanosis) but was still hypothermic. He was placed in a warmer and transferred to the neonatal ICU. His birth weight was 4 lbs, 1 oz. His gestational age was estimated at 36 weeks.

Further history obtained at the hospital revealed that approximately 8 months before, Holly had a bad case of the flu, with diarrhea and vomiting for approximately 7 to 10 days. Her physician guessed that it was during this time that Holly's birth control pills were probably not effective and ovulation occurred.

Holly was dismissed later that day and the infant, who was named for the medic who cared for him, was dismissed 2 days later.

BIBLIOGRAPHY

Berkow, R. & Fletcher A. J. (Eds.). (1992). Normal pregnancy, labor. In R. Berkow & A. J. Fletcher, (Eds.). *The Merck Manual,* (16th ed.). Rahway, NJ: Merck Research Laboratories.

Berkow, R. & Fletcher A. J. eds. (1992). Delivery and disturbances in newborns and infants. In R. Berkow & A. J. Fletcher, (Eds.). *The Merck Manual,* (16th ed.). Rahway, NJ: Merck Research Laboratories.

Bloom, R. S., Cropley, C. S., & Chameides, L. (1994). *Textbook of neonatal resuscitation,* (2nd ed.). Elk Grove Village, IL: American Academy of Pediatrics.

Chameides, L. & Hazinski, M. F., (Eds.). Newborn resuscitation. (1994). In *Pediatric advanced life support,* Dallas, TX: American Heart Association and American Academy of Pediatrics.

Nichols, D. G., Yaster, M., Lappe, D. G., & Haller, J. A. (Eds.). Neonatal emergencies. (1996). In *Golden hour: The handbook of advanced pediatric life support,* (2nd ed.). St Louis, MO: Mosby.

8

OB/GYN Emergencies

OVERVIEW

Emergencies that affect the pregnant patient are particularly stressful to many care providers because of the presence of two patients, the mother and the unborn infant. Fortunately, many of these emergencies involve normal childbirth, where both the mother and infant have a good outcome. However, this is not always the case. With advances in medicine and the application of technology to the field of obstetrics, more and more women who previously would be unable to conceive and carry a child to maturity are now able to do so. Subsequently, with the increase in high-risk pregnancies comes the increase in emergent situations that occur outside a hospital setting. Out-of-hospital care providers are expected to perform as competently in these situations as in an adult trauma situation. The basic principles of care are the same with one addition; the best way to care for the unborn fetus is to care for the mother. When caring for the pregnant patient, knowledge of the changes of pregnancy will help guide the application of those principles to best effect a positive outcome for both mother and baby.

Anatomy and Physiology

Normal changes of pregnancy begin at the time of conception, when hormones designed to promote the growth and development of the placenta and the fetus suddenly increase. Those same hormones contribute to a generalized state of vasodilatation that lasts throughout pregnancy. This pregnancy induced vasodilation causes the circulating blood volume to increase accordingly, until at the time of birth, the mother has increased her total blood volume by as much as 30% to 50% and decreased her systolic blood pressure by 5 to 15 mm Hg. To accommodate the increase in volume, her heart rate increases by as much as 15 to 20 bpm. The growth of the fetus also increases the mother's oxygen demand until, by the third trimester, it has increased by 20% to 30% resulting in an increase in respiratory rate but a decrease in tidal volume resulting from the growth of the fetus exerting pressure on the lungs. By the third trimester, stretching of the peritoneum interferes with normal perception of peritoneal irritation and pressure on the GI tract results in delayed gastric emptying. By the third trimester, pelvic and hip joints have relaxed and all joints have loosened to prepare for childbirth.

Pathophysiology and Treatment

Pathophysiologically, the normal changes of pregnancy result in a delay in recognizing signs and symptoms of shock, a tendency to develop hypoxia and a predisposition for muscu-

155

loskeletal injury (primarily dislocation), as well as aspiration. Positioning is also an important factor. As the pregnant uterus grows, the supine position exerts pressure from the uterus on the vena cava and aorta, interfering with blood return to the heart. This phenomenon is called supine hypotensive syndrome. To avoid this syndrome, the pregnant patient is positioned on her left side.

In traumatic injuries, regardless of the type of trauma, if it involves the abdomen, the assumption is that the fetus is involved and the potential for severity of injury has just increased. A pregnant patient may lose one third to one half of her total blood supply before any signs and symptoms occurring. High flow oxygen is usually required because of the increase in oxygen demand. Positioning on her left side to increase blood return to the heart is necessary. Blunt trauma to the abdomen may also stimulate contractions. These contractions may be painless and not recognized. Pregnant patients who suffer traumatic injuries, especially to the abdomen, should be evaluated at the nearest appropriate medical facility.

Medical emergencies involve infection, dehydration, bleeding (including ectopic pregnancy, placenta previa, and abruptio placenta), hypertensive episodes with or without seizures, abdominal or chest pain, hypoglycemic episodes if the mother is diabetic, and uterine rupture (rare). History is very important, especially the duration of pregnancy. The duration of pregnancy along with assessment findings often determines the most probable cause of the patient's problem. It is vital that this information be communicated to the hospital.

The basic priorities of care (airway, breathing, and circulation) do not change. Administration of high flow oxygen, IV access with fluid replacement, and maintenence of a calm environment are usual standard care procedures. However, priorities also include positioning to increase blood return to the heart (on her left side) and promote clot formation (hips elevated). If the patient is bleeding, clots should be examined for tissue fragments; therefore all clots and expelled tissue should be taken to the hospital with the patient. The rate of bleeding is important to assess. Usually this is done by counting the number of pads used.

Pregnancy induced hypertension is another emergency. Complaints related to hypertension range from headache to abdominal pain, chest pain, blindness, and seizures. Assessment findings include hypertension and may include hyperreflexia. Management of hypertensive episodes includes limiting environmental stimuli (no sirens) and considering magnesium sulfate to prevent or stop seizures.

Normal childbirth is not usually considered a true emergency. However, excessive bleeding before, during, or after childbirth is not normal and is considered an emergency. Excessive bleeding is managed by IV fluid replacement and if the baby has been born, allowing the baby to nurse. Uterine massage and, in some systems, oxytocin (Pitocin) is considered to control bleeding from uterine atony after the baby is born.

Other emergencies include prolapsed cord, limb presentation, or breech birth. Breech deliveries and limb presentations are managed conservatively with oxygen, IV access, and the patient placed on her left side with hips elevated during transport.

A prolapsed cord is a threat to the life of the fetus. As long as the presenting part is pressing on the cord, blood is not getting to the fetus. Treatment includes placing the mother in a supine position and inserting a gloved hand into the vaginal vault to lift the presenting part off the cord. Once in place, the care provider must continue to keep the presenting part off the cord until relieved at the receiving hospital.

During care for the mother, providers should also remember that the father of the infant, if present, is also considered a "patient" and should be given all the consideration that any other patient is given. Answering questions, explaining procedures, and notifying him where the patient will be taken are all pertinent and appropriate actions to take.

CASE 1

Dispatch: 20:30 hrs; a 20 y/o female, possible miscarriage

On Arrival: You find 20 y/o Pella lying on the couch of her apartment. She is awake, appears pale, and seems anxious. Her boyfriend is with her.

Initial Assessment Findings

Mental Status—Awake, anxious, obeys command
Airway—Open and clear
Breathing—R 20, talking in complete sentences; lung sounds clear bilaterally
Circulation—Skin pale, cool, and dry
        Radial pulse 90 and regular
        BP 112/84
Chief Complaint—Abdominal cramping with vaginal bleeding

Focused History

Events—She tells you she started having abdominal cramping this morning with spotting starting this afternoon. About half an hour ago she went to the bathroom and noticed bright red blood in the toilet. She called her boyfriend, and he called EMS.
Previous Illness—None
Current Health Status—Good; pregnancy determined by home test done 3 days ago.
Allergies—Erythromycin
Medications—None

Focused Physical

Current Set of VS—P 90, R 20, BP 112/84
Other Pertinent Findings—Abdomen soft and tender to palpation in lower abdomen; bright red blood on sanitary pad, which she stated she changed about four times this afternoon; pulse oximetry 99%; previous miscarriage a year ago, no other children; admits to occasional recreational drug use but denies any used in last 3 days; no other abnormalities noted.
Diagnostic Tests—Orthostatic hypotension present, P 110, BP 80/62 when placed in sitting position; blood sugar 112

ECG

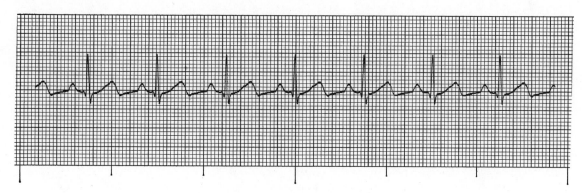

Figure 8-1

QUESTIONS

1. What is significant about Pella's history?

2. What body systems are affected?

3. What is the significance of abdominal cramping followed by spotting?

4. What is indicated by her history of changing a sanitary pad four times in the afternoon?

5. What precaution must you take when estimating blood loss by blood in the toilet?

6. What is significant about her history of recreational drug use?

7. What is implied by her pregnancy being confirmed by a home test?

8. What is implied by a positive orthostatic change?

9. Why does Pella have normal vital signs when lying down but become tachycardic and hypotensive when in an upright position?

10. How would you describe Pella's ECG?

11. Are Pella's signs and symptoms related to her ECG?

12. Is there any other information, either by history or by physical assessment, that you need?

13. What is Pella at risk for?

14. If Pella is pregnant, what do you think is wrong?

15. What conditions could cause vaginal bleeding in a nonpregnant woman?

16. How serious is Pella's situation?

17. How would you begin treatment?

18. Your partner inspects the toilet and finds a small ball of tissue in the bottom of the bowl. What is significant about that tissue, and what should you do?

19. What is the accepted medical term for a miscarriage?

20. What is the theory behind why a miscarriage occurs?

QUESTIONS AND ANSWERS

1. What is significant about Pella's history?

Abdominal cramping is followed by spotting; previous miscarriage a year ago; recreational drug use; bright red blood and change of sanitary pad four times this afternoon; confirmation of pregnancy done by a home test.

2. What body systems are affected?

Cardiovascular—active bleeding, presence of orthostatic hypotension

3. What is the significance of abdominal cramping followed by spotting?

This is a typical progression of symptoms that suggests a miscarriage, or spontaneous abortion.

4. What is indicated by her history of changing a sanitary pad four times in the afternoon?

This implies a frequency of bleeding that needs to be examined more closely.

5. What precaution must you take when estimating blood loss by blood in the toilet?

The actual amount of blood is very difficult to determine. It can be either grossly over or under estimated. The point is this, if there is blood in the toilet, bleeding has occurred. You just can't tell how much.

6. What is significant about her history of recreational drug use?

Recreational drug use can predispose to miscarriages and congenital malformations, as well as other complications of pregnancy.

7. What is implied by her pregnancy being confirmed by a home test?

Potential inaccuracy with being pregnant; inaccuracy with estimation of gestational age; and no prenatal care.

8. What is implied by a positive orthostatic change?

Hypotension that occurs when there is a change in body position (from a lying position to sitting or sitting position to standing) implies a volume deficit.

9. Why does Pella have normal vital signs when lying down but become tachycardic and hypotensive when in an upright position?

Pella's body is able to compensate for volume deficit when lying down. The epinephrine/norepinephrine response to decreased cardiac output causes vasoconstriction, increased heart rate, increased ventricular contractility, and fluid conservation by the kidneys. Together these actions maintain cardiac output and sufficient blood pressure to perfuse the vital organs. This compensatory effort is greatly assisted by putting the body in a horizontal position with the head, chest, and abdomen on the same plane as the heart. As long as perfusion is maintained in this manner, she will not have other overt signs of shock.

10. How would you describe Pella's ECG?

She has a regular sinus rhythm without ectopy.

11. Are Pella's signs and symptoms related to her ECG?

We don't know what her normal heart rate is, but a rate of 90 in a young woman is slightly fast for a resting rate, even though it is not outside the bounds of normal. This rate is probably due to volume deficit but because we don't know her normal rate it is impossible to tell how much it has had to change to generate a systolic pressure of 112.

12. Is there any other information, either by history or by physical assessment, that you need?

What drug(s) is/are used recreationally? When was the last time she used drugs? How far along does she think she is? Or when was her last normal period? Get more specific about her vaginal bleeding—when this afternoon did it start? What is the total number of sanitary pads used since the bleeding started? What was the color of the blood? Has it changed at all? Has she passed any tissue?

13. What is Pella at risk for?

A greater degree of shock. She already has orthostatic changes and is still bleeding.

14. If Pella is pregnant, what do you think is wrong?

There is a high probability of a miscarriage.

15. What conditions could cause vaginal bleeding in a nonpregnant woman?

There are relatively few conditions. Trauma is the most common with lacerations of the vaginal wall or labia, but they usually do not have cramping associated with them. Tumors of the uterus can cause bleeding but usually occur in older women.

16. How serious is Pella's situation?

Pella is unstable due to the presence of orthostatic hypotension.

17. How would you begin treatment?

Apply oxygen by a mask non-rebreather and reservoir at 12 to 15 lpm. Start an IV of NS or LR and administer a fluid bolus of 300 to 500 ml and reassess. Apply a perineal dressing or large trauma dressing to the vaginal area to more closely monitor blood flow.

18. Your partner inspects the toilet and finds a small ball of tissue in the bottom of the bowl. What is significant about that tissue and what should you do?

This is most likely tissue that has been passed and may be placental tissue. If it is intact it contains the fetus. If it is not intact, there is a high probability of retained placental fragments, and Pella will continue to bleed until they are passed. All tissue should be saved.

19. What is the accepted medical term for a miscarriage?

A spontaneous abortion. *Spontaneous* implies that it occurred suddenly for no known reason. *Abortion* means the termination (spontaneous or deliberate) of a pregnancy. A *threatened abortion* is spotting and cramping without tissue expulsion.

20. What is the theory behind why a miscarriage occurs?

More than 10% of pregnancies end as spontaneous abortions, almost all caused by defective eggs.

OUTCOME

Pella was given oxygen by mask non-rebreather at 15 lpm and an initial bolus of 500 ml of NS. She arrived at the ED with a total of 800 ml NS and VS of P 102, RR 24, BP 92/72. She admitted to the ED staff "occasional" marijuana use and was worried that her miscarriage was caused by her marijuana use. After initial blood work and tissue examination in the ED, a unit of blood was started and she was taken to the surgery for a D&C (dilation and curettage) for suspected retained fragments. Pella had an uneventful recovery and, after initial drug abuse counseling, was dismissed to go home.

CASE 2

Dispatch: 11:00 hrs; a 25 y/o female with syncopal episode

On Arrival: You find 25 y/o Cheryl lying on the couch in her living room. She is awake, appears to have good skin tones, and is alone.

Initial Assessment Findings

Mental Status—Alert and oriented, obeys command
Airway—Open and clear
Breathing—R 16 and talking in complete sentences; lung sounds clear bilaterally
Circulation—Skin appears to have good color, has an even tan, cool, and dry
      Radial pulse 80 and regular
      BP 96/78
Chief Complaint—Felt like she was going to faint when she got up to go to the bathroom

Focused History

Events—She felt nauseated and got up to go the bathroom. She then became very dizzy so she lay back down on the couch and called EMS.
Previous Illness—Has not been feeling well for last 3 days with intermittent, "crampy" abdominal pain that has gotten worse until today when the pain is constant but gets worse at times with occasional episodes of nausea; denies vomiting.
Current Health Status—Good, completed a local athletic event a week ago; states she has had a tubal ligation a year ago; menses is normally irregular and began yesterday, but this cramping is different.
Allergies—None known
Medications—Penicillin

Focused Physical

Current Set of VS—P 80, R 16, BP 96/78
Other Pertinent Findings—Abdomen slightly distended with guarding, tender to palpation; when Cheryl turned to allow better access to her abdomen, she suddenly complains of right shoulder pain, which quickly resolves, but denies pain on palpation of shoulder; pulse oximetry 98% to 99% on room air; no other abnormal findings.
Diagnostic Tests—Blood sugar 84

ECG

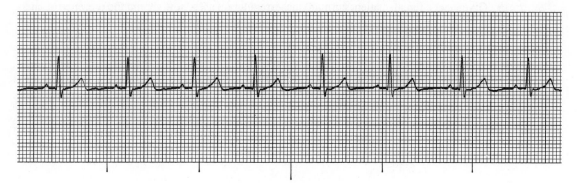

Figure 8-2

1. What is significant about Cheryl's history?

2. What body systems are affected?

3. What is implied by her history of participating in an athletic event, and how is this important?

4. What is the significance of intermittent abdominal pain described as "crampy"?

5. What is the significance of right shoulder pain in a nontrauma patient complaining of abdominal pain?

6. What is the significance of dizziness with a change in position, especially in the presence of abdominal pain with associated shoulder/neck pain?

7. When patients have darker skin tones, where is a good place to look for color changes and why?

8. During your assessment you check Cheryl's mucous membranes and discover her tongue is almost white. What is implied?

9. How would you describe Cheryl's ECG?

10. Are Cheryl's signs and symptoms related to her ECG?

11. Is there any other information, either by history or by physical assessment, that will help you?

12. What is Cheryl at risk for?

13. What do you think is wrong?

14. Does Cheryl's history of having a tubal ligation influence your opinion of what is wrong?

15. How would you begin treatment?

16. When you transfer Cheryl to your stretcher she suddenly complains of a recurrence of right shoulder pain, becomes noticeably pale, breaks out in a sweat and tells you she is going to vomit, which she does. She vomits clear stomach contents. What will you do, and how would you continue treatment?

17. How serious is Cheryl's situation?

18. Is it abnormal for female athletes to suffer from irregular menses?

19. Given that a female patient normally has irregular menses, how should the presence of an irregular menses in a woman of childbearing age with signs and symptoms of internal bleeding be regarded?

20. When a female patient complaining of abdominal pain states she is having her menses, how important is it to determine whether the amount and character of bleeding is normal?

QUESTIONS AND ANSWERS

1. ***What is significant about Cheryl's history?***

    Her description of the onset and progression of abdominal pain (intermittent abdominal pain, described as "crampy" with nausea, becoming increasingly worse for the last 3 days), syncope when getting up, childbearing age, tubal ligation, being an athlete.

2. ***What body systems are affected?***

    Cardiovascular—syncope when rising

    GI—"crampy" abdominal pain, nausea

3. ***What is implied by her history of participating in an athletic event and how is this important?***

    The implication of being an athlete is that she is in good physical shape and that her normal heart rates and blood pressure are probably much lower than a nonathlete of comparable age. Therefore a pulse of 80 may be much faster than normal. Her BP is more difficult, this may be a normal pressure for her.

4. ***What is the significance of intermittent abdominal pain described as "crampy"?***

    She is describing pain that is more typical of hollow organ spasms (intermittent and crampy) than solid organ stretching.

5. ***What is the significance of right shoulder pain in a nontrauma patient complaining of abdominal pain?***

    The shoulders and immediate neck area are sites for referred pain caused by peritoneal irritation. The irritation may be resulting from chemicals of inflammation that occur because of ruptured viscus or swelling and distention of organ capsules that lie close to a shared central afferent nerve pathway (a nerve going toward the spinal cord). Shoulder/neck pain is a common site for referred pain from the liver (on the right), the spleen (on the left), and ovaries or fallopian tubes (on either the right or left).

6. ***What is the significance of dizziness with a change in position, especially in the presence of abdominal pain with associated shoulder/neck pain?***

    This suggests orthostatic hypotension (dizziness with change in position) resulting from abdominal bleeding from a ruptured viscus (abdominal pain with radiation to shoulder or neck).

7. ***When patients have darker skin tones, where is a good place to look for color changes and why?***

    The mucous membranes of the mouth and inside of the lower eyelid are both good places. These areas are typically not pigmented and have a good blood supply with capillaries close to the surface. Mucous membranes are easily checked and show evidence of vasoconstriction early.

8. ***During your assessment you check Cheryl's mucous membranes and discover her tongue is almost white. What is implied?***

    Since the mucous membranes are so good at indicating vasoconstriction, an extremely pale tongue implies an extreme degree of vasoconstriction or anemia.

9. ***How would you describe Cheryl's ECG?***

    A regular sinus rhythm without ectopy.

10. ***Are Cheryl's signs and symptoms related to her ECG?***

    This rhythm can support perfusion and gives no indication of being the source of syncope or pain.

11. ***Is there any other information, either by history or by physical assessment, that will help you?***

    Has this pain happened before? Is her menses normal? If not, how does it differ? Are there any other symptoms that she has noticed? Has she fallen or suffered any trauma 3 to 4 days ago? Do an orthostatic check of her pulse and blood pressure.

12. ***What is Cheryl at risk for?***

    Further blood loss in the abdomen with profound shock.

13. What do you think is wrong?

Cheryl is suffering from fluid loss, most likely blood, and she is bleeding in the abdomen (abdominal pain, referred pain to shoulder, and clear lung sounds). The most likely cause is a tubal pregnancy or ruptured ovarian cyst.

14. Does Cheryl's history of having a tubal ligation influence your opinion of what is wrong?

A history of a tubal ligation is a risk factor for a tubal pregnancy, making that a higher probability than an ovarian cyst. In the field it does not matter which it is; what matters is that you can recognize the indicators for an internal bleed and treat accordingly.

15. How would you begin treatment?

Oxygen, mask non-rebreather with a reservoir at 12 to 15 lpm, start an IV of normal saline or lactated Ringer's and administer a bolus of 300 to 500 ml, then reassess vital signs.

16. When you transfer Cheryl to your stretcher she suddenly complains of a recurrence of right shoulder pain, becomes noticeably pale, breaks out in a sweat, and tells you she is going to vomit, which she does. She vomits clear stomach contents. What will you do, and how would you continue treatment?

Rapidly reassess pulse and BP, lay her flat, elevate her feet, and administer another fluid bolus.

17. How serious is Cheryl's situation?

This is a life threat and is very serious.

18. Is it abnormal for female athletes to suffer from irregular menses?

No, female athletes frequently suffer from irregular menses because of a decrease in the critical amount of estrogens produced that are needed to ovulate or from an extreme loss of weight. As a consequence, menses may be shortened in duration, irregular, or absent altogether.

19. Given that a female patient normally has irregular menses, how should the presence of an irregular menses in a woman of childbearing age with signs and symptoms of internal bleeding be regarded?

Don't let the history of normal irregularity cloud the issue. It is the signs and symptoms of internal bleeding that are the priority; the cause is irrelevant. Causes are taught to emphasize certain recognizable patterns in patient presentation. Either a ruptured tubal pregnancy or ruptured ovarian cyst can cause a woman to think she is having a delayed or absent menses. It is the bleeding that can be life threatening.

20. When a female patient complaining of abdominal pain states she is having her menses, how important is it to determine whether the amount and character of bleeding is normal?

It is very important in terms of trying to determine the amount of blood loss and a probable cause. However, the amount that is exiting the vaginal vault depends on what the problem is and where it is located. Ruptured fallopian tubes may have scant bleeding that is darker than normal, whereas ruptured ovarian cysts may have no vaginal bleeding. A spontaneous abortion may have considerable bleeding that is bright red.

OUTCOME

Before moving Cheryl, oxygen by mask non-rebreather with a reservoir at 15 lpm was started. An IV of normal saline was also started at kvo. When Cheryl was moved to the stretcher she became very pale, dizzy, and vomited clear stomach contents. A quick recheck of her vital signs showed a weak radial pulse with a BP of 70/56. A fluid bolus of 500 ml was administered. En route to the ED, her feet were elevated and she was kept warm. On arrival blood tests including a type and cross for packed RBCs was done. An ultrasound was suspicious for a tubal pregnancy. She was taken to surgery within 45 minutes of arrival. A right-sided ruptured fallopian tube was discovered, along with a liter of blood. Cheryl recovered and was dismissed to home.

CASE 3

Dispatch: 04:30 hrs; 38 y/o pregnant female, abdominal pain

On Arrival: You find 38 y/o Cherise sitting in a recliner in her basement apartment. She is awake, appears very pale and very pregnant. Her husband is with her and is quite upset.

Initial Assessment Findings

Mental Status—Alert and oriented, obeys command
Airway—Open and clear
Breathing—R 24 and regular, talking in complete sentences but seems out of breath; lung sounds diminished in the bases, clear bilaterally
Circulation—Skin pale, cool, and clammy
　　　　　Radial pulse weak and thready, carotid 120
　　　　　BP 98/62
Chief Complaint—Acute abdominal pain

Focused History

Events—Two days ago Cherise, who is 8 months pregnant, was in an automobile accident. Even though Cherise and her husband were not seriously hurt, the baby died. She and her husband were sent home for her to have labor occur naturally. Tonight she didn't feel good and went to bed but was uncomfortable lying down, so she decided to spend the night in the recliner. She describes the abdominal pain as an intermittent "ache" involving her entire abdomen, which has steadily gotten worse. She called her physician and he told her to call EMS.
Previous Illness—None
Current Health Status—Otherwise good; there are three other children in the family, they were sent to stay with relatives.
Allergies—None known
Medications—Prenatal vitamins, no other medications

Focused Physical

Current Set of VS—P 120, R 24, BP 98/62
Other Pertinent Findings—You note a seat-belt bruise across her chest and at the level of the midabdomen; her abdomen is distended and consistently rigid; pulse oximetry reads ERROR
Diagnostic Tests—None done

ECG

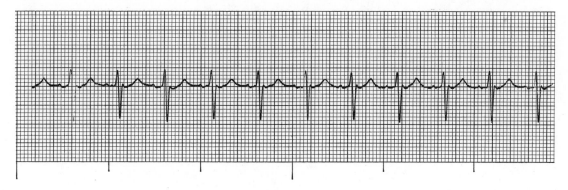

Figure 8-3

QUESTIONS

1. What is significant about Cherise's history?

2. What body systems are affected?

3. How would you describe Cherise's ECG?

4. Does her cardiac rhythm suggest a possible cause for any of her signs and symptoms?

5. What are normal vital sign changes associated with the third trimester of pregnancy?

6. What do Cherise's skin vitals (color, temperature, and moisture) suggest?

7. Is this supported by her vital signs?

8. Why is body position an important consideration when obtaining a blood pressure on any pregnant women past the first trimester?

9. What normal change of pregnancy interferes with the perception of abdominal pain?

10. What is significant about her description of abdominal pain?

11. What is the significance of the seat-belt bruise that is midabdomen?

12. Is there any information, from either her history or your physical, that might be helpful?

13. How serious is Cherise's situation?

14. What is Cherise at risk for developing?

15. How would you begin treatment?

16. What is your priority concerning Cherise's husband?

17. En route to the hospital, Cherise suddenly complains of circumoral numbness and tingling. Shortly thereafter she complains of sharply increased abdominal pain. What is the significance of these changes, and what would you do?

18. What effect does pregnancy have on signs and symptoms of shock?

19. It is often difficult to tell whether a pregnant woman is bleeding internally. What signs would you look for other than changes in vital signs?

20. What is the most desirable position of transport for a third trimester woman and why?

QUESTIONS AND ANSWERS

1. What is significant about Cherise's history?

8 months pregnant, MVC 2 days ago, baby dead, abdominal pain of at least 4 to 6 hours duration

2. What body systems are affected?

Cardiovascular—pale, cool, clammy skin; tachycardia; BP 98/62
GYN—distended, rigid abdomen; consistent with pregnancy

3. How would you describe Cherise's ECG?

Sinus tachycardia without ectopy

4. Does her cardiac rhythm suggest a possible cause for any of her signs and symptoms?

No, her rhythm is most likely an attempt to compensate for whatever is wrong.

5. What are normal vital sign changes associated with the third trimester of pregnancy?

Normal vital signs change with pregnancy and by the third trimester the changes are fairly obvious. Because the total blood volume increases, stroke volume also increases and so does the heart rate, by about 15% or 10 to 15 beats per minute. Cardiac output increases 30% to 50% during pregnancy. To better accommodate the cardiac output, total peripheral vascular resistance relaxes so both systolic and diastolic pressure falls (about 5 mm Hg for systolic pressure and 5 to 10 mm Hg for diastolic pressure).

6. What do Cherise's skin vitals (color, temperature, and moisture) suggest?

Normally, pale, cool, clammy skin suggests an epinephrine/norepinephrine response.

7. Is this supported by her vital signs?

Yes, even with the normal changes of pregnancy a pulse of 120 is still too fast. In Cherise's case, it takes a rate of 120 along with increased peripheral vascular resistance (pale, cool, clammy skin) to support a systolic pressure of 98. This implies that she is compensating for hypotension.

8. Why is body position an important consideration when obtaining a blood pressure on any pregnant women past the first trimester?

A condition known as supine hypotensive syndrome occurs when, in the supine position, the weight of the pregnant uterus lies on top of the vena cava and aorta.

9. What normal change of pregnancy interferes with the perception of abdominal pain?

Normally the peritoneum is sensitive to irritation; however, in the pregnant abdomen the peritoneum gradually stretches to the point where it no longer is as sensitive to irritation as it was in the nonpregnant state.

10. What is significant about her description of abdominal pain?

Her description of abdominal pain is not typical of contractions and suggests another problem.

11. What is the significance of the seat-belt bruise that is midabdomen?

The significance of the bruise is the amount of force involved. The location is significant because a seat belt is not in the correct position at midabdomen. A significant force midabdomen could cause bruising of the uterus itself, which in the last two months of pregnancy is dangerous.

12. Is there any information, from either her history or your physical that might be helpful?

Find out if the midabdomen bruise is from the seat belt or from hitting something else such as the dash. What is her due date? Has she taken any medication for the pain?

13. How serious is Cherise's situation?

This is a life threat.

14. What is Cherise at risk for developing?

A ruptured uterus, shock, a precipitous delivery, or, as a later consequence, DIC (disseminated intravascular coagulation).

15. How would you begin treatment?

Oxygen with a mask non-rebreather and reservoir at 15 lpm, have her lay on her left side to relieve the pressure on the vena cava, start two large bore IVs of NS or LR, administer a fluid bolus of 500 ml and reassess.

16. What is your priority concerning Cherise's husband?

Cherise's husband is your patient too. While he may have issues of his own that may be unknown, considering the history, we do known that he is having to deal with the death of his baby, as well as with what is happening to his wife. His behavior and your program's policy will dictate how he will be transported to the hospital. Offer to call someone to take or meet him there. Keep in mind that his wife may be experiencing a threat to her own life and if the baby should be born in the back of your vehicle, you can't be sure of the condition of the fetus. This atmosphere may not be conducive to supporting her husband.

17. En route to the hospital, Cherise suddenly complains of circumoral numbness and tingling. Shortly thereafter she complains of sharply increased abdominal pain. What is the significance of these changes, and what would you do?

The presence of circumoral numbness and tingling are more often found in patients that hyperventilate. With a rate of 24, Cherise does not appear to be hyperventilating. Because of the normal changes that occur with pregnancy, a chronic compensated respiratory alkalosis is present, which may impede blood-buffering capacity. Instead of circumoral numbness and tingling indicating respiratory alkalosis, her complaint may be resulting from extreme peripheral vasoconstriction in that area. When the body needs to vasoconstrict, the extremities and the skin are the first areas to do so. The face is considered an extremity. The sharply increased abdominal pain is significant and worrisome. The abdomen should be reassessed along with her vital signs and mental status.

18. What effect does pregnancy have on signs and symptoms of shock?

A pregnant woman usually has no clinical signs of shock until about 30% of circulating volume is lost.

19. It is often difficult to tell whether a pregnant woman is bleeding internally. What signs would you look for other than changes in vital signs?

If possible the assessment should be done with the patient lying on her left side. This ensures the best blood return to the heart. If this is done, one of the first signs of internal bleeding is an increase in anxiety or altered mental state. Pallor along with cool, clammy skin are also signs. Complaints of abdominal pain may be present but not typical. Be suspicious of any complaints of vague or diffuse pain. They may indicate a more serious problem is occurring.

20. What is the most desirable position of transport for a third trimester woman and why?

The most desirable position is the left lateral recumbent position to take the pressure of the gravid uterus off the vena cave and aorta. This position promotes the best possible preload and therefore, optimal cardiac output.

OUTCOME

Cherise had oxygen by a mask non-rebreather with a reservoir at 15 lpm and two large bore IVs started. En route she suddenly complained of circumoral numbness and tingling with sharply increased abdominal pain. Her color became rapidly worse, her radial pulse disappeared, and she became disoriented and in extreme pain. Her abdomen was very rigid and vaginal bleeding was observed. VS were: P 136, R 28, BP 70/56. On arrival at the ED she was examined, blood was drawn and she was immediately taken to the OR where a partially ruptured uterus with male fetus was found. Repair of the uterus was unsuccessful, and a hysterectomy was performed. Cherise eventually recovered and was dismissed to home.

CASE 4

Dispatch: 08:00 hrs; 36 y/o with difficulty breathing, possible delivery in progress

On Arrival: You find 36 y/o Raine propped up in bed; a man is next to her, supporting her. She appears very pale, anxious, and is gasping for breath, clutching at the man's arm. A midwife is also there and is holding a newborn infant.

Initial Assessment Findings

Mental Status—Awake, alert, obeys command

Airway—Open and clear

Breathing—R 34 with accessory muscle use; lung sounds have basilar fine rales with wheezes bilaterally

Circulation—Skin very pale, lips cyanotic, cool, and diaphoretic

Radial pulse rapid and irregular

BP 80/68

Chief Complaint—Difficulty breathing

Focused History

Events—The midwife tells you that Raine and her husband have had their last three children at home with no problem. This was a normal delivery until just shortly after the baby was born when Raine suddenly began complaining of shortness of breath and became very pale. The midwife called EMS and called the patient's physician who will meet you at the ED. The midwife tells you the baby appears to be healthy with a 1 minute APGAR of 8 and a 5 minute APGAR of 10. The midwife will continue to take care of the infant.

Previous Illness—None

Current Health Status—Pregnancy was normal, has had four pregnancies with four children, including the one just born. This delivery was very fast but appeared normal until Raine began having difficulty breathing.

Allergies—None

Medications—Prenatal vitamins

Focused Physical

Current Set of VS—P irregular at 136, R 34, BP 80/64

Other Pertinent Findings—Abdomen soft, uterus firm and size of grapefruit at 4 fingers above the pubis, the scant flow of blood from the vagina appears insignificant, the placenta has not yet delivered, pulse oximetry reads ERROR.

Diagnostic Tests—None done

ECG

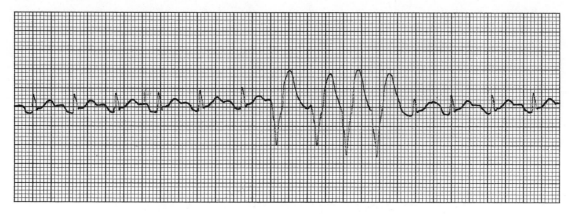

Figure 8-4

QUESTIONS

1. What is significant about Raine's history?

2. What body systems are affected?

3. Why would the pulse oximetry read ERROR?

4. How would you describe Raine's ECG?

5. Is her cardiac rhythm the cause or the result of any of Raine's signs and symptoms?

6. What is the significance of the size of her post delivery uterus?

7. Is there any other information, either from her history or your physical, that could help you?

8. How serious is Raine's condition?

9. What is Raine at risk for?

10. Her husband looks very anxious. What is your priority with him?

11. What do you think is wrong?

12. How would you begin treatment?

13. What types of problems can result in cardiac dysrhythmias in the perinatal period?

14. After your initial treatment you note that Raine has begun shivering and is complaining of feeling cold. You also note jugular venous distension (JVD) and although her circumoral cyanosis did seem to get better after oxygenation, it has not disappeared. What could explain this collection of signs and symptoms?

15. How would you continue treatment?

16. Why would it be very important to monitor vaginal bleeding?

QUESTIONS AND ANSWERS

1. **What is significant about Raine's history?**

Sudden onset of difficulty breathing immediately after birth of the infant, no previous history of any physical problem, previous home deliveries were uncomplicated, age is 36.

2. **What body systems are affected?**

Respiratory—rate is 34, with basilar fine rales and wheezes bilaterally

Cardiovascular—irregular pulse; PVCs; pale, cool, diaphoretic skin; hypotension

3. **Why would the pulse oximetry read ERROR?**

Pulse oximetry is inaccurate in shock states. Raine is hypotensive with peripheral vasoconstriction present.

4. **How would you describe Raine's ECG?**

Sinus tachycardia with a run of ventricular tachycardia (4 PVCs in a row). The PR interval is a 0.20 msec. At a rate this fast, the P wave will appear immediately after the T wave.

5. **Is her cardiac rhythm the cause or the result of any of Raine's signs and symptoms?**

Her PVCs do not perfuse and could possibly interfere with her cardiac output and contribute to her hypotension. However, the PVCs themselves are evidence of irritability in the heart that is unusual in a woman this age, and abnormal after birth. The irritability is from another cause and most likely not cardiac in origin. (Because she had three other children, the possibility of an unrecognized cardiac defect is not likely.)

6. **What is the significance of the size of her post delivery uterus?**

Post delivery the uterus normally clamps down to expel the placenta and control bleeding. To feel a firm uterus the size of a grapefruit about 4 fingers above the pubis is normal and a good sign.

7. **Is there any other information, either from her history or your physical that could help you?**

Is there any cardiac history? Has she ever had any cardiac problems?

8. **How serious is Raine's condition?**

This is very serious and a threat to life.

9. **What is Raine at risk for?**

Cardiac arrest, respiratory failure and arrest, disseminated intravascular coagulation (DIC), and excessive uterine bleeding.

10. **Her husband looks very anxious. What is your priority with him?**

Her husband is your patient also. He needs to know what you are doing and why. His wife is seriously ill and he needs to come to the hospital. Follow your program policy for passengers. The midwife may be able to help by caring for the baby.

11. **What do you think is wrong?**

Raine currently has pulmonary edema with severe hypoxia and hypotension. A preexisting cardiac problem is unlikely since she has had three previous pregnancies with no problem. An amniotic fluid embolus is possible. The sudden onset of shortness of breath in the immediate perinatal period, presence of pulmonary edema and hypotension out of proportion to the amount of blood lost, and cardiac irritability suggest an embolus.

12. **How would you begin treatment?**

Oxygen by mask non-rebreather with a reservoir at 15 lpm, an IV of normal saline or Ringer's lactate, administer a 300 to 500 ml bolus of fluid, and reassess.

13. **What types of problems can result in cardiac dysrhythmias in the perinatal period?**

An underlying cardiac problem can predispose to dysrhythmias, as well as pulmonary edema. Any cause of hypoxia or hypoxemia, such as hypotension or pulmonary emboli, can cause cardiac dysrhythmias in the perinatal period.

14. *After your initial treatment you note that Raine has begun shivering and is complaining of feeling cold. You also note jugular venous distension (JVD) and although her circumoral cyanosis did seem to get better after oxygenation, it has not disappeared. What could explain this collection of signs and symptoms?*

The JVD is a sign of right-sided heart failure, consistent with pulmonary emboli. That would also explain why she still has a degree of cyanosis. It is interesting to note that shivering and chills are also frequently present with amniotic fluid emboli; however, the explanation is speculative. Peripheral vasoconstriction causes a person to feel cold and shock states interfere with the body's heat production. The birth process is one that generates high body heat in the mother. If she suffered peripheral vasoconstriction soon after a high production of body heat, it may be that she feels the absence of body heat more acutely.

15. *How would you continue treatment?*

Cover her with blankets to keep her warm. If the oxygen did not affect the PVCs or hypotension, lidocaine (50 to 150 mg) would be appropriate. The normal dose of lidocaine is 1 to 1.5 mg/kg so go by her body weight, keeping in mind that she just lost about 20 to 25 pounds.

16. *Why would it be very important to monitor vaginal bleeding?*

She hasn't delivered the placenta yet so that must be collected and transported. Because of her age, history of multiple births, and current problem, she is at risk for uterine atony and prolonged, excessive bleeding. If she is covered, you need to frequently check for bleeding or you won't see it.

OUTCOME

There was no appreciable change by the time Raine arrived at the ED. Blood gases were immediately drawn: pH 7.46, PA O_2 60, PA CO_2 30, HCO_3^- 24. She was rapidly assessed by her physician and admitted to the ICU with the diagnosis of a pulmonary embolus. Shortly after arrival, her placenta delivered and she began bleeding. The diagnosis of DIC was made. She developed ARDS and after an extremely rocky course finally began to recover. After 3 weeks in the hospital she was dismissed to home.

CASE 5

Dispatch: 23:30 hrs; 24 y/o pregnant woman, abdominal pain

On Arrival: You find 24 y/o Allie lying on the couch. She appears pale and has a tear-streaked face. She also looks pregnant. There are several other people, about her age, with her.

Initial Assessment Findings
     Mental Status—Awake, alert, and obeys command
     Airway—Open and clear
     Breathing—R 22 and not labored; lung sounds clear bilaterally
     Circulation—Skin pale, cool, and dry
          Radial pulse rapid at 116
          BP 176/100
     Chief Complaint—Abdominal pain

Focused History
     Events—Allie states that she was trying to have "some fun" with her friends when she suddenly experienced a sharp, stabbing pain in the right side of her abdomen about 30 minutes ago. The pain is now described as "something ripping me apart." There is nothing that makes it better. She denies radiation. She ranks the current pain as a 9 on a 1 to 10 scale. When she started bleeding she called EMS.
     Previous Illness—Flu and "stuff like that," she does state that this is her third pregnancy but the previous two pregnancies ended in miscarriages.
     Current Health Status—"Okay." She states she thinks she is 7 or 8 months along, she saw a doctor at the clinic who told her she was pregnant but she hasn't been back since.
     Allergies—None
     Medications—None

Focused Physical
     Current Set of VS—P 116, R 22, BP 176/100
     Other Pertinent Findings—Her uterus is tender and hard to palpation with the fundus midway to the zyphoid from her umbilicus; vaginal bleeding is dark red, and she has used one pad since the pain started; she is also complaining of a headache; you note track marks on her arms, though none look recent; pulse oximetry is 99%.
     Diagnostic Tests—Blood sugar 76

ECG

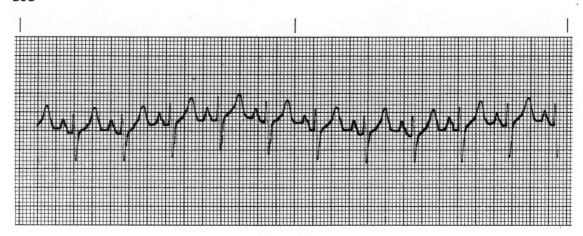

Figure 8-5

QUESTIONS

1. What is significant about Allie's history?

2. What body systems are affected?

3. Is Allie's fundal height consistent with her estimate of gestation?

4. What is significant regarding her vital signs and headache?

5. What other information, either from her history or your physical examination, do you need to know?

6. Where would you listen for fetal heart tones, and what would a normal fetal heart rate be?

7. How would you know if the fetus is in distress?

8. What are the causes of bleeding that can occur in the second trimester; in the third?

9. What is the difference, in terms of signs and symptoms, between abruptio placental and placenta previa?

10. What is the difference between Allie's signs and symptoms and the onset of premature labor?

11. What are the risk factors for a ruptured uterus? Does Allie have any of these risk factors?

12. What do you think is Allie's current problem?

13. What is Allie at risk for?

14. How serious is Allie's current situation?

15. How would you begin treatment?

16. Fetal heart tones were assessed at a rate of 90. After initial treatment and immediately moving Allie to the vehicle, you question her further and discover that she had been snorting cocaine with her friends when the pain started. She also admits to occasional use of marijuana to "calm" her nerves. How does this information contribute to your impression of what is wrong and affect your treatment?

17. What do you particularly need to reassess?

QUESTIONS AND ANSWERS

1. What is significant about Allie's history?

Essentially no prenatal care; estimate of gestational age questionable; previous pregnancies terminated in miscarriages; sudden onset; describing the pain as "tearing;" evidence of past recreational drug use

2. What body systems are affected?

CNS—headache

Cardiovascular—pale, cool, dry skin; tachycardia with hypertension

Reproductive—tender, hard uterus with vaginal bleeding

3. Is Allie's fundal height consistent with her estimate of gestation?

Yes, a fundal height at the level of the umbilicus is about the fifth month and at the level of the zyphoid is about the ninth month. A fundal height midway to the zyphoid is somewhere between the seventh and eighth month.

4. What is significant regarding her vital signs and headache?

Tachycardia and hypertension are not normal, regardless of whether or not she is pregnant. A headache in the presence of hypertension implies a CNS effect, most likely from the hypertension.

5. What other information, either from her history or your physical examination, do you need to know?

Does she have any edema, pedal or facial? Exactly what was she doing when the pain started? What does "having some fun" mean? Has she been doing any drugs? If so, what drug(s) did she take and how long ago? Has she had any problems with this pregnancy—any bleeding, abdominal pain or cramping, headaches, any swelling? Has she felt the baby move today? Has the baby moved since the pain started? When is the baby due?

6. Where would you listen for fetal heart tones, and what would a normal fetal heart rate be?

In the third trimester the best place to hear fetal heart tones is usually below the mother's umbilicus. The closer to delivery time the more likely the baby is in the head-down position with the baby's back to the mother's belly. The fetal heart rate is normally faster than the mother's pulse, between 140 to 160 beats per minute. If the medic has one hand on the mother's pulse while listening for fetal heart tones, it will be easier to distinguish between the echo of the maternal pulse and fetal heart tones.

7. How would you know if the fetus is in distress?

By listening to fetal heart tones. Fetal heart tones less than 120 indicate fetal distress. Changes in movement of the fetus can increase your index of suspicion. An increase in fetal movement followed by no activity is cause for concern.

8. What are the causes of bleeding that can occur in the second trimester? In the third?

Causes of bleeding in the second trimester include a threatened abortion or miscarriage or bleeding resulting from another unrelated cause, such as a clotting disorder. Causes of bleeding in the third trimester, directly related to the pregnancy, include abruptio placental, placenta previa, ruptured uterus, and premature labor.

9. What is the difference, in terms of signs and symptoms, between abruptio placental and placenta previa?

Abruptio placental results in the placenta being abruptly pulled away from the uterine wall. This is painful and results in a hard, tender uterus. Bleeding may or may not occur, depending on whether or not an edge of the placenta has been loosened. If bleeding is present, it usually appears dark.

Placenta previa occurs when the placenta has implanted too low in the uterus and is affected by cervical effacement or thinning. As the cervix thins, it pulls away from the placental attachment and bleeding occurs. Because the cervix has relatively few nerve endings for pain, the process is painless. The bleeding tends to be bright red, with the amount of bleeding in direct proportion to the amount of placental attachment disrupted.

10. What is the difference between Allie's signs and symptoms and the onset of premature labor?

In labor, whether or not the labor is premature, contractions have a gradual onset and are regular and rhythmic. In this instance Allie had a sudden onset, is not experiencing regular contractions, and her uterus is painful to palpation. The description of pain is not typical of a description of a contraction.

11. What are the risk factors for a ruptured uterus? Does Allie have any of these risk factors?

The risk factors for a ruptured uterus are prolonged labor with prolonged contractions, labor in a mother with a previous C-section, and trauma to the uterus. Allie has a hard uterus with no change in the consistency of the uterus to resemble contractions. If she is having a sustained contraction then there is a risk for uterine rupture.

12. What do you think is Allie's current problem?

She definitely is having an abnormal presentation. This is not placenta previa because she is having too much pain. Abruptio placental and ruptured uterus are the more likely choices. She doesn't appear to be in enough shock for a ruptured uterus, although that may be developing. Abruptio placental has a higher probability because of its sudden onset, hard and tender uterus, and dark bleeding.

13. What is Allie at risk for?

Death of the fetus, premature birth, maternal shock, or a ruptured uterus.

14. How serious is Allie's current situation?

This is a life threat to the fetus and a potential life threat to Allie.

15. How would you begin treatment?

Oxygen by non-rebreather mask with a reservoir at 15 lpm; if possible, two IVs of crystalloid, either normal saline or lactated Ringer's; assess for fetal heart tones, and place her on her left side.

16. Fetal heart tones were assessed at a rate of 90. After initial treatment and immediately moving Allie to the vehicle, you question her further and discover that she had been snorting cocaine with her friends when the pain started. She also admits to occasional use of marijuana to "calm" her nerves. How does this information contribute to your impression of what is wrong and affect your treatment?

The use of cocaine would suggest abruptio placental. A sudden, sustained rise in blood pressure is a contributing factor to abruptio and would help explain her headache and hypertension. The use of cocaine may also have aggravated a preexisting problem such as pregnancy induced hypertension, further contributing to her present problem. This, however, is speculation.

Tachycardia, while also an effect of cocaine, may be a factor of pain, as well as an abruptio placenta.

Use of drugs during pregnancy and lack of prenatal care predisposes to birth defects, premature labor, low birth weight infants and infants that may require resuscitation after birth. Get the delivery kit ready.

17. What do you particularly need to reassess?

Any change in Allie's perception of pain or mental status, degree and amount of bleeding, vital signs, presence of crowning.

OUTCOME

En route to the hospital, Allie's condition remained the same with no appreciable change in vital signs. On arrival she was immediately taken to the labor and delivery suite and reassessed. Ultrasound confirmed abruptio placental. Fetal heart tones were absent and there was no movement. The vaginal bleeding increased and an emergency C-section was performed. The male infant died. Allie had a brief episode of respiratory difficulty but rapidly recovered. Three days post surgery Allie left the hospital, AMA.

CASE 6

Dispatch: 16:30 hrs; 18 y/o, headache and eye problem

On Arrival: You find 18 y/o Connie, lying on the couch with a washcloth over her eyes. Connie is lying on her side; you note the even rise and fall of her chest. Her mother is there and is very anxious.

Initial Assessment Findings

Mental Status—Confused but obeys command
Airway—Open and clear
Breathing—R 28 and regular; lung sounds clear in upper lobes, absent in lower lobes
Circulation—Skin pale, warm, and dry
   Radial pulse 110 and slightly irregular
   BP 206/110
Chief Complaint—"Worst headache I've ever had"

Focused History

Events—Connie came home from school with a headache and told her mother she was going to lie down. When her mother came in to check on her, Connie stated she couldn't see and her headache was worse. Her mother called EMS.
Previous Illness—Connie had an elective abortion 2 years ago.
Current Health Status—Connie is about 8 months pregnant. She has had frequent headaches and swelling in her ankles, face, and hands for about the last month.
Allergies—Ragweed and goldenrod
Medications—Midol (OTC medication for PMS)

Focused Physical

Current Set of VS—P 110 and slightly irregular, R 28 and shallow, BP 206/110
Other Pertinent Findings—Abdomen is firm but without contractions; mother tells you Connie's face and lips are swollen; she states she is unable to see but you could not check her pupils because of complaints of pain from the light; pulse oximetry is 98%; you see no other abnormalities; mother also tells you that, after much argument over unexplained weight gain, Connie finally confirmed to her that she was pregnant just 2 weeks ago and has not been to see a doctor yet.
Diagnostic Tests—None done

ECG

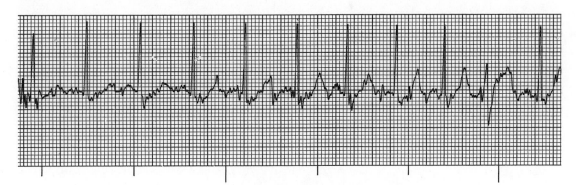

Figure 8-6

QUESTIONS

1. What is important about Connie's history?

2. What body systems are affected?

3. What is the significance of her description of her headache as being the "worst headache . . ."?

4. Is there a relationship between her BP and her chief complaint?

5. What is the relationship between her inability to see and her BP?

6. Is there a relationship between her facial swelling, photophobia, and her BP?

7. How would you describe Connie's ECG?

8. Is her cardiac rhythm responsible for any of Connie's signs or symptoms?

9. What is Midol used for, and why do you think Connie was taking it?

10. Is there any other information, either from her history or your physical, that could help you?

11. What do you think is the cause of Connie's current problem?

12. How serious is Connie's current situation?

13. What is Connie at risk for?

14. Connie's mother began crying and asking many questions regarding what you are doing and whether Connie will be all right. She is so agitated that she is beginning to interfere with your treatment of Connie. How would you handle Connie's mother?

15. How would you begin treatment?

16. While taking Connie's BP the second time, you note a jerking motion of her thumb and forefinger of the hand in the same arm when you pump up the pressure in the cuff. What is the significance of this?

17. How would you continue treatment and what modifications would you make to your transport?

18. En route to the hospital Connie has a grand mal seizure. How would you treat her?

19. How would you document Connie's pregnancy history in terms of gravida and para?

QUESTIONS AND ANSWERS

1. **What is important about Connie's history?**
   She is 8 months pregnant and has had no prenatal care; frequent headaches, swelling in face and hands for last month, photophobia.

2. **What body systems are affected?**
   CNS—complains of "worst headache I've ever had," photophobia
   Cardiovascular—irregular pulse, hypertension
   Other—swelling in extremities and face

3. **What is the significance of her description of her headache as being the "worst headache . . ."?**
   Her description is more common with headaches that occur because of increased intracranial pressure or hemorrhagic strokes.

4. **Is there a relationship between her BP and her chief complaint?**
   Her BP is 206/110, which is extremely hypertensive and could be causing her complaint of headache. However, most hypertensive headaches are not described in this manner unless associated with increased intracranial pressure.

5. **What is the relationship between her inability to see and her BP?**
   Her inability to see, particularly her complaint of photophobia, implies irritation of the optic nerve with interference of the function of the optic nerve. This complaint in the presence of hypertension implies increased intracranial pressure, which explains her particular description of her headache as being the "worst headache I've ever had."

6. **Is there a relationship between her facial swelling, photophobia, and her BP?**
   These are components of a pattern of signs and symptoms that usually occur with toxemia of pregnancy, sometimes known as preeclampsia/eclampsia, and more currently known as one of the types of pregnancy-induced hypertension (PIH).

7. **How would you describe Connie's ECG?**
   This rhythm has a lot of 60-cycle interference, enough so you cannot see clear P or T waves. The only identifiable waveforms are the QRS and one possible PVC (complex 10). Because the QRSs are all (with the exception of complex 10) within normal limits and have equal R to R intervals, it is fair to assume that they are supraventricular or atrial in origin.

8. **Is her cardiac rhythm responsible for any of Connie's signs or symptoms?**
   Probably not, her rhythm is a result of her condition, rather than the cause.

9. **What is Midol used for and why do you think Connie was taking it?**
   Midol is a popular OTC (over the counter) medication used for PMS (premenstrual syndrome). It contains a mild diuretic, among other things. She may have been taking it for fluid reduction for her swelling.

10. **Is there any other information, either from her history or your physical that could help you?**
    Once away from her family you could ask when her last period was so you could confirm the gestational age of the fetus. Determine the height of the fundus by how many fingerwidths below the zyphoid it lies. Assess fetal heart tones and ask about fetal movement. Does she have any vaginal bleeding? Does she have any other complaints of pain or discomfort? Have Connie explain her weight gain. Did it happen suddenly or more gradually? Sudden weight gain is more typical of toxemia.

11. **What do you think is the cause of Connie's current problem?**
    Connie sounds as if she has pregnancy-induced hypertension and is toxemic (PIH).

12. **How serious is Connie's current situation?**
    This is a life threat. She is getting ready to have a seizure.

13. *What is Connie at risk for?*

Grand mal seizures, abruptio placental, an explosive delivery, and a ruptured uterus.

14. *Connie's mother began crying and asking many questions regarding what you are doing and whether Connie will be all right. She is so agitated that she is beginning to interfere with your treatment of Connie. How would you handle Connie's mother?*

If the information regarding Connie is factual, Connie's mother just found out Connie was pregnant 2 weeks ago. If Connie kept it a secret, then Connie's mother is having to deal with that and the fact that her daughter is very ill. She obviously is having trouble coping. If possible, assign one person to Connie's mother to explain everything that is going on. Tell her what hospital you are taking Connie. Ask whether there is a neighbor, friend, or clergyman you can call to drive Connie's mother to the hospital.

15. *How would you begin treatment?*

Oxygen by a mask non-rebreather with a reservoir at 12 to 15 lpm. Start an IV of normal saline in the forearm as opposed to the wrist or antecubital space. In case of a seizure you do not want the catheter bent. Place Connie on her left side and transport without light and sirens. Get the diazepam and magnesium sulfate ready.

16. *When you take Connie's BP the second time, you note a jerking motion of her thumb and forefinger of the hand in the same arm, when you pump up the pressure in the cuff. What is the significance of this?*

This is evidence of hyperreflexia, a sign of impending seizures.

17. *How would you continue treatment, and what modifications would you make to your transport?*

According to local protocol, you might administer magnesium sulfate. Local protocols will dictate when to administrate. An initial bolus of 2 to 4 mg, slow IV push, followed by an IV drip for those with long transport times, is fairly common. If lights and sirens weren't eliminated before they should be now. Lights in the back of the rig should also be dimmed. This will cut down on sensory stimulation to prevent seizures.

18. *En route to the hospital Connie has a grand mal seizure. How would you treat her?*

Keep Connie on her left side, administer diazepam, 5 to 10 mg, slow IV push until the clinical event has ceased. Immediately suction and ventilate. Check for vaginal drainage or crowning. If she has not been given magnesium sulfate before this, give her 2 to 4 gms slow IV push now.

19. *How would you document Connie's pregnancy history in terms of gravida and para?*

Connie has no living children but has had two pregnancies, this one and one 2 years ago. Her pregnancy history would be documented as para 0, gravida 2.

OUTCOME

Connie was initially managed with oxygen by non-rebreather mask with a reservoir at 12 lpm, and an IV of normal saline was started at kvo. En route, Connie's hand reaction of twitching when the BP was taken was reported by radio. The receiving physician ordered 2 g of magnesium sulfate to be given, slow IV push. On arrival at the ED, Connie suffered a grand mal seizure when being lifted from the squad gurney to the ED stretcher. Another 4 g of magnesium sulfate and 5 mg diazepam was given sequentially with a 20 ml bolus of fluid between. Connie went into active labor and delivered twins within 15 minutes of arrival at the ED. The twins were premature and depressed. After vigorous resuscitation and administration of surfactant, the twins were placed in the neonatal ICU. Connie did well and was dismissed after 4 days. Her babies had a rocky course and were dismissed 6 weeks after delivery.

BIBLIOGRAPHY

Bledsoe, B. E. (1994). Gynecological emergencies. In B.E. Bledsoe, R. S. Porter, & B. R. Shade (Eds.). *Paramedic emergency care.* Englewood Cliffs, NJ: Brady, A Prentice Hall Divison.

Bledsoe, B. E. (1994). Obstetrical emergencies. In B.E. Bledsoe, R. S. Porter, B. R. Shade (Eds.). *Paramedic emergency care.* Englewood Cliffs, NJ: Brady, A Prentice Hall Divison.

Burke, M. E. & Medford, L. K. (1991). Hypertension in pregnancy. In C. J. Harvey (Ed.). *Critical care obstetrical nursing.* Gaithersburg, MA: Aspen Publishers.

Fontanarosa, P. B. (1997). Abdominal, genitourinary and back pain. In P. Pons & D. Cason (Eds.). *Paramedic field care: A complaint based approach.* St. Louis, MO: Mosby.

Harvey, M. G. (1991). Physiologic changes of pregnancy. In C. J. Harvey (Ed.). *Critical care obstetrical nursing.* Gaithersburg, MA: Aspen Publishers.

Pozaic, S. (1991). Hemorrhagic complications in pregnancy. In C. J. Harvey (Ed.). *Critical care obstetrical nursing.* Gaithersburg, MA: Aspen Publishers.

Mears, G. (1997). Pregnancy and childbirth. In P. Pons & D. Cason (Eds.). *Paramedic field care: A complaint based approach.* St. Louis, MO: Mosby.

Sanders, M. J. (1994). Obstetrical emergencies and neonatal resuscitation. In *Mosby's paramedic textbook.* St. Louis, MO: Mosby.

Silen, W. (Ed). (1996). *Cope's early diagnosis of the acute abdomen* (19th ed.). New York: Oxford University Press.

9

Gastrointestinal/Genitourinary Emergencies

OVERVIEW

Patients with gastrointestinal/genitourinary (GI/GU) problems can be some of the most challenging because of the lack of observable organ systems. Most patients will present with abdominal pain as their chief complaint. Understanding the physiology and pathophysiology of the organ systems and the physiology of pain helps the care provider to determine whether an immediate, potential, or low probability for a threat to life is present life.

Anatomy, Physiology, and Pathophysiology

The GI/GU system can be divided into solid and hollow organs. When irritated, both hollow and solid organs have a tendency to stretch, distend, and/or bleed. When bleeding is involved, solid organs bleed within their capsules, occasionally so much so that the capsule will rupture. Hollow organs may also bleed but usually will bleed within the organ itself resulting in blood within the substance produced, such as bloody urine, melena, or hematemesis. The color of blood in the intestinal tract depends on the amount of blood and the degree of digestion that has occurred. Generally, melena is produced when approximately 200 ml of blood is present and the blood is well digested. If blood is present in the stomach, digestive enzymes there will cause it to appear like "coffee grounds" if vomited. Vomiting usually occurs if the irritation is above the ligament of Treitz (in the duodenum). If the bleeding occurs past that ligament, diarrhea is stimulated and melena is produced.

Irritation, either from chemicals causing inflammation or inflammation related to infection, has a tendency to cause stretching of the organ capsule. Stretching tends to cause pain, usually perceived in the immediate area, especially if that area is palpated. Pain associated with solid organs tends to be dull and steady in nature, whereas the pain associated with hollow organs tends to be colicky or intermittent. All abdominal organs are covered with the peritoneum (visceral peritoneum) as is the inner wall of the abdomen (parietal peritoneum). The peritoneum is also sensitive to distention, as well as chemicals of inflammation, either related to infection, chemicals released from ruptured viscus, or normal body chemicals that have escaped their natural organ systems, such as pancreatic enzymes. Pain from peritoneal irritation tends to be sharp, well localized, and sensitive to any activity that causes movement of the peritoneum, such as coughing, deep breathing, or straightening the legs.

Radiating pain is another phenomenon of organs found in the GI/GU system. Distention of the gallbladder may be perceived as right sided subscapular pain, whereas distention of the splenic capsule may be perceived as pain in the left shoulder and neck. Pain in hollow organs may be perceived as following the path of the "tube." For example, a kidney stone may cause radiating pain to the groin, whereas the pain of an abdominal aneurysm may be perceived as low back or abdominal pain radiating to the flank (if around the renal artery) or down the legs (if extending down the iliac arteries).

Pain from extraabdominal sites may also radiate pain to the abdomen. For example, cardiac pain may cause unrelenting indigestion, and a patient in diabetic ketoacidosis may complain of abdominal pain.

There are also patients with chronic diseases involving these systems who may need assistance because of their disease process or an unrelated problem. One of the most frequent chronic diseases that involved the GU system is kidney failure with resultant dialysis. Additional problems related to dialysis include hypovolemia, hypoglycemia, anemia, and electrolyte imbalances. Chronic diseases involving the GI tract include ulcer disease, cirrhosis of the liver, Crohn's disease, and diverticulitis, as well as others.

Treatment

Because of the wide variety of causes of emergencies involving the gastrointestinal tract and genitourinary tract, the care provider makes a determination of the seriousness of the situation based on history and physical findings. Most of the probability of cause is based on an accurate, thorough history. Diagnostic tests, related to these systems are limited. A fluid challenge may be one of the most useful diagnostic tests that can be used in the field. Additional diagnostic tests include blood glucose determination and evaluation of the ECG.

Treatment of GI/GU emergencies is usually symptomatic, with the presence of an immediate or potential life threat dictating actions. The priorities of airway, breathing, and circulation do not change. Airway and breathing are supported by positioning, oxygen administration, and suctioning, if indicated. IV access and fluid administration are additional measures to be taken if assessment findings indicate they are appropriate. Pharmacologic therapy is usually not indicated unless cardiac involvement or a contributing chronic disease process is present and requires treatment. Positioning and keeping the patient warm are additional important treatment measures.

CASE 1

Dispatch: 21:00 hrs; 56 y/o male, difficulty breathing

On Arrival: You find 56 y/o Fred sitting in a recliner. He is awake and his face appears flushed. What is striking about his appearance is his abdomen, which is huge. His abdomen and arms appear to have a yellow tinge to the skin.

Initial Assessment Findings

Mental Status—Awake and alert; spontaneous eye opening; obeys command

Airway—Open and clear

Breathing—R 28 and shallow, is panting when he talks; faint audible wheezing. Lung sounds very difficult to hear; posterior lobes inaccessible, patient is unable to lean forward

Circulation—Skin pale, cool, and moist; yellow tinge to skin and sclera

   Radial pulse rapid and regular at 116

   BP 164/100

Chief Complaint—Difficulty breathing

Focused History

Events—Difficulty breathing began yesterday and has steadily been getting worse

Previous Illness—History of alcoholism with cirrhosis

Current Health Status—Last hospitalization was 2 months ago when "they drained fluid off my belly;" missed his last two appointments, the last one 3 days ago.

Allergies—Morphine, sulfa drugs

Medications—Aldactone (spironolactone), Lasix (furosemide), Slow-K (potassium supplement), folic acid, ferrous sulfate, and vitamins

Focused Physical

Current Set of VS—P 116, R 28, BP 164/100

Other Pertinent Findings—Distended veins branching from the umbilical area across upper abdomen; Fred is a very large man, about 6 ft 4 in, weighing about 230 lbs, but his legs appear very thin and wasted; pulse oximetry 82%

Diagnostic Tests—Blood sugar 82 mg/dl

ECG

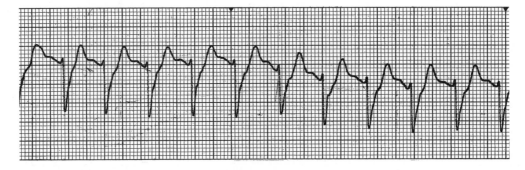

Figure 9-1

QUESTIONS

1. What is significant about Fred's history?

2. What body systems are involved?

3. What is Fred's Glasgow Coma Score?

4. What is cirrhosis, and what causes it?

5. What is the relationship between Fred's cirrhosis and the yellow tinge to his skin and sclera?

6. What is significant about Fred's cirrhosis and his "large" abdomen?

7. What is the cause of Fred's distended veins across his upper abdomen, and what does its presence imply?

8. How would you describe Fred's ECG?

9. Is there a relationship between Fred's ECG and his history of cirrhosis?

10. What is the significance of the ferrous sulfate and the folic acid?

11. Fred is complaining of difficulty breathing and his pulse oximetry is 82%. What are possible causes?

12. Is there any information, either from his history or your physical examination that might be helpful?

13. How serious is Fred's situation?

14. How would you begin treatment?

15. What is Fred at risk for?

16. How would you continue treatment?

QUESTIONS AND ANSWERS

1. What is significant about Fred's history?

Alcoholism with cirrhosis; missed last appointment; drained abdominal fluid last time in hospital; difficulty breathing since yesterday.

2. What body systems are involved?

Respiratory—R 28 with faint audible wheezes
Cardiovascular—tachycardia; pale, cool, moist skin, BP 164/100
GI/GU—yellow color to skin and sclera

3. What is Fred's Glasgow Coma Score?

GCS 15 (4 spontaneous eye opening, 6 motor response, 5 verbal response)

4. What is cirrhosis, and what causes it?

A condition where injury has occurred to the liver and normal repair processes (affected by the extent of injury, the presence of continuing damage, and the liver's reaction to these agents) distort large areas of the liver through scarring and extensive bands of fibrous tissue. The liver eventually becomes nodular, normal liver function is disrupted, and blood flow becomes obstructed. When blood flow becomes obstructed, pressure backs up in the portion of the venous system (portal vein) that drains the liver.

The causes of cirrhosis include infection (such as hepatitis B and hepatitis C), toxins (such as alcohol), altered immune response, biliary obstruction, and vascular disturbance. In the United States, most cases are secondary to alcohol abuse.

5. What is the relationship between Fred's cirrhosis and the yellow tinge to his skin and sclera?

When the scar tissue, liver nodules, and bands of fibrous tissue obstruct bile flow, bile salts build up in the blood. They are eventually deposited in the skin and sclera. This causes jaundice and pruritus. One of the causes of cirrhosis is hepatitis. Both hepatitis B and advanced cirrhosis cause jaundice. The assumption here is that Fred has cirrhosis only from alcoholism. Do not make that assumption. Body substance isolation precautions are especially in order.

6. What is significant about Fred's cirrhosis and his "large" abdomen?

Eventually the process of cirrhosis will cause such a back-up of blood in the portal system that vascular pressure increases to the point where fluid is forced from the vascular space to the surface of the liver. Fluid then literally drips into the peritoneal space, accumulates, and eventually distends the abdomen.

7. What is the cause of Fred's distended veins across his upper abdomen, and what does its presence imply?

Because of the presence of increased portal vein pressure, vessels close to the surface of the abdomen also enlarge and protrude (abdominal varices). The typical pattern is a branching from the umbilicus up toward the sternum and ribs. The medical term for them is caput medusae. The presence of these varices implies that Fred also has varices in his esophagus (esophageal varices).

8. How would you describe Fred's ECG?

Sinus tachycardia with a wide QRS (possible bundle branch block) and is suspicious for an elevated S-T segment.

9. Is there a relationship between Fred's ECG and his history of cirrhosis?

Normally, cirrhosis does not affect the heart or the cardiac conduction system. However, Fred is an admitted alcoholic. It is possible that cardiac myopathy has occurred because of factors other than cirrhosis.

10. What is the significance of the ferrous sulfate and folic acid?

Ferrous sulfate is an iron compound frequently used for patients who have iron deficiency anemia. Folic acid is indicated in the treatment of macrocytic anemia associated with alcoholism. The significance is the indication that Fred is anemic.

11. Fred is complaining of difficulty breathing and his pulse oximetry is 82%. What are possible causes?

Causes include an inability to fully ventilate. With a severely distended abdomen, the diaphragm is unable to fully contract, leading to an impaired tidal volume and reduced arterial O_2 saturation. Resulting intrapulmonary shunting and ventilation-perfusion mismatch along with a reduction in O_2 diffusing capacity are all highly likely.

Another cause for difficulty breathing and low pulse oximetry could be related to his cardiac status. Fred has a suspicious ECG in Lead II for a bundle branch block and elevated S-T segment. There could be some congestive failure involved.

It is also possible that his hypoxemia has contributed to his cardiac condition, thus leading to a cyclic pattern of symptoms.

Because the liver is involved in cirrhosis and because of the medications (ferrous sulfate and folic acid) it is fair to assume that Fred has anemia. Anemia may also contribute to his difficulty breathing, may precipitate congestive failure and could lead to an inaccurate reading for the pulse oximetry.

12. Is there any information, either from his history or your physical examination that might be helpful?

Ask about any other complaints such as chest pain, pressure, or discomfort. Ask if this has happened before, that is, before his last hospitalization. Does he have any other problems? Has he ever been told that he had a heart problem? How does Fred sleep in the recliner?

13. How serious is Fred's situation?

Fred is hypoxic; this is serious.

14. How would you begin treatment?

Place Fred in as much of an upright position as possible to help him breathe. Use a mask non-rebreather with reservoir at 10 to 15 lpm and start an IV crystalloid, kvo or saline lock, and reassess respirations/respiratory status.

15. What is Fred at risk for?

Progressive respiratory distress, developing an acute MI, or bleeding from his esophageal varices. Because the liver is involved, Fred probably also has an increased tendency for bleeding anyway.

16. How would you continue treatment?

For most transport times further treatment would probably be unnecessary. Use of a bronchodilator might be tried if respiratory status does not change. A bronchodilator with relatively little cardiac effect, such as metaproterenol, would be the most desirable.

OUTCOME

En route to the hospital, Fred's pulse oximetry improved to 92% with the mask non-rebreather and reservoir at 15 lpm. On arrival at the ED a chest x-ray was taken. After the x-ray was read an IV of albumin was begun and an abdominal paracentesis was performed, which, over a period of time, drained approximately 4500 ml of fluid. Fred also was anemic with a hemoglobin of 8 and a hematocrit of 32. After the peritoneal tap and albumin infusion, his O_2 sats improved to 96% on a mask non-rebreather. Fred was admitted to the hospital. Two days later he developed an esophageal bleed and expired 7 days after admission.

CASE 2

Dispatch: 18:30 hrs; 54 y/o male, abdominal pain

On Arrival: You find 54 y/o Juan, lying on his side in the fetal position, on the living room couch. He appears pale and is awake. As you enter the room he is vomiting.

Initial Assessment Findings

Mental Status—Alert, oriented, and anxious; obeys command
Airway—Open and able to clear on his own
Breathing—R 32 and shallow; lung sounds clear bilaterally
Circulation—Skin pale, cool, and dry
　　　　　　　Radial pulse regular at 100
　　　　　　　BP 106/70
Chief Complaint—Abdominal pain

Focused History

Events—Abdominal pain began suddenly after eating dinner (lamb and pasta); is constant, and described as "a knife in the pit of my stomach." The pain radiates to his back, ranks as a 9 on a scale of 1 to 10, lying in the fetal position lessens the pain, and coughing or moving makes the pain worse.
Previous Illness—Ulcers 12 years ago that required surgery
Current Health Status—Good, but has been under a lot of stress at work
Allergies—None
Medications—None prescribed, wife states he "drinks Maalox like water and takes Pepcid (famotidine) and Tagamet (cimetidine) like candy." (Pepcid and Tagamet are now available OTC.)

Focused Physical

Current Set of VS—P 100, R 32, BP 106/70
Other Pertinent Findings—Vomitus is approximately 300 ml undigested food; abdomen is firm, distended, and tender to palpation, particularly in the epigastric area; pulse oximetry is 98% on room air; note a porch full of empty beer cans, wife states he drinks one to two 6-packs every weekend; denies black, tarry diarrhea.
Diagnostic Tests—None done

ECG

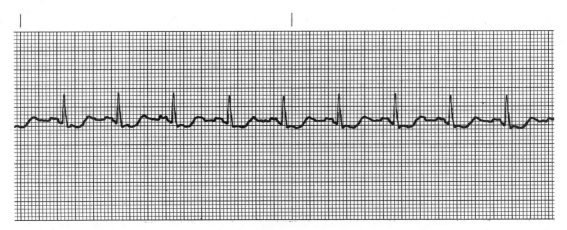

Figure 9-2

QUESTIONS

1. What is significant about Juan's history?

2. What body systems are affected?

3. What is the significance of the wife's description of Juan's drinking "Maalox like water and takes Pepcid and Tagamet like candy?"

4. Is the comment regarding his alcohol ingestion relevant to his current problem?

5. What is the significance of a respiratory rate of 32 and shallow respirations in a person with abdominal pain?

6. What is the relationship between his heart rate and blood pressure?

7. What can cause an elevated heart rate in a patient with abdominal pain?

8. Is there a relationship between Juan's skin color, temperature, and moisture and his VS?

9. How would you describe Juan's ECG?

10. Is there any other information, either from his history or your physical examination, that might help?

11. What do you think is probably causing Juan's current problem?

12. What is Juan at risk for developing?

13. How severe is Juan's problem?

14. How would you begin treatment?

15. What would you include in your full treatment?

16. What is the significance of a patient complaining of abdominal pain and lying in the fetal position?

17. Can you tell the difference between a perforated ulcer, pancreatitis, and severe gallbladder attack in the field?

18. If Juan has a GI bleed caused by an ulcer, wouldn't he have blood in his vomit?

19. What is the pathophysiology of pancreatitis?

QUESTIONS AND ANSWERS

1. What is significant about Juan's history?

Juan's pain began after eating, is constant, and described as knifelike with radiation to his back; has been taking OTC meds, Maalox, Pepcid, and Tagamet; history of steady alcohol ingestion; stress at work; previous history of ulcers.

2. What body systems are affected?

Respiratory—R of 32 and shallow
Cardiovascular—pulse of 100 and BP 106/70; skin pale, cool, and dry
GI—vomiting, abdomen firm, distended, and tender to palpation

3. What is the significance of the wife's description of Juan's drinking "Maalox like water and takes Pepcid and Tagamet like candy?"

These meds are common OTC antacids taken for indigestion, heartburn, and gas. The description of taking them so frequently is especially significant because it implies that his indigestion or heartburn was not relieved, severe, or both.

4. Is the comment regarding his alcohol ingestion relevant to his current problem?

There is a high probability that it is. Alcohol is a gastric irritant, leading to gastritis, ulcer formation, pancreatitis, cirrhosis, and a host of other problems. It is definitely worth documenting and relaying to the receiving hospital.

5. What is the significance of a respiratory rate of 32 and shallow respirations in a person with abdominal pain?

When this occurs, suspect peritoneal irritation. The peritoneum lies just under the diaphragm. When the peritoneum is irritated, any movement by the diaphragm may be perceived as pain. When normal tidal volume causes increased abdominal pain (resulting from movement of the diaphragm), respirations become shallow to decrease the pain. When shallow respirations result in decreased tidal volume, the body compensates by increasing the rate. Thus shallow respirations at a rate of 32 are a logical result.

6. What is the relationship between his heart rate and blood pressure?

The blood pressure is a very rough gauge of cardiac output. Cardiac output is determined by stroke volume (the amount of blood reaching the left ventricle) and heart rate ($CO = SV \times HR$). When stroke volume is normal, an increase in heart rate will increase cardiac output, thus increasing blood pressure. If Juan's stroke volume is normal, a heart rate of 100 should result in a systolic pressure higher than 106.

7. What can cause an elevated heart rate in a patient with abdominal pain?

Fluid loss, anxiety, or pain.

8. Is there a relationship between Juan's skin color, temperature, and moisture and his VS?

Pale, cool, dry skin implies peripheral vasoconstriction. In the presence of a heart rate of 100, a systolic pressure of 106, and abdominal pain, the relationship is most likely one of a sympathetic response to fluid or blood loss.

9. How would you describe Juan's ECG?

Sinus rhythm.

10. Is there any other information, from either his history or your physical examination that might help?

Has he seen a physician for his indigestion/heartburn? When was the last time he saw his physician? Has he been vomiting? If so, how frequently and what did it look like? Is this episode like the last time he had an ulcer?

11. ***What do you think is probably causing Juan's current problem?***

Severe gastritis or a perforated ulcer are both consistent with his complaints and physical assessment. Pancreatitis is another possibility because of the description and type of radiating pain. Pancreatitis is also common with a history of chronic alcohol use. Both a perforated ulcer and pancreatitis can cause peritoneal irritation and shock.

A gallbladder attack is another possibility as is an acute MI. Both a gallstone and an MI can mimic each other. Juan has a history of chronic indigestion and, in this case, an onset of pain after eating that is typical of both problems, especially an MI. The things that don't quite fit include the current distinct complaint of abdominal pain, not indigestion and the signs of peritoneal irritation (lying in the fetal position, steady pain, rapid shallow respirations).

An aortic aneurysm is also a possibility, though the history of indigestion is not commonly associated with a dissecting aneurysm.

12. ***What is Juan at risk for developing?***

Progressive shock. The sudden onset abdominal pain that results in a distended, tender abdomen; pale, cool skin; and increased heart rate in the presence of a systolic BP that is lower than expected all indicate a high probability for an internal bleed or third spacing of body fluid.

If Juan is a chronic alcohol user, portal hypertension may also be a problem and esophageal varicosities may be present. Esophageal varicosities may rupture with the trauma of vomiting. Juan is at risk for a GI bleed if he doesn't already have one.

13. ***How severe is Juan's problem?***

This is a severe problem because of the combination of history and physical signs and symptoms. Juan has signs of peritoneal irritation, and his physical assessment is suspicious for compensated shock.

14. ***How would you begin treatment?***

Keep Juan on his side for comfort. Begin oxygen per a mask non-rebreather and reservoir at 15 lpm and start an IV of normal saline kvo.

15. ***What would you include in your full treatment?***

Consider administering a fluid bolus and reevaluating lung sounds and blood pressure. If his systolic pressure increases, his heart rate decreases, and his lung sounds stay clear, a fluid deficit may be assumed.

16. ***What is the significance of a patient, complaining of abdominal pain, lying in the fetal position?***

The significance of that position is the suspicion of peritoneal irritation. In the fetal position the peritoneum is relaxed. If the patient is forced to lie on his back or with his legs straight when the peritoneum is irritated, those positions will stretch the peritoneum, causing pain. The patient will assume the position of least pain, thus lying in the fetal position and not moving.

17. ***Can you tell the difference between a perforated ulcer, pancreatitis, and severe gallbladder attack in the field?***

A severe gallbladder attack is not usually associated with a lower blood pressure although it can cause tachycardia and severe pain. Neither is it usually associated with signs of peritoneal irritation, although in severe attacks it can happen.

A perforated ulcer and pancreatitis have many similar symptoms, including peritoneal irritation. If a perforated ulcer results in a GI bleed with vomiting or melena then what is important is to recognize the GI bleed. Otherwise you may not be able to tell the difference. But correct treatment does not depend on your being able to do so. What is most important is to recognize the presence of compensated shock and to choose correct treatment to support body systems.

18. ***If Juan has a GI bleed caused by an ulcer, wouldn't he have blood in his vomit?***

Not necessarily, not all ulcers result in extensive bleeding. Usually only those that perforate a blood vessel will result in enough blood to stimulate vomiting. If there is extensive bleeding but the blood collects beyond the Treitz ligament, then melena will occur.

19. What is the pathophysiology of pancreatitis?

Pancreatitis is an inflammation of the pancreas. Over 80% of cases are caused by either an obstruction causing pooling of pancreatic juices within the pancreas or by chronic alcohol use, which causes the protein of pancreatic enzymes to precipitate randomly within small pancreatic ductules. Either way, digestive enzymes within pancreatic juice become activated, digesting the tissues of the pancreas itself. Edema, tissue necrosis, and/or hemorrhage are the result. In most cases the inflammatory response is limited to the pancreas itself; however, that is not always the case. Because the pancreas lies in both the retroperitoneal space and the anterior peritoneal space, pancreatic exudate containing toxins and activated enzymes can permeate both cavities, inducing a chemical burn, increasing blood vessel permeability resulting in third spacing, and autodigesting surrounding tissues. Pain is usually severe, steady, and boring in quality, radiating through to the back. This description of pain is very similar to the description of pain with a perforated ulcer.

OUTCOME

Oxygen by mask non-rebreather with reservoir at 15 lpm was started as was an IV normal saline at 100 ml/hr. A second set of VS showed: P 106, R 36, and BP 98/66. A bolus of 500 ml normal saline was infused with no change in respiratory status, VS were P 90, R 30, BP 110/78. On arrival at the ED Juan had a second IV started, lab work and x-rays done, and was admitted to the ICU with a diagnosis of acute pancreatitis with peritonitis. Three hours later he was taken to surgery for evacuation of pancreatic cysts and necrotic tissue. He developed adult respiratory distress syndrome and cardiac failure. Juan died 7 days later.

CASE 3

Dispatch: 14:00 hrs; 67 y/o male, abdominal pain

On Arrival: You find 67 y/o Marcos, lying supine across a bare mattress. He is awake, appears pale, is moaning and stating ". . . do something, I'm dying, it hurts so bad . . ."

Initial Assessment Findings

Mental Status—Awake, alert, and anxious; obeys command
Airway—Open and clear
Breathing—R 26, talking in complete sentences; lung sounds clear in all lobes
Circulation—Skin pale, cool, and diaphoretic
        Radial pulse weak at 76
        BP hard to hear at 70/42
Chief Complaint—Abdominal pain

Focused History

Events—Marcos woke up this morning not feeling well with a vague low backache that increased in its intensity throughout the day, spreading to the abdomen, until he couldn't stand it any more and called EMS. He describes the pain as constant, sharp, "killing" his back, and "boring" through his abdomen. He ranks it as a 10 on a scale of 1 to 10. There is nothing that makes it better, moving makes it worse.
Previous Illness—Hypertension and ventricular irritability
Current Health Status—Did not feel well this morning
Allergies—None known
Medications—Tenormin (atenolol), Tonocard (tocainide hydrochloride)

Focused Physical

Current Set of VS—P 76, R 26, BP 70/42
Other Pertinent Findings—Marcos is 6'6'', 300 lbs; his abdomen is distended and mottled, tender to palpation with no masses; legs are pale with no pedal pulses
Diagnostic Tests—BS 156, fluid challenge of 500 ml had no change in BP or lung sounds

ECG

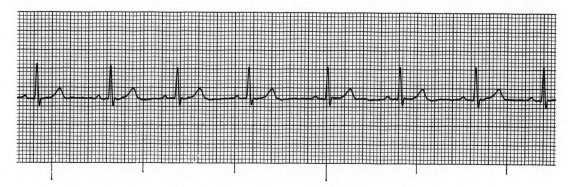

Figure 9-3

QUESTIONS

1. What is significant about Marcos' history?

2. What body systems are affected?

3. What is significant about Marcos' description of his pain?

4. What is tocainide hydrochloride?

5. What is atenolol?

6. It is unusual to find a low BP with a normal pulse rate. What might be the cause?

7. What is the significance of his mottled abdomen?

8. What is the most likely cause of his mottled abdomen?

9. How would you describe Marcos' ECG?

10. Is there any other information, either from his history or your physical examination that might help?

11. What do you think is probably causing Marcos' current problem?

12. How serious is Marcos' problem?

13. What is Marcos at risk for developing?

14. How would you begin treatment?

15. When Marcos' abdomen was palpated, no masses were felt. Is that what you might expect to find?

16. Recommendations for fluid replacement in cases of internal bleeding often have limits put on the amount of fluid to give in the field. What is the reasoning behind this?

17. A fluid challenge of 500 ml in this patient did not appear to make any difference. What is/are the most likely reason(s) for that?

QUESTIONS AND ANSWERS

1. What is significant about Marcos' history?

Marcos has a history of hypertension and ventricular irritability, did not feel well when he got up, pain has steadily increased all day, duration approximately 7 to 8 hours, description of pain (location, character, radiation)

2. What body systems are affected?

Respiratory rate 26

Cardiovascular—"normal" heart rate in presence of hypotension; skin pale, cool, and diaphoretic; mottled abdomen

3. What is significant about Marcos' description of his pain?

His pain started as vague low back pain that spread to his abdomen, now describing it as "sharp," constant, and radiating through to abdomen. Vague pain in one body region that then becomes sharp, constant, and more localized is typical of visceral pain that has become somatic or parietal. Somatic or parietal pain is indicative of peritoneal or diaphragmatic irritation. The pattern of radiation is typical of an aneurysm.

4. What is tocainide hydrochloride?

Tocainide is similar to lidocaine, is taken orally, and is effective in treating ventricular dysrhythmias. However, tocainide has some serious side effects involving pulmonary edema, blood disorders, and blood clots. Its presence implies that the patient has had ventricular dysrhythmias.

5. What is atenolol?

Atenolol is a beta$_1$-selective antagonist that is devoid of intrinsic sympathomimetic activity. More simply put, atenolol is a beta-blocker, selective for the heart that prevents an increase in heart rate and decreases inotropic heart action thereby decreasing oxygen demand. All of these are effects that commonly occur with sympathetic stimulation. Beta blockers, in this case atenolol, are commonly used to control hypertension and angina. Its significance is with the history of hypertension.

6. It is unusual to find a low BP with a normal pulse rate. What might be the cause?

Marcos is definitely hypotensive. Normally his sympathetic response would be evident. However, atenolol is a beta blocker that prevents normal response to sympathetic stimulation. Thus atenolol may be a cause for his slow heart rate and/or hypotension. However, in most people a sufficient sympathetic response will eventually over-ride the effects of normal doses of beta blockers. The question is how much of a sympathetic response will it take?

It is also possible that Marcos has a slower rate normally. In such cases, a rate of 80 might be significantly elevated from a normal rate of perhaps 60.

7. What is the significance of his mottled abdomen?

Mottled skin in an adult is an indication of stasis of blood. Stasis of blood in an extremity usually indicates peripheral capillary bed shut down. In this case, a mottled abdomen may indicate peripheral shut down to the abdominal wall.

8. What is the most likely cause of his mottled abdomen?

There are probably two mechanisms working here. First, Marcos has hypotension and pale, cool, diaphoretic skin, which is consistent with peripheral vasoconstriction. Because he is taking a beta blocker that is specific for beta$_1$ receptors, peripheral vasoconstriction (under alpha receptor control) still occurs but the corresponding increase in heart rate and contractility may be compromised. Because normal compensatory mechanisms are incomplete, even more sympathetic stimulation occurs leading to further increase in vasoconstriction. Severe peripheral vasoconstriction leads to peripheral capillary bed shut down with stasis of blood in those capillary beds.

The second likely cause is the underlying pathology of his abdominal pain. The abdominal aorta has arterial roots that branch off and supply the peripheral abdominal wall. When circulation through the part of the aorta that contains those arterial roots is impaired, perfusion through those arterial roots is also impaired, leading to tissue hypoxia, venous stasis, and mottled skin.

9. How would you describe Marcos' ECG?

Sinus rhythm with no ectopy.

10. **Is there any other information, either from his history or your physical examination that might help?**

    Does he take his medication regularly? Did he take it today? How much did he take? Are his stools normal?

11. **What do you think is probably causing Marcos' current problem?**

    His pattern and description of pain is fairly typical of an abdominal aortic aneurysm.

    Other possibilities include diverticulitis where a diverticulum has ruptured. This frequently leads to blood in the stool. Although that might not be obvious in the field, questions regarding presence of blood, and/or melena are important to ask.

12. **How serious is Marcos' problem?**

    This is very serious and a potential life threat. His pattern of pain, even if his problem is not an aneurysm, is indicative of a surgical abdomen (duration of time, increasing severity of pain, pattern of visceral characteristics to somatic characteristics).

13. **What is Marcos at risk for developing?**

    Profound shock (ruptured aneurysm and exsanguination) and/or ventricular dysrhythmias.

14. **How would you begin treatment?**

    Oxygen by non-rebreather mask and reservoir at 10 to 15 lpm; IV normal saline at tko status, and transport rapidly.

15. **When Marcos' abdomen was palpated, no masses were felt. Is that what you might expect to find?**

    Marcos is such a big man that to feel a pulsating mass, with such a low BP, would probably be difficult.

16. **Recommendations for fluid replacement in cases of internal bleeding often have limits put on the amount of fluid to give in the field. What is the reasoning behind this?**

    Replacing large amounts of blood with crystalloid such as normal saline or lactated Ringer's does not replace the oxygen carrying power or clotting ability of whole blood. The goal is to supplement existing whole blood with enough volume to maintain perfusion but at a pressure that does not destroy existing clots. Perfusion to the brain, in a normal adult, lying supine, is approximately 60 to 70 mmHg. Research studies have suggested that field providers should be administering fluids only enough to maintain a pressure of around 90 to 100 systolic or, if the patient is alert and oriented, to maintain a pressure of 80 systolic. However, research is based on trauma patients and the decision is up to your local medical director.

17. **A fluid challenge of 500 ml in this patient did not appear to make any difference. What is/are the most likely reason(s) for that?**

    There might be two reasons. First, it could be that the amount of blood that he has already lost is significantly more than 500 ml, and therefore the amount is much too small. Second, this is a big man. His body mass is such that his total blood volume could easily be double that of the "normal" 70 kg man (Marcos weighs 136 kg). Either way, 500 ml was probably not enough to make much of a difference.

OUTCOME

Marcos was given repeated fluid challenges to a maximum of 1500 ml of normal saline before arrival. On arrival VS were: P 74, R 24, BP 76/54. An abdominal film showed a large 8 cm fusiform aneurysm and he was taken immediately to the OR. A 10 cm length of his aorta was repaired and 3 liters of blood removed from his retroperitoneal space. Three days post-op Marcos developed delirium tremens. He was managed with lorazepam, Librium, and thiamine supplements. Recovery was rocky with a bout of ARDS and renal failure. Five weeks from admission Marcos was dismissed to home.

CASE 4

Dispatch: 21:30 hrs; 46 y/o male, vomiting blood

On Arrival: You find 46 y/o Tom lying supine on the floor in his living room. He is awake and appears pale. His wife is present.

Initial Assessment Findings

Mental Status—Alert but confused, follows command with spontaneous eye opening
Airway—Open and clear, blood present on tongue
Breathing—R regular at 22, talking in complete sentences; lung sounds clear in all lobes
Circulation—Skin extremely pale, cold, and dry
       Radial pulse weak at 88
       BP 106/76
Chief Complaint—Vomited blood

Focused History

Events—Was watching TV when felt nauseated, got up, and vomited in bathroom, then became dizzy and slumped to the floor, wife then called EMS.
Previous Illness—History of ulcers and high blood pressure
Current Health Status—Has had intermittent abdominal pain for last several days, described as "crampy" indigestion, did not feel well this morning, described as "achy" with no appetite
Allergies—None known
Medications—Vasotec (enalapril)

Focused Physical

Current Set of VS—P 88, R 22, BP 106/76
Other Pertinent Findings—Generalized abdominal tenderness to palpation, especially in epigastric region; pulse oximetry reads 98% on room air; no cuts noted in mouth; bright red blood obvious on tongue; denies melena; no other obvious abnormalities noted
Diagnostic Tests—Orthostatic change noted when put in sitting position, became diaphoretic, complained of dizziness, systolic BP 82, radial pulse disappeared

ECG

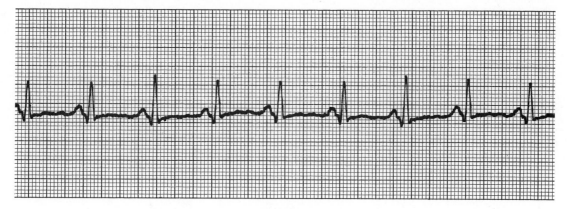

Figure 9-4

QUESTIONS

1. What is significant about Tom's history?

2. What body systems are affected?

3. What is Tom's Glasgow Coma Score?

4. How would you describe Tom's ECG?

5. What is the significance of dizziness after vomiting?

6. What is the significance of his pale, cool, dry skin?

7. Why was Tom's initial pulse rate not any higher?

8. Tom is confused; what is/are the likely causes?

9. What does intermittent abdominal pain described as "crampy" indigestion most likely indicate?

10. What is enalapril, and how does it work?

11. Is there any special significance regarding Tom's being on enalapril?

12. Is there a relationship between enalapril and Tom's signs and symptoms?

13. Is there any other information from either Tom's history or your physical examination that might help you?

14. What is the significance of the orthostatic change noted when Tom was put in the sitting position?

15. What do you think is causing Tom's current problem?

16. How would you begin treatment?

17. If Tom's second set of VS was P 120, R 26, BP 78/56, how would your treatment change?

18. If Tom had peritonitis, how would his signs and symptoms change?

19. Tom vomited blood; is it possible that he has not had melena?

QUESTIONS AND ANSWERS

1. What is significant about Tom's history?

Dizziness after vomiting; history of abdominal pain with indigestion for several days; hypertension; history of ulcers

2. What body systems are affected?

Cardiovascular—pale, cold skin; BP and pulse appear normal while supine
CNS—confused

3. What is Tom's Glasgow Coma Score?

GCS 14 (4 eye opening, spontaneous; 6 motor response, follows command; 4 verbal response, confused)

4. How would you describe Tom's ECG?

Sinus rhythm without ectopy.

5. What is the significance of dizziness after vomiting?

The act of vomiting results from pressure on the duodenum, proximal jejunum, and stomach against a tensed diaphragm. Because most of the force comes from a powerful expiratory movement that elevates intraabdominal pressures, carotid artery bodies in the neck are also affected. Stimulation of those areas often triggers bradycardia that can drop blood pressure and cause dizziness and confusion among other things.

6. What is the significance of his pale, cool, dry skin?

Pale skin is usually a result of peripheral vasoconstriction. This seems to be supported by the fact that his skin is cool. Skin usually is cool due to shunting of body heat that occurs with vasoconstriction. Dry skin in the presence of vasoconstriction may be caused by several mechanisms. There may be something interfering with the body's ability to sweat (e.g., medication), or the person was cold and vasoconstriction was to prevent loss of body heat, or the condition causing the vasoconstriction occurred relatively slowly. In this case it is reasonable to assume that the condition occurred relatively slowly, over a period of days.

7. Why was Tom's initial pulse rate not any higher?

There may be several reasons. Remember, patients do not read the textbook and do things their own way. However, there is a reason for everything the body does and in this case several are possible. Consider that Tom's resting pulse rate may be lower, around 60 to 65. If so, a rate of 88 is 20-plus beats per minute greater than usual. Another reason that is more common concerns the disease process and his position. This problem is not sudden. With a slow onset the body has had time to compensate. Combine that with lying supine and his heart rate would probably remain within normal limits.

8. Tom is confused; what is/are the likely causes?

Confusion in a 46 y/o is not normal. The most common causes are hypoxia and hypoxemia with lack of perfusion to the brain. Even though his initial VS are within normal limits, peripheral vasoconstriction indicates altered perfusion is present.

9. What does intermittent abdominal pain described as "crampy" indigestion most likely indicate?

Intermittent abdominal pain with a description of colic or cramping is more frequent with hollow organ irritation. Indigestion is more indicative of stomach irritation.

10. What is enalapril, and how does it work?

Enalapril is an ACE inhibitor. ACE inhibitors inhibit angiotensin converting enzyme from converting angiotensin I into angiotensin II, a powerful vasoconstrictor. It also prevents aldosterone (conserves sodium and thus water) from being formed.

11. Is there any special significance regarding Tom's being on enalapril?

Yes, since it is an ACE inhibitor and limits aldosterone production, his normal body compensatory mechanisms for loss of blood and body fluids are compromised.

12. *Is there a relationship between enalapril and Tom's signs and symptoms?*

The relationship is most likely with his blood pressure. Because enalapril interferes with two of the body's normal compensatory mechanisms to support blood pressure (cannot convert angiotensin I to angiotensin II and interferes with sodium and water retention in the kidney), the resulting reduction in preload and reduction in afterload is seen as low BP. Because enalapril does not interfere with alpha stimulation to vasoconstrict, Tom is pale and cool. However, without the addition of angiotensin II and conservation of sodium and water, Tom is worse than he would be otherwise.

13. *Is there any other information from either Tom's history or your physical examination that might help you?*

Send someone to check the bathroom. If there is blood on the floor it might give an idea of how much was lost. However, blood in the toilet is misleading in amount. Has he had melena or black, tarry stools? How many times has he vomited, and what did it look like? How long ago did he have ulcer problems? What was done for them? Has he continued to take his meds?

14. *What is the significance of the orthostatic change noted when Tom was put in the sitting position?*

This change of lowered systolic BP, disappearing radial pulse, and complaint of dizziness suggests the presence of internal bleeding or fluid loss and is diagnostic for hypovolemia, regardless of the cause.

15. *What do you think is causing Tom's current problem?*

Tom most likely has a GI bleed. The presence of orthostatic changes together with his abdominal pain, indigestion, and history of ulcers suggests a bleeding ulcer. However, the presence of an acute myocardial infarction must also be considered.

This collection of signs and symptoms could just as easily be caused by an MI with cardiogenic shock, especially with a heart rate that is within normal limits. The significant difference here is the presence of vomiting blood. If cardiogenic shock were a factor, look for the presence of pulmonary edema with further fluid boluses.

Another equally understandable cause could be peritonitis with a perforated ulcer. The thing to watch for here is a rigid, boardlike abdomen with signs of peritoneal irritation.

16. *How would you begin treatment?*

High flow oxygen with a mask non-rebreather at 15 lpm and IV of crystalloid, either normal saline or lactated Ringer's with a fluid bolus of 300 to 500 ml and reassess lung sounds.

17. *If Tom's second set of VS was P 120, R 26, BP 78/56, how would your treatment change?*

Repeat fluid boluses of 300 to 500 ml with reassessment of blood pressure and respiratory status would be the field treatment of choice. The goal would be to attain a systolic BP of 90 to 100 mm Hg.

18. *If Tom had peritonitis, how would his signs and symptoms change?*

Peritoneal irritation tends to be a steady, severe pain that increases in intensity as time goes on. The pain usually begins as a localized pain that then becomes generalized as the entire peritoneal membrane is effected.

Other signs of peritoneal irritation are seen with body position and movement. A side-lying position with knees drawn up, otherwise known as the fetal position, lessens tension on the peritoneum and reduces pain. Actions or movement that stretch the peritoneum are avoided, such as coughing, deep breathing, extending legs, and so on.

19. Tom vomited blood, is it possible that he has not had melena?

Yes, although it usually depends on the amount of blood present. There is a ligament known as the ligament of Treitz that is distal to the duodenum that is a landmark of sorts for what gets vomited and what is eliminated through the bowel. Free blood within the GI tract is highly irritating to the mucous membranes. If the irritation occurs above the ligament of Treitz then the substance will probably be vomited. On the other hand, if the irritation occurs past the ligament of Treitz then the irritating substance will be eliminated through the bowel. Depending on the amount of blood and its location, vomiting will probably not eliminate all the blood present and some will be eliminated as melena. In this case either the melena was not noticed or there hasn't been time for a noticeable amount to appear. It takes about 200 ml of blood in the GI tract for melena to be noticed.

OUTCOME

After the orthostatic changes, Tom's VS were: P 120, R 26, BP 78/56. Fluid boluses of normal saline were repeated to a total of 1 L. On arrival at the local ED admission BP was 92/78. An NG tube was inserted, a Foley and a second IV started. Lab was drawn and an H/H was 8/28. A sudden episode of involuntary and uncontrollable melena triggered a precipitous drop in systolic pressure. After two units of packed cells and another liter of normal saline, his VS continued to be unstable. After his fourth unit of packed RBCs he was transferred to surgery. Tom had a perforated duodenal ulcer that ruptured through a portion of the gastric artery. He suffered peritonitis after surgery but eventually recovered and was dismissed to home.

CASE 5

Dispatch: 18:30 hrs; 64 y/o female, diabetic, syncopal episode

On Arrival: You find 64 y/o Juanita supine on the living room floor. She appears pale, is awake, and her husband is with her.

Initial Assessment Findings

Mental Status—Awake, alert and oriented; obeys command

Airway—Open and clear

Breathing—R 18, talking in complete sentences but seems to be out of breath; lung sounds clear in all lobes

Circulation—Skin pale, cool, and dry

Radial pulse slightly irregular at 74

BP 100/56

Chief Complaint—"Light-headed" when getting up

Focused History

Events—Had dialysis treatment this morning, normal events for dialysis, felt okay remainder of day but this evening when she stood up from couch felt "light-headed" and "almost blacked out"

Previous Illness—Insulin-dependent diabetic; hypertension; has been on hemodialysis for kidney failure for 2 years

Current Health Status—Chronic weakness, but relatively good

Allergies—None known

Medications—Regular and ultra lente insulin, timolol, EPO (erythropoietin), Feosol (ferrous sulfate), and a vitamin/mineral supplement

Focused Physical

Current Set of VS—P 74, R 18, BP 100/56

Other Pertinent Findings—Mucous membranes pale; dialysis fistula site in left forearm; pulse oximetry reads "ERROR"; abdomen nontender; states black stools are caused by iron supplement, denies any recent change; denies vomiting; denies any pain; no other abnormal findings

Diagnostic Tests—Blood sugar 112; orthostatic change when put into sitting position, radial pulse disappeared, patient lost consciousness, systolic BP 60; she was immediately placed supine with legs elevated and consciousness returned

ECG

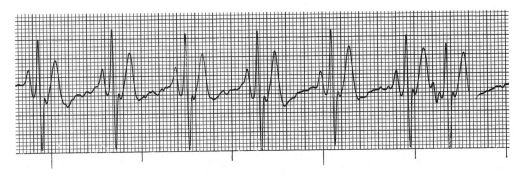

Figure 9-5

QUESTIONS

1. What is significant about Juanita's history?

2. What body systems are affected?

3. What is Juanita's Glasgow Coma Score?

4. How would you describe Juanita's ECG?

5. What changes in your actions does the presence of a hemodialysis site require, and why?

6. What is the significance of Juanita's becoming out of breath when talking, and what treatment is indicated?

7. What is the term for becoming hypotensive when going from a sitting to a standing position?

8. What is the significance of Juanita becoming hypotensive when going from a sitting to a standing position?

9. Is there a relationship between Juanita's becoming out of breath when talking and her change in BP when moving to a sitting position?

10. What are possible side effects of long-term kidney failure/hemodialysis?

11. What are possible short-term side effects (those that occur during or immediately after) hemodialysis?

12. Which of the short- or long-term side effects is/are most likely present now?

13. Juanita is an insulin-dependent diabetic. What types of medical conditions, more typical of diabetics, could explain Juanita's syncopal episode with orthostatic hypotension?

14. What is timolol, and how does it work?

15. How is the history of timolol relevant to Juanita's assessment findings?

16. What do you think is causing Juanita's current problem, and why?

17. After 5 minutes in the supine position, Juanita was alert and oriented, still with no complaints of pain or discomfort. Another set of VS showed P 70, R 22, BP 96/60. How serious is Juanita's problem?

18. Is Juanita's problem serious enough to warrant using her fistula as an IV site?

19. How would you begin treatment?

20. If you gave a fluid bolus, how much would you give and why?

21. What is Juanita at risk for?

22. How would you assess for that/those risk factors?

QUESTIONS AND ANSWERS

1. ***What is significant about Juanita's history?***

   Insulin-dependent diabetic; on hemodialysis; hypertension; on timolol and Feosol; chronic weakness; became light-headed after standing from a sitting position

2. ***What body systems are affected?***

   Respiratory—seems out of breath after talking
   Cardiovascular—pale, cool skin; radial pulse low end of normal; BP low end of normal

3. ***What is Juanita's Glasgow Coma Score?***

   Her initial GCS was 15 (spontaneous eye opening, oriented verbal response and obeys command) but after she was moved to the sitting position and lost consciousness her GCS probably was about 3

4. ***How would you describe Juanita's ECG?***

   Sinus rhythm with one PAC. Extra complex coming sooner in the cycle with clear P wave.

5. ***What changes in your actions does the presence of a hemodialysis site require, and why?***

   A blood pressure will not be taken in that arm, nor will an IV be started in the site unless a life threat is present and that is the only site for an IV that is available. The reason for this is that it takes a surgical procedure and a maturation time period to establish an effective site for hemodialysis. Consequently anything that could "ruin" the site, such as a blood clot or infection, could effectively eliminate access for hemodialysis. Taking a blood pressure disrupts flow to the area and could theoretically cause a site of irritation or inflammation leading to clot formation. Starting an IV at the site or giving medications through the IV could cause irritation leading to clot formation and/or infection. Thus another site would need to be selected and the process for establishing access started all over again.

6. ***What is the significance of Juanita's becoming out of breath when talking and what treatment is indicated?***

   Inadequate tidal volume at rest. She needs oxygen.

7. ***What is the term for becoming hypotensive when going from a sitting to a standing position?***

   There are several. One is orthostatic hypotension; another is a positive "tilt" test.

8. ***What is the significance of Juanita becoming hypotensive when going from a sitting to a standing position?***

   Something is causing her blood pressure to drop precipitously. The most likely cause is fluid related.

9. ***Is there a relationship between Juanita's becoming out of breath when talking and her change in BP when moving to a sitting position?***

   There most likely is a relationship. Hypotension when moving to a sitting position indicates a lack of volume. When occurring in conjunction with shortness of breath, a corresponding lack of red blood cells or anemia is highly probable.

10. ***What are possible side effects of long-term kidney failure/hemodialysis?***

    Consequences of long-term kidney failure/dialysis include anemia, susceptibility to fractures, vitamin deficiencies and electrolyte imbalances, recurring infection, in addition to hepatitis B.

    Anemia results from an interference with the production and secretion of erythropoietin, the hormone that stimulates red blood cell production. Most dialysis centers routinely measure a hemoglobin and hematocrit for each patient, and EPO is prescribed as a routine medication.

    There is a susceptibility to fractures caused by an inability of the kidney to activate vitamin D, resulting in an inability to use calcium, even though it is mobilized from the bones. Movement of calcium, its mobilization and deposit, is closely tied to the phosphate ion which is also affected by kidney failure. Electrolytes also shift across the filter, not always in appropriate amounts, thus leading to excesses or deficiencies. Vitamin and mineral supplements are routinely given to dialysis patients.

Infection is always a threat when the body's vascular system is violated on a regular basis. Hemodialysis is usually done three times a week. The incidence of hepatitis B was cut dramatically when filters were limited to one patient only. However, the overall incidence of infection is higher because of a reduced immune function, probably a result of the kidney failure itself.

11. What are possible short-term side effects (those that occur during or immediately after) hemodialysis?

Air embolism may occur during dialysis or immediately after. This is due to air entering the IV line.

Hypoglycemia is common because hemodialysis is unable to regulate the filtration of glucose. This is why after a treatment most patients choose to eat a meal.

Hypovolemia is another common side effect. Sometimes too much body water is dialyzed out. This is why patients are encouraged to wait 10 to 15 minutes after a treatment and get up gradually to ensure orthostatic hypotension is not present before driving home.

Bleeding is also possible because dialyzed blood is treated with heparin during the dialysis treatment to prevent clotting. Normally the heparin is discontinued about 20 minutes before the end of the treatment to ensure that blood will clot normally before dismissal. GI bleeds are possible and usually painless or "silent."

Hyperkalemia is possible because of a build-up of potassium just before dialysis or just after. Cardiac dysrhythmias are common results of hyperkalemia.

12. Which of the short- or long-term side effects is/are most likely present now?

With her 2-year history of being on dialysis, Juanita is at risk for all these side effects. However, with her history of having dialysis this morning and now it is the evening, the most likely side effects related to dialysis that are currently affecting her include anemia and bleeding.

13. Juanita is an insulin-dependent diabetic. What types of medical conditions, more typical of diabetic patients, could explain Juanita's syncopal episode with orthostatic hypotension?

Diabetics are prone to developing peripheral neuropathies that alter pain sensation. Therefore the pain of an aneurysm, abdominal pain from a GI bleed, or even a "silent" heart attack could explain her current problem. Diabetics are also prone to sepsis, which might also explain her current episode.

14. What is timolol, and how does it work?

Timolol is a selective B_1 blocker with no intrinsic sympathomimetic activity. This means the drug is specific for the heart, decreasing heart rate and ventricular contractility, thus lowering blood pressure and limiting oxygen demand. It is used for Juanita because it is metabolized by the liver, with only a small amount of unchanged drug in the urine. Thus it does not build up in the blood as easily as other antihypertensives.

15. How is the history of timolol relevant to Juanita's assessment findings?

It may explain why her pulse is no faster than it is in the presence of possible hypovolemia.

16. What do you think is causing Juanita's current problem, and why?

Hypovolemia with anemia is most likely the problem. This is supported by her breathlessness, orthostatic hypotension, and dialysis. However, hypovolemia from too much body water removed from the dialysis treatment is not likely. The time frame is too long (the body compensates with fluid shifts relatively quickly). Hypovolemia from blood loss is much more likely. She already has black stools but has explained them by the iron supplement she already takes. A "silent" GI bleed is just as likely as an aneurysm.

Another likely cause is sepsis. Dialysis patients are prone to infection anyway and considering that this patient is a diabetic, infection resulting in sepsis is a definite possibility. However, there isn't anything in her history to lead you to suspect an infection is present.

A "silent" heart attack is also possible. Diabetics are prone to myocardial infarctions and cardiogenic shock could explain her assessment findings.

17. After 5 minutes in the supine position, Juanita was alert and oriented still with no complaints of pain or discomfort. Another set of VS showed P 70, R 22, BP 96/60. How serious is Juanita's problem?

As long as she is supine, Juanita perfuses her brain. But you don't know for how long. Juanita is potentially unstable.

18. Is Juanita's problem serious enough to warrant using her fistula as an IV site?

The answer to this depends on your transport time, your local protocols and your "feel" of the patient. The external jugular vein would probably be your best access site for an IV; however, look at the right antecubital space too. Save the fistula for a last resort when she becomes frankly unstable.

19. How would you begin treatment?

Oxygen by mask, non-rebreather and reservoir at 12 to 15 lpm. Keep her supine, head elevated if necessary. Start an IV of normal saline or Ringer's lactate. Monitor cardiac activity closely.

20. If you gave a fluid bolus, how much would you give and why?

She needs volume but the hazard is overloading her system. Start low, with 200 to 250 ml, monitoring respirations and tidal volume along with vital signs.

21. What is Juanita at risk for?

Abruptly decompensating. She could bleed out internally or have a sudden onset of cardiac dysrhythmias and arrest.

22. How would you assess for that/those risk factors?

Watch her abdominal girth, listen to lung sounds, observe the cardiac monitor, compare radial pulse with the ECG, and continually assess mental status, pulse rate, blood pressure, and any complaints Juanita may develop.

OUTCOME

Paramedics were able to start an external jugular IV and infused two boluses of normal saline to a total of approximately 500 ml. Juanita's vital signs on arrival were P 70, R 16, BP 100/68. She remained out of breath when she talked despite the oxygen. However, Juanita remained stable en route to the hospital. When the medics attempted to transfer her to the ED cart, Juanita had a sudden, involuntary episode of a dark red mixed with black, jellylike stool. She remained conscious but her BP dropped to 80 systolic. Another 500 ml of NS was given along with vitamin K. She finally admitted to having this type of stool for the last several days but did not want to go to the hospital so did not tell anyone. Her physician thought that her dialysis treatment, with the administration of heparin, exacerbated a previously existing GI bleed. Two units of packed cells were administered in the ED before she was transferred to the ICU with a lower GI bleed. She was eventually dismissed to home.

BIBLIOGRAPHY

Alexander, D. (1996). New concepts in shock management. *Air Medical Journal,* 15(2) 85-91.

Berkow, R. & Fletcher, A. J. (Eds.). (1992). *The Merck manual.* Rahway, NJ: Merck Research Laboratories.

Bickell, W. H., Wall, M. J., Pepe, P. E., Martin, R. R., Ginger, V. F., Allen, M. K., & Mattox, K. L. (1994). Immediate versus delayed fluid resuscitation for hypotensive patients with penetrating torso injuries. *New England Journal of Medicine,* 331(17) 1105-1109.

Bledsoe, B. E. (1994). Gastrointestinal, genitourinary, and reproductive system emergencies. In B. E. Bledsoe, R. S. Porter, & B. R. Shade (Eds.). *Paramedic emergency care,* (2nd ed.). Englewood Cliffs, NJ: Brady, A Prentice Hall division.

Capone, A. C., Safar, P., Stezoski, W., Tisherman, S. & Peitzman, A. B. (1995). Improved outcome with fluid restriction in treatment of uncontrolled hemorrhagic shock. *Journal of the American College of Surgeons,* 180: 49-56.

Fontanarosa, P. B. (1997). Abdominal, genitourinary, and back pain. In P. Pons & D. Cason (Eds.). *Paramedic field care.* St. Louis, MO: Mosby.

Guyton, A. C. (1992). The gastrointestinal tract. In *Human physiology and mechanisms of disease.* Philadelphia: W. B. Saunders.

Heuther, S. E. (1994). Structure and function of the digestive system. In K. L. McCance & S. E. Huether (Eds.). Pathophysiology: *The biologic basis for disease in adults and children.* (2nd ed.). St. Louis, MO: Mosby.

Heuther, S. E. & McCance, K. L. (1994). Alterations of digestive function. In *Pathophysiology: The biologic basis for disease in adults and children,* (2nd ed.). St. Louis, MO: Mosby.

Kaweski, S. M. et. al. (1990). The effect of prehospital fluids on survival in trauma patients. *Journal of Trauma,* 30(10) 1215.

Martini, F. H. & Bartholomew, E. F. (1997). The digestive system. In *Essentials of anatomy and physiology.* Upper Saddle River, NJ: Prentice Hall.

McQuaid, K. & Knauer, C. M. (1994). Alimentary tract. In L. M. Tierney, S. J. McPhee, & M. A. Papadakis (Eds.). *Current medical diagnosis and treatment: A Lange medical book.* Norwalk, CT: Appleton & Lange.

10

Environmental Emergencies

OVERVIEW

Environmental emergencies usually involve those physical conditions that result when the environmental temperature is abnormally hot or cold. Providers in most areas of the country may encounter both types of patient conditions. Depending on the area of the country, some conditions may be seen more frequently than others.

HEAT RELATED EMERGENCIES
Anatomy, Physiology, and Pathophysiology

Heat related emergencies are generally divided into two types, those that involve fluid and electrolyte disturbance (heat cramps and heat exhaustion) and hyperthermia, which is a result of a failure of the thermoregulating mechanism in the brain (heat stroke).

Heat cramps frequently occur when an individual is engaging in vigorous physical activity in a hot environment. Sweating is the body's mechanism to help keep it cool, but with sweating comes loss of body water and associated electrolytes, specifically sodium and chloride. Painful muscle contractions occur as a result of salt depletion since sweat losses are replaced with water alone. Muscle cramping is the most frequent complaint. Skin is often moist and cool and there may be muscle twitching. Mental status is intact with stable vital signs, but the patient is in pain and may be agitated.

Heat exhaustion results from prolonged heavy exercise with inadequate salt intake in a hot environment. Dehydration, along with sodium depletion, contributes to cardiovascular changes. Body temperature may rise over 100° F (37.8° C), tachycardia and moist skin are usual signs. Heat cramps may be present along with complaints of thirst, weakness, headache, and fatigue. Mental status may be altered with confusion, impaired judgment, and sometimes psychosis.

Heat stroke is an acute life threat, resulting from a failure of the thermoregulatory mechanism. In heat strokes body temperatures frequently exceed 106° F (41° C). This extreme increase in body temperature results in a corresponding increase in the metabolic rate that, in turn, increases oxygen demand. The increased oxygen demand rapidly exceeds the body's ability to supply oxygen and results in metabolic acidosis. This puts a severe demand on all organ systems. The heat itself can be associated with cell breakdown. At temperatures of 108° F (42.2° C) protein breakdown and cellular lipid membrane disruption occurs. The cells most sensitive to heat are those of the brain.

There are two forms of heat stroke. Classic heat stroke occurs in patients with compromised homeostatic mechanisms, such as the very young, the elderly, or those taking certain medications (phenothiazines, anticholinergics, or antihistamines). Exertional heat stroke occurs in previously healthy persons undergoing strenuous exertion in hot environments, such as unconditioned amateurs in strenuous athletic activities. Impaired mental status with high body temperature and the absence of sweating is typical of classic heat stroke. In exertional heat stroke, clothing may be damp from earlier sweating, but at the time of heat stroke, sweating has ceased. Signs of shock are usually present, and multiple organ failure is frequent.

Treatment

Treatment begins with removal of the patient to a cool environment, airway control, and oxygen therapy. Replacement of fluids and electrolytes in patients with heat cramps can be done orally with an electrolyte solution (1 teaspoon per quart of water). In heat exhaustion, IV therapy of an electrolyte solution of normal saline will avoid GI upset and vomiting. In the case of heat stroke, rapid cooling is necessary, along with vigorous support of the respiratory and cardiovascular systems. Move the victim to a cool environment and begin cooling procedures. Evaporative cooling is effective and easily performed. Remove all clothing and wet the skin. Evaporation may be enhanced if fans or an air conditioning unit is used in the back of the transport vehicle. Caution should be used to prevent shivering. Airway access by endotracheal intubation may be necessary. Controlling ventilations with a bag-valve-mask will help manage tidal volume and ineffective respiratory rates. IV access and fluid replacement with normal saline by repeated fluid boluses is also necessary. Checking for blood glucose levels and treating with D_{50} is also appropriate.

COLD RELATED EMERGENCIES
Anatomy, Physiology, and Pathophysiology

Cold related emergencies are divided into two types: frostbite and hypothermia. Frostbite is localized freezing of tissue, and hypothermia is generalized lowering of body temperature. During frostbite tissue damage occurs in two ways, mechanical and chemical. Mechanical damage occurs through the formation of ice crystals. Water expands roughly 7% during ordinary freezing and cell membranes are destroyed in the process. Chemical damage occurs because of the process of ice crystal formation. When ice crystals are formed, within or between cells, the sodium pump is destroyed, thus rupturing cell walls. As a result, red blood cells clump and platelet microemboli form to cause thrombosis and a loss of vascular integrity occurs. During rewarming, local edema becomes evident, and disruption of nutritive blood flow contributes to ischemia. Ischemia often produces the most damaging effects of frostbite.

In mild cases of frostbite only the skin and subcutaneous tissues are involved with numbness, a prickling sensation, and itching being evident. With increased severity, deep frostbite involves deeper structures, and along with numbness and tingling, stiffness may be present. Skin that has suffered frostbite may appear pale, then waxy or yellowish in appearance, and firm to the touch.

Hypothermia is defined as a generalized loss of body heat where the core temperature is below 95° F (35° C). As body temperature begins to drop, immediate vasoconstriction in the peripheral vessels and simultaneous increase in sympathetic nervous discharge along with a catecholamine release increases basal metabolism producing heat for the body but requiring glucose for energy. As cold exposure continues, preshivering muscle tone increases, generating heat for the body. Shivering puts a great demand on all available glucose and glycogen reserves. Shivering does not stop until either the core temperature reaches approximately 86° F (30° C), glucose or glycogen is depleted, or insulin is no longer available for glucose transfer. Variations between available glucose, the amount of glycogen stores, and functioning insulin help explain why some patients stop shivering at 90° F (32° C) although others are still shivering at 87° F (30.5° C). As a general rule, most textbooks state that shivering stops between 89° F and 87.8° F (31° C).

As the state of hypothermia continues, energy stores are rapidly depleted. The body's temperature regulating mechanism fails and the body rapidly loses heat. Electrolyte and endocrine imbalances are common. Enzyme systems necessary for metabolic function fail because of the cold temperature. Muscles stiffen, reflexes are lost, and pupils dilate. The metabolic rate falls and the heart cannot keep up, because of expended energy and/or because of enzyme systems that cannot work. The respiratory rate slows, cardiac output drops, and the heart rate goes from the tachycardia of early hypothermia to the bradycardia of severe hypothermia. Atrial fibrillation can occur at any time although bradycardia is considered a late sign of hypothermia.

Hypothermia can be mild, moderate, or severe. The exact temperatures at which these occur vary between authorities. In general, hypothermia begins at a core temperature of 95° F (35° C). Mild hypothermia is considered when the core temperature drops to >91.4° F (33° C); moderate to severe hypothermia occurs at temperatures less than 90° F (32° C). Hypothermic patients may appear cold, stiff, and blue with fixed, dilated pupils and no spontaneous breathing or palpable pulses. The ability to predict patient viability is not accurate until the patient has been rewarmed. *No patient is considered dead until he or she is warm and dead.*

Treatment

For frostbite, rapid rewarming in a controlled environment, usually in an emergency department, is the treatment of choice. During transport remove all wet, constricted clothing from the affected body part and cover with dry dressings. Immobilize the frostbitten part, taking care not to break any blisters that may have formed. Wrap gently and elevate. Do not manipulate or rub the tissue and do not expose to further cold. If a frostbitten area is allowed to thaw and refreeze, greater tissue destruction results than if the tissue had remained frozen until arrival at the hospital.

For generalized hypothermia, initial treatment is designed to prevent further heat loss. Other considerations may be suggested by the history. Trauma may be a factor although pedestrian accidents may be more difficult to realize when discovered after the fact. Medical conditions such as hypoglycemia, intracranial hemorrhage, or systemic infections may predispose to hypothermia as does alcohol and drug abuse. The patient should be moved to a warm environment and have any wet clothing replaced with warm blankets. Heat packs should be placed around the head, neck, axilla, and groin. It is important that the patient be treated as gently as possible to avoid stimulating ventricular fibrillation. Airway management is controversial. Generally it is recommended that when respirations are spontaneous, administer 100% oxygen with assistance from a bag-valve-mask device if necessary. Use warmed and humidified oxygen if possible. Endotracheal intubation should be reserved for apneic patients or patients where the airway cannot be protected by other means. All hypothermic patients require ECG monitoring. As the core temperature approaches 90° F, any dysrhythmia may be seen. However, atrial fibrillation is common early in the condition, deteriorating to a bradycardic rhythm as the body continues to lose heat. The J wave (Osborne wave or hypothermic hump) is frequently seen in lead II and is described as a "hump" or elevation of the ST segment at the junction of the QRS complex and the ST segment. Pharmacologic therapy, as well as defibrillation, at body temperatures less than 82° F (28° C) are usually ineffective. The percentage of a drug that is protein bound is increased with hypothermia. Repeated drug doses to a hypothermic patient will predispose to a toxic dose during the rewarming process.

Hypothermic patients also require IV access with normal saline or Ringer's lactate (warmed if possible). Most hypothermic patients are dehydrated and will require volume expansion. Many patients with hypothermia present with altered mental status. Because hypoglycemia may occur as a result of the hypothermia, testing blood glucose levels is appropriate. For the moderate to severely hypothermic patient, transport to the nearest facility with cardiopulmonary bypass capability is the best option. Cardiopulmonary bypass is the ideal technology to control the active rewarming process in the hypothermic patient who is unresponsive to usual rewarming techniques.

CASE 1

Dispatch: 15:30 hrs; unconscious 2 y/o male

On Arrival: You find 2 y/o Nathan lying across the hood of a car in a parking lot. He is extremely flushed and appears to be sleeping. His father is there and is hysterical.

Initial Assessment Findings

Mental Status—Unresponsive to voice and pain
Airway—Open, with some foamy saliva present
Breathing—R extremely shallow at 70 with sternal and substernal retractions
Circulation—Skin hot, dry, and red; extremities mottled; lips are gray
Apical Pulse—Weak and too fast to count
Chief Complaint—Unresponsive

Focused History

Events—Father left the child in the car, with the windows rolled up, while he went in the store "for a few minutes," but was delayed an estimated 90 minutes. When he came back he found his son unresponsive and started yelling for help. A passerby called EMS. The ambient temperature is 90° F with 88% humidity. The child is dressed in a tee shirt, shorts, and a diaper.
Previous Illness—none
Current Health Status—good
Allergies—none known
Medications—none

Focused Physical

Current Set of VS—P over 200, R 70
Other Pertinent Findings—There is a blue-gray color to the child's lips; lung sounds are very faint but clear; extremities are red and mottled with delayed capillary return (> 2 sec); tympanic thermometer reads 107° F (41.7° C); pulse oximetry reads ERROR; weight is 30 lbs.
Diagnostic Tests—none

ECG

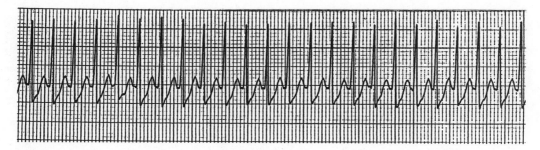

Figure 10-1

QUESTIONS

1. What is significant about Nathan's history?

2. What body systems are affected?

3. What is Nathan's Glasgow Coma Score?

4. Given Nathan's history and your physical assessment findings, what do you think is wrong?

5. How serious is Nathan's condition?

6. What is the significance of a respiratory rate of 70?

7. How would you describe Nathan's ECG?

8. What is the significance of a heart rate of 270?

9. What would be your immediate treatment?

10. What is Nathan at risk for?

11. What is the significance of a fever of 41.7° C (107° F)?

12. How would you continue to treat Nathan?

13. If a crystalloid is administered, how much would be given?

14. A blood pressure was not taken on Nathan. However, capillary return was delayed. How does delayed capillary return relate to blood pressure?

15. What precautions need to be taken when externally cooling a patient, child or adult?

16. What is the difference between heat exhaustion and heat stroke including signs and symptoms?

17. After oxygenating and cooling procedures had been started, Nathan began posturing by extending his arms and legs. What does that response indicate?

QUESTIONS AND ANSWERS

1. What is significant about Nathan's history?

He was in a hot car for about 90 minutes with no ventilation; no previous history.

2. What body systems are affected?

CNS—unresponsive, temperature 107° F (41.7° C)
Respiratory—rapid rate at 70, faint lung sounds
Cardiovascular—extremely rapid heart rate; red, mottled skin with cyanotic lips

3. What is Nathan's Glasgow Coma Score?

GCS 3 (1, no eye opening, 1, no motor response, 1, no verbal response)

4. Given Nathan's history and your physical assessment findings, what do you think is wrong?

The pattern of a history of being in an enclosed car in hot weather; unresponsive and unconscious; hot, dry, red skin; and an extreme fever in the absence of a history of illness are consistent with dehydration and heat stroke. It is unlikely that the cause is infection.

5. How serious is Nathan's condition?

This is an immediate life threat.

6. What is the significance of a respiratory rate of 70?

Nathan is in respiratory failure. The rate is too fast for adequate tidal volume and is too fast for Nathan to keep going for long. Because of the inadequate tidal volume, confirmed by very faint lung sounds, there is inadequate exchange of oxygen and carbon dioxide and a high probability of respiratory acidosis. Because Nathan's rate is 70, he will likely tire and quit breathing altogether.

7. How would you describe Nathan's ECG?

SVT at a rate of 270 by monitor.

8. What is the significance of a heart rate of 270?

This rate is too fast for an adequate cardiac output. This rate also puts an incredible strain on the heart and greatly increases the oxygen demand of the heart. Nathan has a high probability for cardiac failure.

9. What would be your immediate treatment?

Move him to the medic unit, strip him of his clothing, and start assisting ventilations with a pediatric bag-valve-mask and reservoir with 100% oxygen at a rate of 30 per minute. Turn up the air conditioner, soak a towel with cool water or saline and start cooling him down.

10. What is Nathan at risk for?

Seizures, brain damage, respiratory failure or arrest, cardiac failure, and full arrest.

11. What is the significance of a fever of 41.7° C (107° F)?

Any fever increases the metabolic demands of the body. An extreme fever, such as this one, exerts a severe demand on all organ systems. Fevers increase the metabolic rate that then increases oxygen demand. This increase in oxygen demand rapidly exceeds the body's ability to supply oxygen, resulting in metabolic acidosis. In addition to the metabolic demand, the heat itself is harmful. A core temperature of 42.2° C (108° F) is associated with protein denaturation and cellular lipid membrane breakdown.

When a temperature high enough to predispose cellular damage itself is present, along with acidosis, which further contributes to cellular damage, a threat to life rapidly develops. The most sensitive cells to this life threat are those of the brain.

12. How would you continue to treat Nathan?

After oxygenating and beginning external cooling, try and find an IV access route. It is likely that the only route available will be an interosseous route. An external jugular is sometimes accessible in a 2 y/o, but for many their necks are still too chubby. Regardless of which route you find, administer a crystalloid bolus of normal saline or Ringer's lactate, at 20 ml/kg.

13. *If a crystalloid is administered, how much would be given?*

The standard dose is 20 ml/kg, reassess and repeat. Reassessment is critical because of the probability of congestive heart failure. Because of this, many systems may limit prehospital administration of fluids to children to a maximum of 60 ml/kg.

14. *A blood pressure was not taken on Nathan. However, capillary return was delayed. How does delayed capillary return relate to blood pressure?*

Both are indicators of perfusion. However, delayed capillary return is an early indicator of inadequate perfusion, whereas low blood pressure is a late indicator of inadequate perfusion. Thus it is possible to have a patient in shock with delayed capillary return and yet have an adequate blood pressure because of compensatory mechanisms. In children, capillary refill is (in normal ambient temperatures) considered a more accurate indicator of actual perfusion status than blood pressure.

15. *What precautions need to be taken when externally cooling a patient, child or adult?*

Do not let the patient shiver. The presence of shivering indicates body temperature is being lowered too fast for the body to adjust thus causing shivering. The process of shivering will raise the body temperature.

16. *What is the difference between heat exhaustion and heat stroke including signs and symptoms?*

The two are markedly different. Heat exhaustion is the result of excessive fluid and electrolyte loss. Heat stroke is a failure of heat loss mechanisms resulting a failure of the body's thermoregulating mechanism. Most of our knowledge and information regarding these two conditions comes from adults. In the adult, the presence of flushed, dry skin with fever is typical of the heat stroke patient, whereas pale, cool, clammy skin is typical of the heat exhaustion patient. Exertional heat stroke can result in sweating and both conditions may result in altered mental status.

Because the sweating mechanism in children differs according to age (the very young do not have reliable sweating mechanisms) and skin color varies greatly depending on the age of the child, the only consistent reliable indicators of heat stroke in children are a history of exposure, the presence of a fever, and altered mental status.

17. *After oxygenating and cooling procedures had been started, Nathan began posturing by extending his arms and legs. What does that response indicate?*

His mental status is improving. When the medics first arrived, Nathan was completely unresponsive (GCS 3). Now, after treatment has started, there is a response (GCS 4). Care must be taken to differentiate posturing from seizures, since tonic seizures can present in a similar fashion. No further conclusions can really be made.

OUTCOME

Nathan was ventilated by a bag-valve-mask with a reservoir and 100% O_2 at 30/min. His clothing was removed and cool towels were applied and the air-conditioner in the back of the squad was turned on full force. Attempts to intubate were unsuccessful. An IV of normal saline was started in his L proximal tibia and 300 ml was infused rapidly. During transport, posturing by extension was noted. A second bolus of 300 ml was infused. Repeat VS were: P 250, R 60, bagging at 30; capillary return $>$ 3 sec. On arrival at the ED he was sedated, paralyzed and rapidly intubated, and placed on a ventilator, and a central line was started. He received another 600 ml of lactated Ringer's. Core temperature was 106.2° F (41.2° C). Initial ABGs showed a pH of 6.8, $PaCO_2$ 72, PaO_2 125, HCO_3^- 18, BE -17. A cooling blanket was applied and IV Valium was given to control any shivering. He was admitted to the pediatric ICU. Three hours later his core temperature was down to 102° F (38.8° C). Five hours later he was beginning to open his eyes and obey command. Twenty-four hours later he was off the ventilator and appeared to be responding normally to his parents. His core temperature was 99° F. Social Services and Child Protective Services were involved in this case. Nathan was dismissed 2 days after the incident. Pediatricians pointed out to Nathan's parents that when children are this young, detecting brain damage is relatively impossible. His full outcome is unknown.

CASE 2

Dispatch: 17:45 hrs; 72 y/o unconscious woman

On Arrival: You find 72 y/o Cleo, lying on her right side on her kitchen floor. She is very pale and appears to be sleeping. There is bread dough rising on the counter. Her oven door is open and it is extremely hot in the room. You note a cut on her ankle with dried blood and no active bleeding. Her son is present.

Initial Assessment Findings

Mental Status—Unconscious and unresponsive to voice, flexes to painful stimuli
Airway—Open and clear
Breathing—R 36 and shallow; lung sounds rales, wheezes, and rhonchi upper and lower lobes left side of chest, no sounds upper and lower lobes right side of chest
Circulation—Skin very pale with gray color; hot and dry
      No radial pulse, weak and rapid carotid pulse
      BP unable to hear
Chief Complaint—Unconscious and unresponsive

Focused History

Events—Son had talked to her earlier in the day because her air-conditioner had stopped working. Her son stopped by after work to check on her and found her on the floor with the oven on. He turned the oven off and called EMS.
Previous Illness—AMI about 3 years ago, Type II diabetic for 5 years.
Current Health Status—Had problems with swollen feet since beginning of summer, son said mother blamed it on the heat and refused to see her physician.
Allergies—None known
Medications—Digoxin (digitalis), Lasix (furosemide), Glucotrol (glipizide)

Focused Physical

Current Set of VS—P 160-170 irregular; R 36; BP undetectable; tympanic thermometer 106° F (41° C); pulse oximetry reads ERROR
Other Pertinent Findings—Clothing dry; pitting edema to mid-shin bilaterally; nail beds cyanotic with mottled skin on extremities; abdomen distended but soft and no masses; ankle laceration is approximately 4 cm long and caked with dried blood, there is no immediate evidence as to how it happened; pupils are constricted and nonreactive.
Diagnostic Tests—BS 34

ECG

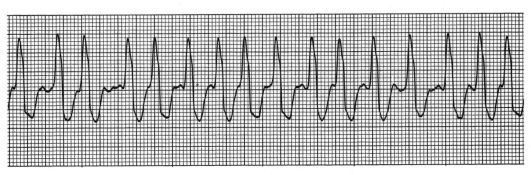

Figure 10-2

QUESTIONS

1. What is significant about Cleo's history?

2. What body systems are affected?

3. What is Cleo's Glasgow Coma Score?

4. What is the significance of and relationship between, Cleo's respiratory rate, lung sounds, and difference between her right and left lung sounds?

5. What is the significance of Cleo's temperature in relation to her age?

6. What is the significance of a history of NIDDM, previous AMI, digitalis, and furosemide?

7. How would you describe Cleo's ECG?

8. What is the relationship between Cleo's temperature and her ECG?

9. What is the relationship between Cleo's vital signs and her temperature?

10. What is Cleo at risk for?

11. What is the relationship between Cleo's signs and symptoms, blood sugar value, and hyperthermia?

12. Is there any other information, from either a history or physical examination that might help you?

13. Given Cleo's history and your physical assessment findings, what do you think is wrong?

14. How serious is Cleo's condition?

15. What would be your immediate treatment?

16. How much fluid would you administer?

17. After oxygenating and administering IV fluids, Cleo has a grand mal seizure. How would you continue to treat Cleo?

18. Is there a relationship between Cleo's nonreactive pupils and her seizure?

19. When cooling a hyperthermic patient, should it be done quickly or more slowly and controlled?

20. What is the actual effect of shivering and how can it be controlled?

QUESTIONS AND ANSWERS

1. **What is significant about Cleo's history?**

   Prolonged exposure to high temperatures; NIDDM and heart problems; some months of increased fluid retention; and not monitored by a physician

2. **What body systems are affected?**

   CNS—unconscious, unresponsive; nonreactive pupils
   Respiratory—tachypneic; rales, wheezes, and rhonchi; unequal lung sounds
   Cardiovascular—pale, gray color; undetectable BP, tachycardic; poor perfusion
   Other—fever (hot, dry skin)

3. **What is Cleo's Glasgow Coma Score?**

   GCS 3 (1 no verbal response; 1 no motor response; 1 no eye opening)

4. **What is the significance of and relationship between, Cleo's respiratory rate, lung sounds, and difference between her right and left lung sounds?**

   A rate of 36 is too fast for an adequate tidal volume. But the increased rate is an indicator of the body's attempt to compensate, usually for an increased oxygen demand and/or a need to "blow off" accumulated CO_2. She has rales, wheezes, and rhonchi, indicating pulmonary edema. The pulmonary edema causes hypoxia and predisposes to acidosis (first respiratory as carbon dioxide is retained, then metabolic as the cells, in the absence of sufficient oxygen, are forced to engage in anaerobic metabolism).

   The absence of lung sounds on her right side is consistent with her position (lying on her right side). Fluid follows gravity and would be a rough indicator of just how much fluid she has in her lungs (enough to fill an entire side).

5. **What is the significance of Cleo's temperature in relation to her age?**

   Fever increases the metabolic demands of the body. An extreme fever, such as this one, exerts a severe demand on all organ systems. Fevers increase the metabolic rate, which then increases oxygen demand. This increase in oxygen demand rapidly exceeds the body's ability to supply oxygen, resulting in metabolic acidosis. In addition to the metabolic demand, the heat itself is harmful. A core temperature of 42.2° C (108° F) is associated with protein breakdown and cellular lipid membrane disruption. A temperature high enough to predispose to cellular damage, in the presence of acidosis, is an indicator of a life threat. All body systems and all body cells are affected by extremes in heat. The most sensitive cells to this condition are those of the brain.

   The difference between an older person and a younger person is the amount of reserve present to withstand this type of stress. The older person has less reserve in the heart, lungs, brain, and kidneys as a process of aging. Although the very young and very old are more susceptible, in general, the older the patient, the more frequent the complications and the worse the outcome.

6. **What is the significance of a history of NIDDM, previous AMI, digitalis, and furosemide?**

   Adult onset diabetics are prone to arteriosclerotic heart disease and AMI. Sequelae of AMI frequently includes congestive heart failure (CHF). Meds such as digitalis and furosemide are commonly prescribed for patients with CHF. Patients with a history of diabetes, CHF, and those taking diuretics are at high risk for heat-related illnesses.

7. **How would you describe Cleo's ECG?**

   Atrial fibrillation with a wide QRS. At first glance, it might seem like ventricular tachycardia; however, while the rate is 180 and consistent with VT, it is also grossly irregular and perfuses enough for a carotid pulse to be felt. The 7th complex has enough time before the complex for a P wave, if it were present, to be seen. Keep in mind that although there are cases of prolonged VT that generate a pulse, most cases of VT degenerate into v-fib rather rapidly. If VT were triggered by the irritability of ischemia, acidosis, and extreme temperature, it would be very likely to degenerate into v-fib. This rhythm does not change.

8. *What is the relationship between Cleo's temperature and her ECG?*

An extremely high body temperature, especially in an older patient, puts an extreme stress on the heart. We don't know if atrial fibrillation with a conduction defect was a preexisting rhythm or not. Atrial fibrillation is reasonable with her history but ventricular tachycardia is likely with this temperature. However, her temperature may also be a contributing factor to another cause. Extreme body heat contributes to electrolyte loss, through sweating, and breaks down the body's enzyme systems. The SA node, to generate an impulse, depends on enzyme systems to precipitate an electrolyte exchange (sodium leaks out faster). This enzyme system is sensitive to temperature extremes in both directions. In an already compromised heart where sodium stores are depleted and an enzyme system is compromised, atrial fibrillation may be a result.

Her conduction defect, while it may have been preexisting, is also a casualty of extreme fever for the same reasons. To conduct impulses, enzyme systems, and electrolyte exchange processes must be intact.

9. *What is the relationship between Cleo's vital signs and her temperature?*

Her extreme temperature explains all her vital signs. Cleo's heart rate is a reflection of both her body's attempt to cool off and the effect of hypoxia and ischemia on her heart. Her extreme hypotension is a reflection of vasodilation and loss of body fluid. The respiratory rate is a reflection of her body's attempt to use the respiratory system to cool off and a stimulus to increase the respiratory rate from hypoxia and acidosis.

10. *What is Cleo at risk for?*

Stroke, AMI, seizures, dysrhythmias such as VT and v-fib, coagulation problems, and multiorgan systems failure

11. *What is the relationship between Cleo's signs and symptoms, blood sugar value, and hypothermia?*

While some of her signs and symptoms could be related to her low blood sugar, her signs, symptoms, *and* low blood sugar are a result of her heat-related illness, complicated by her diabetes. The metabolic demands of trying to cool off, as well as the severely increased energy demands of a high metabolic rate, induced by her hyperthermic state, rapidly deplete the body's glucose stores. Her underlying diabetes compounds the problem.

12. *Is there any other information, from either a history or physical examination that might help you?*

Most of the information you need is already there. The son may be able to add additional information. The hospital might appreciate knowing if she takes her medication regularly and when she last saw her physician.

13. *Given Cleo's history and your physical assessment findings, what do you think is wrong?*

This is most likely heat stroke. Even though meningitis or sepsis are possibilities, the history and conditions at the scene are more suggestive for heat stroke.

14. *How serious is Cleo's condition?*

This is a threat to life; her condition is of the highest priority. Cleo is dying.

15. *What would be your immediate treatment?*

Intubate her and ventilate at 30/min with a BVM and reservoir at 15 lpm oxygen. IV access with NS or LR. Administer 25 gms of D_{50} as soon as IV access is available. Strip her down and cover with cool towels. Get her into the squad and turn the air conditioning up as high as possible.

16. *How much fluid would you administer?*

Even though she has pulmonary edema of cardiac origin, she needs fluids. Keep positive pressure ventilation and administer a 200-ml bolus and reassess. Avoid vasopressors since they tend to interfere with heat loss.

17. *After oxygenating and administering IV fluids, Cleo has a grand mal seizure. How would you continue to treat Cleo?*

Administer diazepam (Valium) 5 to 10 mg, slow IV push, during the clinical event. Valium does not prevent seizures, it only stops them once started. When the seizure stops, ventilate and reassess, continuing cooling measures.

18. Is there a relationship between Cleo's nonreactive pupils and her seizure?

Yes there is. Both nonreactive pupils and seizure activity may be results of cerebral edema. Heat stroke causes cerebral edema resulting from enzyme and cellular membrane disruption. This destroys the natural balance between intracellular and extracellular contents leading to an influx of body water into brain cells. If not controlled, brain cells will rupture and die.

19. When cooling a hyperthermic patient, should it be done quickly or more slowly and controlled?

It should be done relatively quickly for the following reason. It is not the degree of temperature that is as important as the length of time the temperature is allowed to continue. Because cellular membrane disruption and protein breakdown cause exposure of cellular contents to excess water, cells will rapidly expand to the point where they rupture and die. Thus the longer the time of elevated temperature, the greater the potential for cellular destruction.

20. What is the actual effect of shivering and how can it be controlled?

The muscle activity from shivering can increase heat production by as much as 400%. Thus shivering should be avoided and the cooling process accompanied by shivering control. In the field there are two mechanisms. The first is to control the rapidity of the cooling. The second is to administer diazepam. Diazepam is not as effective as lorazepam (Ativan). Which method to be used should be up to local medical control.

OUTCOME

Cleo was intubated, ventilated with a BVM at 15 lpm at a rate of 30, IV access established and approximately 500 ml administered before arrival at the ED. She was stripped down, covered by a wet sheet, and a hand-held fan was directed on her body. Her BP improved to 50 systolic. On arrival VS were P 168, R 30 and assisted with a BVM, BP 58 systolic. She had a core temperature confirmed at 106° F (41° C). She was immediately placed on a cooling blanket and a central line inserted. Fluid resuscitation continued with a careful balance between fluid input and output maintained. A total of 5 liters of crystalloid were infused in the ED. Lorazepam was administered to control shivering and further seizures. Over the next hour her core temperature dropped to 102.2° F (39° C) and she was admitted to ICU. Liver enzymes (indicative of cellular liver damage) were elevated to 20 times the upper limit of normal (AST 792, normal values = 5 to 40; ALT 685, normal values = 5 to 35), clotting times were greatly prolonged and there was myoglobin (a protein released from muscle cell breakdown) in the urine. She developed ARDS along with DIC (disseminated intravascular coagulation) and kidney failure from the myoglobinuria. One month later while still recovering, she suffered a severe stroke and died.

CASE 3

Dispatch: 16:45 hrs; 20 y/o male, medical problem, nature unknown

On Arrival: You find 20 y/o Ivan, wrapped in a blanket, sitting at the kitchen table. He opens his eyes when you speak and appears very drowsy. You note his face is pink but his lips are dusky and he has yellowish, waxy spots on his cheeks and nose.

Initial Assessment Findings

Mental Status—Obeys command, responds verbally but slurred speech and disoriented
Airway—Open and clear
Breathing—R 10 and shallow, talking in complete sentences but seems out of breath; lung sounds clear
Circulation—Skin on arms cold and dry with a gray tinge; yellowish, waxy spots on cheeks and nose
        Pulse irregular at 54
        BP 80/40
Chief Complaint—Confusion

Focused History

Events—He came stumbling home after falling through the ice while out riding his snowmobile. Mother tells you he walked home, approximately 3 miles. Mother states she had him strip down and get into the shower. He was in there about 5 minutes when she heard a noise. He had fallen in the shower so she helped him out, wrapped him in a blanket. He was very drowsy. When he didn't recognize her she called EMS. She has been trying to get him to drink some hot coffee, with little success, while waiting for you to arrive.
Previous Illness—Hay fever
Current Health Status—No current problems
Allergies—Penicillin and pollen
Medications—Hismanal (astemizole) only in the Fall

Focused Physical:

Current Set of VS—P 54 and irregular, R 10, BP 80/40
Other Pertinent Findings—Pulse oximetry 87%; feet and legs are very pale, cold, and dry; blanching of toe nail > 3 sec; abrasions noted on both knees and left shin, left arm and hand; pupils are equal and sluggish; he denies any pain; moves all extremities, movements are weak and uncoordinated.
Diagnostic Tests—Blood sugar 48, fluid bolus of 300 ml normal saline results in BP 86/52 and no change in mental status

ECG

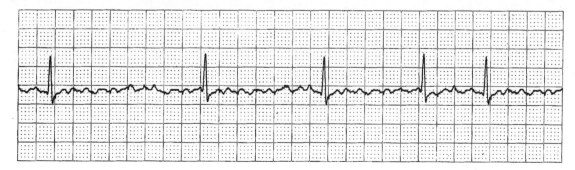

Figure 10-3

QUESTIONS

1. What is significant about Ivan's history?

2. What body systems are affected?

3. What is Ivan's Glascow Coma Score?

4. How would you describe Ivan's ECG?

5. What is important to note about the hot coffee?

6. What is the best explanation for Ivan's yellowish, waxy spots on his cheeks and nose?

7. What is/are possible explanations for Ivan's confusion?

8. Is there any other information either from Ivan's history or your physical assessment that might help you?

9. During questioning you discover that approximately 30 minutes have elapsed from the time Ivan arrived home to when EMS arrived. Why is that important information for you?

10. What do you think is the most likely cause of Ivan's current problem?

11. What is Ivan at risk for developing?

12. How serious is Ivan's condition?

13. What is the most likely reason behind Ivan's blood sugar level? Should it be treated?

14. What is the most likely reason behind Ivan's ECG rate and rhythm? Should it be treated?

15. What is the most likely reason behind Ivan's respiratory rate and BP?

16. What would your initial treatment be?

17. Is C-spine immobilization something you would do? Why or why not?

18. Hypothermic patients should be treated very gently. Why?

19. In this situation, what would be *most* important to reassess and why?

20. Is there any specific treatment for his cheeks and nose?

21. En route to the hospital Ivan begins to shiver; what is the significance of his shivering?

22. What is the difference between a dry cold exposure and a wet cold exposure?

23. What is the "after-drop" phenomenon?

QUESTIONS AND ANSWERS

1. What is significant about Ivan's history?

He fell through the ice, "stumbled" home (3 miles after the incident), and fell during his shower.

2. What body systems are affected?

CNS—lack of coordination, drowsiness, slurred speech, disorientation

Respiratory—rate of 10, seemed to be out of breath

Cardiovascular—pulse 54 and irregular, BP 80/40, delayed capillary refill, dusky lips, and gray tinge to his skin

Skin—yellowish, waxy spots on cheeks and nose; extremities pale, cold, and dry

3. What is Ivan's Glascow Coma Score?

GCS 12 (3 eye opening; 6 motor response; 3 verbal response)

4. How would you describe Ivan's ECG?

Atrial fibrillation with a ventricular response of 54, no discernible P wave, QRS narrow < 0.10 msec and an irregular ventricular response.

5. What is important to note about the hot coffee?

There are two things to note: first, giving someone with an altered mental status something to drink is placing them at risk for aspiration. His mother had been "trying" to get him to drink it. Was there a problem with him taking it or with choking? Second, any drink with caffeine is contraindicated in cold exposure because of the effects of caffeine. Caffeine is a vasoconstrictor, a diuretic, and has an irritant effect on the heart.

6. What is the best explanation for Ivan's yellowish, waxy spots on his cheeks and nose?

The significance is the presence of frostbite. Frostbite is local freezing of tissues. Tissue damage occurs in two ways, mechanical and chemical. Mechanical damage occurs through the formation of ice crystals themselves. Water expands roughly 7% during ordinary freezing, and cell membranes throughout the affected area are destroyed in the process. Chemical damage occurs because of the process of ice crystal formation. When ice crystals are formed, within or between cells, the sodium pump is destroyed, thus rupturing cell walls, RBCs clump and platelet microemboli form to cause thrombosis and loss of vascular integrity occurs. During rewarming, local edema becomes evident, and disruption of nutritive blood flow contributes to ischemia. Ischemia often produces the most damaging effects of frostbite.

7. What is/are possible explanations for Ivan's confusion?

His history suggests that hypothermia is the most likely problem. However, his history also involves falling through the ice and falling in the shower. The suspicion of internal injury and/or head injury is also present. Lack of perfusion (hypotension), hypoxia, and hypoglycemia are also present. Of these possibilities, hypothermia, hypoglycemia, hypoxia and hypotension are the easiest to treat and all may contribute to confusion.

8. Is there any other information either from Ivan's history or your physical assessment that might help you?

Find out if anyone was with him and where are they? Is it possible that he also hit his head? Ask where his clothes are so you can see if he was fully immersed or partially. How long was he in the water? Inspect his head more closely to look for a bump or abrasion. If you have a thermometer, take a temperature. Does he have any abdominal bruising or distention? Gently examine his neck and palpate for pain or irregularity.

9. During questioning you discover that approximately 30 minutes have elapsed from the time Ivan arrived home to when EMS arrived. Why is that important information for you?

Usually if a hypothermic patient is conscious and rewarming methods are begun, they rapidly improve their status. Ivan does not seem to be rapidly improving. There may be another problem.

10. What do you think is the most likely cause of Ivan's current problem?

There are two conditions, hypothermia and hypoglycemia, that are most likely the cause. In terms of hypothermia, Ivan is not unconscious but does have disorientation with ECG changes. He is probably at the moderate to severe stage. He is also hypoglycemic. Hypotension is not unusual for hypothermia but with the suspicion of trauma he may have another problem.

11. What is Ivan at risk for developing?

Dysrhythmias, the most serious is ventricular fibrillation; another injury may be missed because of his hypothermia (especially a head injury); complications from rewarming (acidosis, severe hypotension, cardiac injury); unconsciousness from untreated hypoglycemia.

12. How serious is Ivan's condition?

Ivan's condition is very serious. He is not improving at a rate that would seem normal; his hypothermia predisposes him to cardiac rhythm changes, and he is hypoglycemic. With a history of trauma a head injury is also possible.

13. What is the most likely reason behind Ivan's blood sugar level? Should it be treated?

Glucose and glycogen reserves are rapidly used when the body becomes cold. The immediate vasoconstriction in the peripheral vessels and simultaneous increase in sympathetic nervous discharge along with a catecholamine release increases basal metabolism, producing heat for the body but requiring glucose for energy. As cold exposure continues, preshivering muscle tone increases, and the body generates heat in the form of shivering. Shivering puts a great demand on all available glucose and glycogen reserves. Shivering does not stop until the core temperature reaches approximately 87.8° F (31° C), glucose or glycogen is depleted, or insulin is no longer available for glucose transfer. Hypoglycemia should be treated as soon as an IV can be established.

14. What is the most likely reason behind Ivan's ECG rate and rhythm? Should it be treated?

Atrial fibrillation can occur at any time, while bradycardia is considered a late sign of hypothermia. Hypothermic bradycardia is usually refractory to atropine. The best treatment is to prevent further heat loss and treat gently, monitoring the rhythm all the time.

15. What is the most likely reason behind Ivan's respiratory rate and BP?

As the state of hypothermia continues, energy stores are rapidly depleted. The respiratory rate slows, cardiac output drops (for two reasons, blood is shunted to the core and "hypothermic diuresis" occurs) and heart rate slows.

16. What would your initial treatment be?

The goal is to assure airway, breathing, and circulation and prevent further heat loss. (Active rewarming should take place at the hospital.) Apply oxygen by a mask non–rebreather with a reservoir at 12 to 15 lpm (warmed and humidified if possible). Start an IV of normal saline (warm by a commercial rewarmer or by wrapping IV tubing around a hot towel) and administer another bolus. Place heat packs, covered with a towel, in his groin and axilla. NOTE: These actions do not significantly increase core temperature but, instead prevent continued heat loss and may minimize the severity of the "after drop" phenomenon. Ensure that he is dry and cover him with blankets.

Administer 25 ml of 50% dextrose and water slow IVP. Move to the vehicle and turn the heater on "high."

17. Is C-spine immobilization something you would do? Why or why not?

C-spine immobilization is necessary. He has a mechanism, is disoriented, uncoordinated, and has generalized weakness. He should be immobilized until mentation significantly improves to get an accurate history and physical or c-spines are cleared in the ED.

18. Hypothermic patients should be treated very gently. Why?

A cold heart is very irritable. Rough handling, even though a pulse or rhythm is present, can trigger ventricular fibrillation.

19. In this situation, what would be most important to reassess and why?

Immediately reassess mental status, this will determine further treatment decisions. If mental status improves, continue treatment measures and prevention of heat loss. If mental status did not improve then repeat fluid boluses, continue to prevent heat loss and suspect another problem. Further reassessment would also include vital signs, especially systolic blood pressure; pulse oximetry values; changes in ECG; lung sounds, another blood sugar level, and pupil checks.

20. Is there any specific treatment for his cheeks and nose?

Not really, but they are indicators that his digits are also at risk for frostbite. They should be inspected and carefully wrapped in dry dressings if frostbite is suspected.

21. En route to the hospital Ivan begins to shiver, what is the significance of his shivering?

He is improving. Reassess his mental status to confirm and reassess his pulse. The ECG may be unreadable but look for an increase in rate. Shivering also increases metabolic rate, which could exacerbate electrolyte and endocrine problems. Consider consulting with medical control regarding the use of diazepam to control his shivering.

22. What is the difference between a dry cold exposure and a wet cold exposure?

The rate of loss of body heat. The body will lose heat 17 times faster if exposed to wet compared to dry exposure. (Water conducts heat faster than air.) Thus a person becomes hypothermic much faster. Ivan's 3-mile walk after being immersed in cold water was a double problem. It was good that he got out of the cold water, but the walk exposed him to heat loss from evaporation, as well as conduction. He is lucky he made it home.

23. What is the "after-drop" phenomenon?

The phenomenon refers to the tendency for the body's core temperature to continue to drop, even after the patient's removal from the environment. It is thought to be a result of the combined effects of the deep tissues continuing to lose heat to surrounding tissues and the return of cold blood from the extremities to the trunk. This is why there is no effective way to significantly rewarm a hypothermic patient in the field. It is more important for prehospital care providers to prevent further heat loss.

OUTCOME

Ivan was immobilized and given oxygen by a mask non-rebreather with reservoir at 15 lpm. An IV was started and 25 ml of $D_{50}W$ administered slow IVP. Within minutes Ivan's mental status improved to full orientation and his pulse increased to 110. Violent shivering began shortly thereafter. Diazepam 5 mg slow IV push was administered to control shivering. On arrival at the ED, a warming blanket was ready and rewarming was continued. His core temperature was 88° F (32° C), lab tests were done, and he was admitted for moderate hypothermia. His atrial fibrillation converted when his core temperature reached 90° F (33° C). No other injuries were discovered other than the frostbite of his cheeks and nose. Those areas developed a black eschar, which sloughed off. His nose required plastic repair. He was dismissed without any further problem. However, his face remained extremely sensitive to the cold thereafter.

CASE 4

Dispatch: 00:24 hrs—All available police and fire units in area of 23rd and Montrose Avenue, missing 4 y/o, dressed in robe and pajamas
00:45 hrs—Unconscious 4 y/o female, in alley between 26th and 27th street at Vernon Avenue

On Arrival: You find 4 y/o Callie, curled in the fetal position, dressed in a robe and pajamas. It is bitterly cold out and she is lying on her side in the snow. She is unresponsive.

Initial Assessment Findings

Mental Status—Unresponsive to voice and touch
Airway—Open and clear
Breathing—R none detected; lung sounds none
Circulation—Skin on face white, mottled extremities, cold and hard to the touch
> Pulse faint carotid
> BP none taken

Chief Complaint—Unresponsive, cold exposure

Focused History

Events—Police officers state her mother noticed her missing and when searching through the house noticed the back door open. When she saw footprints outside in the snow and did not see any sign of Callie, she called the police. Police officers and firefighters in the immediate area followed the footprints and found her several blocks from her home. EMS was a block away.
Previous Illness—None
Current Health Status—Good
Allergies—None known
Medications—None known

Focused Physical

Current set of VS—P faint carotid at 30, R none detected, BP none taken
Other Pertinent Findings—Callie was in a fetal position, her legs and arms were flexed, there were no abrasions or signs of trauma noted; pupils were dilated and fixed
Diagnostic Tests—None necessary

ECG

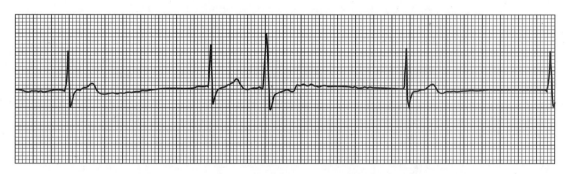

Figure 10-4

QUESTIONS

1. What is significant about Callie's history?

2. What body systems are affected?

3. What is Callie's Glascow Coma Score?

4. How would you describe her ECG?

5. What is the best explanation for Callie's mottled extremities?

6. Is there any other information either from Callie's history or your physical assessment that you need to know?

7. What do you think is the most likely cause of Callie's current problem?

8. What is the best explanation for Callie's ECG?

9. What is Callie at risk for developing?

10. How serious is Callie's condition?

11. Medics did not get Callie's blood pressure. Should that have been obtained?

12. What would your initial treatment be?

13. If you knew her core temperature was 82° F (28° C), would that have changed your treatment?

14. Callie's heart rate was 30, and she was unresponsive. AHA and PALS advocate doing CPR on young children when heart rates are too slow to support perfusion. Should CPR be done on Callie?

15. Why is gentle handling an extremely important consideration?

16. On arrival at the hospital while Callie is moved from the gurney to the ED cart, she fibrillates. What is your immediate response?

17. What is the difference between a pediatric and adult hypothermic patient?

18. If Callie did not have a pulse, should she have been pronounced in the field?

QUESTIONS AND ANSWERS

1. *What is significant about Callie's history?*

Relatively unprotected exposure to extreme cold for an unknown time; previously healthy child

2. *What body systems are affected?*

CNS—unconscious, unresponsive
Cardiovascular—weak carotid pulse, bradycardic; lack of perfusion
Respiratory—none detected

3. *What is Callie's Glascow Coma Score?*

GCS 3 (1 eye opening; 1 verbal response; 1 motor response)

4. *How would you describe her ECG?*

Bradycardia (lack of P wave indicates a probable junctional rhythm) with one premature (probable PVC) beat.

5. *What is the best explanation for Callie's mottled extremities?*

Cold, mottled skin indicates pooling of blood in the capillary beds.

6. *Is there any other information either from Callie's history or your physical assessment that you need to know?*

There is enough information to be able to treat. However, taking a core temperature is a priority. Additional information that will be needed later on will be a thorough explanation of exactly how Callie was exposed to ensure that child neglect or abuse was not involved.

7. *What do you think is the most likely cause of Callie's current problem?*

Her history is consistent with severe hypothermia.

8. *What is the best explanation for Callie's ECG?*

Callie has a junctional bradycardia with a premature beat. Hypothermia predisposes to bradycardia for several reasons. Initial responses to a fall in body temperature causes shivering and increased muscle tone, resulting in increased metabolism to maintain the body temperature. When this additional heat production can no longer keep up with heat lost from the body surface, or the body's stores of energy are used up, the body's temperature regulating mechanism fails and the body rapidly loses heat. Electrolyte and endocrine imbalances are common. Enzyme systems necessary for metabolic function fail, because of the cold temperature. The metabolic rate falls and the heart cannot keep up, either because of expended energy and/or because of enzyme systems that cannot work. Thus the heart goes from the tachycardia of early hypothermia to the bradycardia of severe hypothermia.

9. *What is Callie at risk for developing?*

Ventricular fibrillation

10. *How serious is Callie's condition?*

This is an immediate threat to life.

11. *Medics did not get Callie's blood pressure. Should that have been obtained?*

No. If her arms are flexed and fixed in that position, do not try to force the joints to move. You can cause tissue damage. Obtaining a BP at this point will not aid in treatment.

12. *What would your initial treatment be?*

Initial treatment is designed to prevent further heat loss. Gently move her to the back of the vehicle. Turn up the heater as much as possible. Carefully remove clothing and cover with warm blankets. Use a bag-valve-mask with a reservoir and ventilate at a rate of 20/min, preferably with warm, humidified oxygen. An oral airway or intubation may be necessary to secure the airway. It is important to treat Callie as gently as possible. Follow your local protocols.

13. *If you knew her core temperature was 82° F (28° C), would that have changed your treatment?*

No. Absence of shivering indicates a temperature below 89° to 87° F, fixed dilated pupils indicates severe hypothermia <86° F (<30° C). Your assessment findings already indicated severe hypothermia.

14. *Callie's heart rate was 30, and she was unresponsive. AHA and PALS advocate doing CPR on young children when heart rates are too slow to support perfusion. Should CPR be done on Callie?*

No, she has a pulse, even though it is faint and bradycardic, it is functioning and some perfusion to the brain is occurring. Hypothermia stimulates the body to shunt blood only to the major organs. Such rough handling as CPR will likely irritate the vagal nerve, resulting in asystole or fibrillation.

15. *Why is gentle handling an extremely important consideration?*

Hypothermia causes the heart to become particularly sensitive and very irritable. Increased irritability and increased sensitivity predisposes to asystole or fibrillation. Both of which are resistant to defibrillation until a certain core temperature is reached. This is because enzyme systems necessary for the efficient function of the heart are no longer working.

16. *On arrival at the hospital while Callie is moved from the gurney to the ED cart, she fibrillates. What is your immediate response?*

Begin chest compressions. Defibrillation in the hypothermic patient tends to be unsuccessful until a certain core temperature is reached. Current AHA guidelines advocate attempting up to three shocks with a hypothermic adult patient in ventricular fibrillation. If that fails to convert the rhythm, attempt no additional shocks until the patient is rewarmed. Follow your local protocols.

17. *What is the difference between a pediatric and adult hypothermic patient?*

A pediatric patient is more vulnerable to cold exposure because of a proportionately larger body surface area for their weight than adults. Their temperature regulation mechanism is also less well developed so their heat conservation efforts are less effective. But perhaps one of the biggest differences is the fact that children can survive severe cold exposure better than adults, with less side effects.

18. *If Callie did not have a pulse, should she have been pronounced in the field?*

No, patients aren't dead until they are warm and dead.

OUTCOME

Callie was moved to the vehicle, oxygenated with a bag-valve-mask, clothing removed, and heated blankets applied. On arrival at the hospital, she converted to v-fib when being transferred to the cot. CPR was started while a rectal temperature was obtained and a pediatric bypass machine readied. Callie was intubated and placed on pediatric bypass. Her body temperature was gradually warmed, her heart converted to a sinus rhythm at 88° F (31° C). She continued to improve, responding to touch by flexion. Three days later she was obeying command. Callie suffered frostbite on her toes and fingers but did not have any other serious problem. Ten days after admission she was dismissed to home, neurologically intact.

Her parents stated that Callie had always had a fascination for snow. The day of the incident, her father found her walking out in the snow after dinner. Her mother then hung up Callie's coat thinking that if she put her coat away, that Callie would not go outside. Evidently, Callie woke up in the night and decided to go outside anyway.

BIBLIOGRAPHY

Berkow, R. & Fletcher, A. J. (Eds.). (1992). *Merck manual of diagnosis and therapy.* Rahway, NJ: Merck Research Laboratories.

Chameides, L. & Hazinski, M. F. (Eds.). American Heart Association (1994). *Textbook of pediatric advanced life support.* Dallas, TX: American Heart Association.

Cummins, R. O. (Ed.). American Heart Association. (1994). *Advanced cardiac life support textbook.* Dallas, TX: American Heart Association.

Eichelberger, M. R., Ball, J. W., Pratsch, G. L., & Clark, J. R. (1998). *Pediatric emergencies,* (2nd ed.). Upper Saddle River, NJ: Prentice Hall.

Hofftrand, H. (1997). Environmental problems: Accidental hypothermia and frostbite. In R. M. Barkin (Ed.). *Pediatric emergency medicine: Concepts in clinical medicine.* St. Louis: Mosby.

Kelley, S. J. (1994). *Pediatric emergency nursing,* (2nd ed.). Norwalk, CT: Appleton & Lange.

Kohl, J. (1996). Heat stroke. *American Journal of Nursing,* 96(7), 51.

Ludwig-Beymer, P., Huether, S. E., & Schoessler, M. (1994). Pain, temperature regulation, sleep, and sensory function. In K. L. McCance & S. E. Huether (Eds.). *Pathophysiology: The biologic basis for disease in adults and children,* (2nd ed.). St. Louis, MO: Mosby.

Macho, J. R. & Schechter, W. P. (1994). Care of patients with environmental injuries. In F. S. Bongard and D. Y. Sue (Eds.). *Current: Critical care, diagnosis and treatment.* Norwalk, CT: Appleton & Lange.

Martini, F. H. & Bartholomew, E. F. (1997). *Essentials of anatomy and physiology.* Upper Saddle River, NJ: Prentice Hall.

Parks, F. B. & Calabro, J. J. (1990). Hyperthermia: Performing when the heat is on. *Journal of Emergency Medical Services,* (8), 24-32.

Sanders, M. (1994). Environmental emergencies. In *Mosby's paramedic textbook.* St. Louis: Mosby.

Semenza, J. C., Rubin, C. H., Falter, K. H., Selanikio, J. D., Flanders, W. D., Howe, H. L., & Wilhelm, J. L. (1996). Heat-related deaths during the July 1995 heat wave in Chicago. *New England Journal of Medicine,* 335 (2), 84-90.

Tierney, L. M., McPhee, S. J., & Papadakis, M. A. (Eds.). (1994). *Current: Medical diagnosis and treatment.* Norwalk, CT: Appleton & Lange.

11

Behavioral Emergencies

OVERVIEW

A behavioral emergency implies a behavior pattern that is presenting a threat to the well-being or life of the person exhibiting the behavior. Such a behavior may also present a threat to the well-being or life of another. The dilemma with behavioral emergencies is to define "normal" behavior. There is no clear definition of what normal is or even what it means. Ideas of normal vary by culture/ethnic group and family norms. The concept of abnormal behavior implies behavior that deviates from society's norms and expectations. From a holistic point of view, this behavior then interferes with the patient's well-being and the ability to function. The behavior may also be harmful to the individual or to a group. The concept of a behavioral emergency is one where the behavior that is being exhibited is threatening to the patient or to others. It is unanticipated and requires immediate intervention by emergency responders. Behavioral emergencies cover a wide range of disturbances. In general, most are emotionally painful states that cause suffering.

Anatomy, Physiology, and Psychopathology

Behavioral emergencies can be divided into emotional and psychiatric disorders. This group of disorders covers a broad range of conditions of varying severity, characterized by abnormal or maladaptive behaviors. Causes may be biologic as in diseases, tumors, or toxins; or psychosocial as in childhood trauma or parental deprivation; or sociocultural such as war, rape, or death of a loved one. The result is a disturbance in normal functioning that may be temporary or chronic. Biologic causes are also known as organic or physical. Mental causes are known as psychological.

Some conditions, such as manic-depressive or bipolar syndrome and depression are known to involve imbalances of chemicals important to brain function, such as lithium, dopamine, and serotonin. Other conditions, such as hyperglycemia, hypoglycemia, and hypoxia, are temporary and curable. They are also known for their sometimes bizarre effect on brain function. The dementias, specifically Alzheimer's disease, have an organic cause and are specifically known to affect the older population group. Eating disorders, such as bulimia and anorexia, are thought to have a psychological origin and are known for affecting younger population groups, primarily teenage girls.

Recreational drugs, such as methamphetamines or cocaine, and drug interactions, such as cheese in the presence of an MAO inhibitor, are also known for their effect on brain function and thus may manifest as abnormal behavior. Other conditions, such as schizophrenia have origins that are not so well defined but are thought to also involve biochemical imbalances.

There are also behavioral emergencies that are situationally induced. These may be temporary, such as the sudden shock of a motor vehicle crash, or chronic, such as a phobia or panic attack.

Behavioral emergencies may also exhibit characteristic behaviors. Agitation, disordered thought, thought broadcasting (the belief that thoughts are broadcast aloud), accelerated speech, paranoia, hallucinations, and clouding of consciousness are just some of the behaviors that can be noted. Two of these, hallucinations and clouding of consciousness, bear further explanation.

Hallucinations may occur with any of the five senses. Tactile (touch) hallucinations are more likely to have a medical cause, such as drug withdrawal or overdose. Gustatory (taste) and olfactory (smell) hallucinations are frequently associated with seizures. Auditory hallucinations are more common with psychological conditions. Visual hallucinations may occur with either medical or psychological conditions. Auditory hallucinations have several presentations. Patients may only hear murmuring or the patient may hear relatively distinct voices where the number of voices and gender can be identified but exactly what is being said is not understood. Clear and distinct voices the patient can understand, occur in two types, a running commentary or conversational voice and a command voice. A patient may have both types occurring either simultaneously or independently of one another. It is important to ask if a patient is hearing voices and what the voices are saying. The answers to those questions have a direct bearing on your immediate safety, safety of the scene, and the potential for violence.

Clouding of consciousness is a term used when a patient suddenly seems to lose his or her train of thought in the middle of a sentence. After a short period, the conversation is picked up where it left off. This is considered a sign of a physical or organic problem. One frequent cause is brain injury with a subdural hematoma being a frequent finding.

Assessment

Assessment of the patient with a behavioral emergency begins with scene evaluation. The priority is to determine if a violent or potentially unsafe situation exists. Consider the need for law enforcement. In the absence of obvious danger, observe the scene for information to assist with patient assessment and care. Look for signs of violence, evidence of substance abuse, general environmental conditions, and any clue that might indicate a previously existing medical problem, such as diabetes. The initial assessment includes a rapid assessment of the ABCs, limiting the number of people around the patient, and maintaining alertness to danger. Observe overt behavior of the patient (language, intellect, thought, mood, and activity) and body language (posture and gestures). Note evidence of emotion out of proportion to the event (rage, elation, hostility, depression, fear, confusion). The focused history and physical should center on questions regarding the immediate problem, establishing a rapport using therapeutic interviewing techniques and noting physical findings.

Assessment of cognitive function such as orientation to person, place, and time; perception of reality, presence of disorganized thought, evidence of delusions, hallucinations, and disorganized speech are all significant findings.

Determination of lethality is specifically important with the depressed patient. Asking if a person intends to harm themselves is appropriate and necessary. Asking if a plan has been made and how much has been carried out also impacts your safety and those around you.

It is also important to remember that patients with psychological problems may have physical problems as well. In patients who suffer from delusions or hallucinations, the determination of the presence of a physical problem can be a challenge. Often the patient with a coexisting psychological problem will word the symptoms of the physical problem in terms of their delusion or illusion. For example, a patient who suffers from delusions may word their abdominal pain in terms of the "mice that are eating my guts." It is very important to be alert to any statement that may suggest a physical complaint.

Treatment

Management of a patient with a behavioral emergency centers on maintaining safety, controlling violent situations, treating medical problems (hypoglycemia or hypoxia), and avoiding judgments. Knowing what community resources are available is also helpful. These resources can be utilized when more traditional methods for care and transport are either unnecessary or unsuccessful. This is particularly useful in the case of an emotional crisis such as a sudden death. For example, calling in SIDS counselors for parents grieving the death of their baby may be the most appropriate action.

If a patient is suffering a delusion, it is very important *not* to talk about the delusion as if you can "see" or "hear" what the patient sees and hears. Delusions are extremely complex and serve a purpose. If the caregiver tries to go along with the delusion, the deception will be discovered and, at best, the caregiver risks losing whatever rapport was developed. At its worst, the caregiver may precipitate a violent event. Appropriate statements are the honest ones. The caregiver may state that they cannot see or hear what the patient can, so the caregiver needs the patient's help by telling the caregiver what is being seen or heard.

Decisions need to be made regarding when and where to transport, use of restraints, consent, and other aspects of patient care specific to behavioral emergencies. Local protocols should be followed regarding the use of restraints, implementing emergency protective care orders, and use of law enforcement.

CASE 1

Dispatch: 11:00 hrs; police request; a 50 y/o female, medical problem, nature unknown

On Arrival: Earline answers your knock at the door wrapped in aluminum foil with Christmas lights draped across her shoulders. Police are there because Earline called for help, stating arrows were flying through her windows. Police state there are no arrows and during their conversation with her they noticed that she was talking to herself and occasionally her answers to questions did not make sense to them. They think this is a problem for EMS.

Initial Assessment Findings
Language—Clear, rapid speech with a loud voice
Intellect—Intact, oriented to person, place, and time
Thought—Content is delusional, Martians across the street
Mood—Fearful, afraid of what will happen
Activity—Agitated, pacing, clutching at chest

Physical Assessment
Airway—Open and patent
Breathing—R regular at 20
Circulation—Skin appears pale on her face, cool and dry
      Pulse regular at 96
      BP 156/92
Physical Complaint—When asked if anything hurts, yells "Can't you see those arrows! Stop those damn arrows!"

Focused History
Events—Earline states she noticed the arrows coming in her apartment about an hour ago, they are getting worse and she needs them to stop. As she talks, her rate of speech increases, her voice gets louder, and her agitation increases.
Previous Illness—Schizophrenia, hypertension
Current Health Status—Good
Allergies—None known
Medications—Risperdal (risperidone), Tenormin (atenolol)

Focused Physical
Current Set of VS—P 96, R 20, BP 156/92
Other Pertinent Findings—None found, would not allow pulse oximetry

ECG: Would not allow

QUESTIONS

1. What is significant about Earline's history?

2. What body system(s) is/are being affected?

3. What is the absolute first priority when caring for a patient such as Earline?

4. You ask if you can remove some of the aluminum foil to do a better assessment. She becomes even more agitated and somewhat belligerent, stating she needs it for protection. What should you do?

5. What is the significance of the officer's description of her behavior before your arrival?

6. Earline begins to talk to herself. You listen to what she is saying and it is as if you are listening to a one-sided conversation. What should you do, if anything?

7. What is the implication of Earline's response to being asked if anything hurts?

8. You tell Earline that you can't see the arrows but know that she can, so she needs to help you and tell you where the arrows are. Earline becomes very agitated and tells you, "Can't you see? All 24 are hitting my chest!" Why is this a significant statement?

9. Is there any additional information that might be helpful?

10. What do you think is the cause of Earline's current problem?

11. What is Earline at risk for?

12. What is important to remember about delusions in acutely psychotic patients?

13. How would you get Earline to accept treatment?

14. At one point Earline was asked what the Martians were saying to her. She stated that the Martians were angry at her but she couldn't understand what they were saying. What stage of auditory hallucinations was she demonstrating?

15. Earline is exhibiting illusions and delusions. What is the difference between the two?

QUESTIONS AND ANSWERS

1. **What is significant about Earline's history?**
   Evidence of delusions, previous history of schizophrenia and hypertension

2. **What body system(s) is/are being affected?**
   CNS—The immediate impression is the CNS with impaired cognition.

3. **What is the absolute first priority when caring for a patient such as Earline?**
   Your safety first, then the safety of your partner, then safety of the patient, in that order.

4. **You ask if you can remove some of the aluminum foil to do a better assessment. She becomes even more agitated and somewhat belligerent, stating she needs it for protection. What should you do?**
   Leave it alone. This is part of her delusion. Delusions tend to be very complicated and highly structured. You don't want to become a threat to her, nor do you want to provoke any violence.

5. **What is the significance of the officer's description of her behavior before your arrival?**
   The police officers state that they noticed that she was talking to herself and occasionally her answers to questions did not make sense to them. Earline may be hearing voices.

6. **Earline begins to talk to herself. You listen to what she is saying and it is as if you are listening to a one-sided conversation. What should you do, if anything?**
   This is highly suspicious for auditory hallucinations. It is very important that you ask her if she is hearing someone talk to her. Most patients with this type of condition are honest and will tell you the truth. If the answer is affirmative, then ask what the voice(s) is/are saying. The answer is important for you in determining scene safety. In this case, Earline tells you that the Martians are angry at her but she can't understand what they are saying.

7. **What is the implication of Earline's response to being asked if anything hurts?**
   Her response was "Can't you see those arrows?" This suggests that Earline is also having visual hallucinations and appears to be associating the "arrows" with some type of discomfort.

8. **You tell Earline that you can't see the arrows but know that she can, so she needs to help you and tell you where the arrows are. Earline becomes very agitated and tells you, "Can't you see? All 24 are hitting my chest!" Why is this a significant statement?**
   Earline may be telling you she is having chest pain, with 24 arrows the pain sounds significant. She is describing her symptoms in terms of her delusion.

9. **Is there any additional information that might be helpful?**
   Has she taken her medication? Does she have a social worker or someone who looks in on her? Are the "arrows" striking her anywhere else? In some communities it may be appropriate to ask her which physician/psychiatrist she sees.

10. **What do you think is the cause of Earline's current problem?**
    She is having an acute episode of her chronic schizophrenia that may be complicated by chest pain, which could be angina or an acute MI.

11. **What is Earline is at risk for?**
    Earline is at risk for dysrhythmias or cardiac arrest. Violence is also a risk.

12. **What is important to remember about delusions in acutely psychotic patients?**
    Delusions are created to fulfill a need. They tend to be highly complicated and extremely structured. If you buy into the delusion, for instance tell Earline that you see the Martians too, it will not take long for her to discover that you really don't know anything about the structure she has created. You will lose all credibility with her and may provoke her anger. Instead, respect the delusion but be very honest about what you cannot see or hear. For instance, you can tell her that you believe that *she* can see and hear the Martians, but you cannot, so she will have to tell you what they are saying and where the arrows are.

13. How would you get Earline to accept treatment?

You can present treatment in terms of her delusion. But *do not* buy into the delusion. For instance, you can tell her you have some oxygen that may help her with the pain (or discomfort) she is feeling from those arrows. But you cannot see the arrows so she will have to tell you if it works. You can try the same thing with the nitro. Show it to her and explain it in the same way.

The real challenge will be in getting her to your vehicle. She is the best one to tell you how she will feel protected when you take her outside. Remember, she is feeling chest pain, so to tell her that the Martian's can't get her when she is in your vehicle may mislead her into thinking that once she is there she will feel no pain and/or she will have no arrows. You can't guarantee she will have no chest pain. It may be more accurate to say that you will take her to a place where they can help her with the pain from the arrows she sees.

In situations like this, respect the delusion; don't buy into it; be honest and do the best you can. No technique ever works all the time in all situations. If you follow these simple guidelines, you will have a greater chance of success.

14. At one point Earline was asked what the Martians were saying to her. She stated that the Martians were angry with her but she couldn't understand what they were saying. What is significant regarding this description of auditory hallucinations?

There are five general types of auditory hallucinations. One type is manifested by murmuring; another consists of voices but the gender and number are not distinguished; in a third type the gender and number are distinguishable but what is being said is not understood. The last two types are most important. In the fourth type the number of voices and gender are clear, as is what is being said; however, the voice is typically a running commentary. The last type is most dangerous and is a command voice. The running commentary and command voices can change between one another without warning. It is particularly important to discover if the command voice is suicidal/homicidal. Earline is hearing the third type.

15. Earline is exhibiting illusions and delusions. What is the difference between the two?

An illusion is a misinterpretation of stimuli in the environment. Illusions occur in everyday life (e.g., a magic show consists of illusions). Normally, when evidence is given to correct the misinterpretation, the illusion no longer exists. However, when the evidence is discounted then the illusion is termed a *delusion*. In a psychotic patient, a delusion is an irrational belief that is contrary to reality and persists despite evidence and common sense to the contrary.

OUTCOME

Earline was given oxygen by mask and two doses of nitroglycerin sublingually but refused an IV and the cardiac monitor. She was taken to the medic unit on the stretcher but with her face covered by a black blanket (the oxygen was on so she could breathe) and aluminum foil wrapped around each leg. She had not taken her medication for 3 days, which probably explained her acute psychosis. On arrival at the ED risperidone was administered. She allowed a monitor and eventually an IV. After blood was drawn, she was admitted to the CCU. Earline had developed unstable angina. Her medication was adjusted, and she was dismissed after 3 days, with no delusions.

CASE 2

Dispatch: 19:30 hrs; 36 y/o male, attempted suicide, police en route, unknown if weapons involved

On Arrival: The police arrive the same time as you and enter the apartment first. After about 5 minutes one officer exits and gestures for you to enter. You find 36 y/o Guiseppie, sitting in an overstuffed chair in the living room. The apartment is very clean and almost bare, but there are paper wads scattered on the floor by the kitchen door. Guiseppie is clean but disheveled and looks like he has slept in his clothing.

Initial Assessment Findings

Language—Speaks in a low tone and slowly, words are understandable
Intellect—Oriented to person, place, and time
Thought—States he isn't worth anything, the world would be better off without him
Mood—Depressed
Activity—Slow and measured

Physical Assessment

Airway—Open and clear
Breathing—R 14 and regular
Circulation—Skin normal color, warm, and dry
        Radial pulse regular at 72
        BP 124/72
Physical Complaint—States he is very tired

Focused History

Events—His wife is divorcing him, he lost his job earlier this week, and this morning he discovered that his car was stolen. He decided that he just couldn't take it anymore and came into the house, called his estranged wife and told her she wouldn't have to worry about him, just give his clothes to the Goodwill and there was enough money in the bank account to buy a headstone. Then he said good-bye and hung up. She immediately called 9-1-1.
Previous Illness—Insulin dependent diabetic, diagnosed depression
Current Health Status—Good
Allergies—None known
Medications—Humulin 70/30 (insulin), Paxil (paroxetine)

Focused Physical

Current Set of VS—P 72, R 14, BP 124/72
Other Pertinent Findings—Blood sugar 90, no other pertinent findings

ECG: Not done

QUESTIONS

1. What is your first priority in this situation?

2. What is significant about Guiseppie's history?

3. What body systems are affected?

4. What condition is suggested by his slow speech, low tones, and complaint of fatigue?

5. Differentiation between psychiatric (functional) and organic causes of psychosis is important. What assessment findings could help in this case?

6. What is the importance of the paper wads on the floor? What, if anything, do you do with them?

7. While your partner is questioning Guiseppie, you are casually looking around. What are you looking for?

8. While your partner is getting the rest of the history, you glance in the bedroom and notice a suit of clothes laid out on the bed with a tie, set of underwear, and clean socks beside the suit. What is the implication?

9. After your partner has introduced himself and obtained a history, he asks Guiseppie if he has thought of hurting himself. Explain if this is, or is not, an appropriate question.

10. If Guiseppie admitted to thoughts of suicide, what question should your partner immediately ask?

11. What is Guiseppie at risk for?

12. How serious is this situation for Guiseppie?

13. Guiseppie admitted to thoughts of suicide and planning to inject himself with all his insulin. He refuses to answer questions asking him if he has done that yet and you could find no insulin bottles in the apartment. You have decided to transport and start treatment en route. Should a bolus of $D_{50}W$ be given at this point?

14. If Guiseppie had injected himself with all his insulin, but his initial blood sugar was 90, what signs or symptoms would alert you to a falling blood sugar?

15. What is Paxil (paroxetine), and how does it work?

16. Is diabetes a factor in depression?

QUESTIONS AND ANSWERS

1. *What is your first priority in this situation?*

   Your safety first, the safety of your partner next, and then the safety of your patient, in that order.

2. *What is significant about Guiseppie's history?*

   Divorce, loss of job, and stolen car; content of phone call; insulin dependent diabetic; diagnosed depression.

3. *What body systems are affected?*

   CNS—The immediate impression is the CNS with his affect, slow speech, low tones, slow rate of activity.

4. *What condition is suggested by his slow speech, low tones, and complaint of fatigue?*

   These signs and symptoms are consistent with depression.

5. *Differentiation between psychiatric (functional) and organic causes of psychosis is important. What assessment findings could help in this case?*

   Mental status, particularly orientation to person, place, time, and mentation, as well as blood sugar levels.

6. *What is the importance of the paper wads on the floor? What, if anything, do you do with them?*

   They could be vitally important. Find out what they contain. You may discover suicide notes, to-do lists before committing the suicide, or indicators of intent to do bodily harm. If you find any note or list, give them to the officers. Treat them as you would anything else considered evidence.

7. *While your partner is questioning Guiseppie, you are casually looking around. What are you looking for?*

   Anything that may be out of the ordinary, any other persons there, any weapons, any indication of the intent to do harm or the method to be used.

8. *While your partner is getting the rest of the history, you glance in the bedroom and notice a suit of clothes laid out on the bed with a tie, set of underwear, and clean socks beside the suit. What is the implication?*

   This suggests that he is preparing to go somewhere. He may be preparing the clothing he will wear for his burial.

9. *After your partner has introduced himself and obtained a history, he asks Guiseppie if he has thought of hurting himself. Explain if this is, or is not, an appropriate question.*

   This is a necessary question to establish an intent and the potential for harm. Do not be afraid of suggesting something that he has not already thought. Guiseppie may or may not be truthful; many times people contemplating suicide are more truthful than you would think. Usually an admission of thoughts of suicide is enough to place them under arrest or protective custody.

10. *If Guiseppie admitted to thoughts of suicide, what question should your partner immediately ask?*

    Ask if he has a plan or how he planned on doing it. You need to discover if there is a weapon and where it is, if he has taken any drugs, or if he has arranged something else that could be of harm to you, himself, or to anyone else. Scene safety is the important factor here. The police officers may take over questioning at this point.

11. *What is Guiseppie at risk for?*

    He is at risk for harming himself, harming someone else, or a diabetic reaction.

12. *How serious is this situation for Guiseppie?*

    Just with his affect, Guiseppie is giving evidence of depression. With his actions (clothing laid out, phone call to estranged wife) he suggests that suicide is a definite possibility. Guiseppie is acutely depressed and the situation is serious.

13. Guiseppie admitted to thoughts of suicide and planning to inject himself with all his insulin. He refuses to answer questions asking him if he has done that yet and you could find no insulin bottles in the apartment. You have decided to transport and start treatment en route. Should a bolus of $D_{50}W$ be given at this point?

> This is a situation where consulting medical control would be advisable. Starting an IV and retesting his blood sugar every few minutes, is a reasonable decision. However, by the time a drop is detected, his blood glucose level may be falling precipitously. If there is reason to believe that Guiseppie is telling the truth, an argument could be made for administering a bolus of $D_{50}W$ as a preventive against a precipitous drop, especially since you have no way of knowing how much he took. Reassessing his mental status, vital signs and skin color, temperature, and moisture will be very important. Maintaining the rapport established at the scene and transporting to the nearest appropriate facility would also be necessary.

14. If Guiseppie had injected himself with all his insulin, but his initial blood sugar was 90, what signs or symptoms would alert you to a falling blood sugar?

> Altered mental status and changes in his skin, especially color and sweating. If his blood sugar dropped fast enough, grand mal seizures may occur.

15. What is Paxil (paroxetine), and how does it work?

> Paroxetine is a serotonin-reuptake inhibitor. Serotonin and norepinephrine are neurotransmitters produced in the brain. Serotonin has a depressant effect and induces sleep. Norepinephrine has an excitatory (or inhibitory in some areas) effect and promotes wakefulness and euphoria. One or both neurotransmitters may be involved in depression.

16. Is diabetes a factor in depression?

> It can be. However, the disease process itself is not generally thought to cause depression. Rather the chronicity of the disease is thought to be "depressing" in nature and may be more of a factor. However, although some research suggests that there may be a physiologic link, it is difficult to say whether the link is due to the need for sugar by the brain, physiologic changes that may be induced by the disease diabetes mellitus, or by the knowledge by the patient of the implications of the disease.

OUTCOME

Guiseppie remained quiet and was not talking while en route to the ED. His blood sugar remained stable at 88 mg/dl. Time at the scene and transport time was short, 10 minutes. On arrival at the ED, his blood sugar was 80 mg/dl. Shortly after arrival, he suffered a grand mal seizure. Another blood sugar was immediately obtained, his blood sugar value at that time was 20 mg/dl. His IV had been started in a forearm vein and well secured so it remained patent. One amp of 25 gs of D_{50} administered IVP appeared to stop the seizure activity. After 15 minutes, Guiseppie remained unresponsive and in a postictal state. A repeat blood sugar was 35 mg/dl so a second dose of 25 gms of D_{50} was administered. Guiseppie then became responsive to verbal stimuli. He was subsequently admitted to the ICU. He was transferred 4 days later to a psychiatric institution for acute depression.

12

Communicable Diseases

OVERVIEW

Communicable diseases can present with a wide variety of signs and symptoms, depending on the nature of the infection. It is important to note that not all infections are communicable. For instance, ulcers, gall bladder disease, and pancreatitis are not communicable. However, certain types of hepatitis (Hepatitis A, B, and C), measles, influenza, tuberculosis, certain types of pneumonia, and the common cold are all communicable. As healthcare providers, we are expected to have a high index of suspicion for recognizing the potential for a communicable disease to exist.

Anatomy, Physiology, and Pathophysiology

Communicable diseases are infections generally caused by bacteria, viruses, fungus, or parasites. Once an organism has breached the surface defenses and invaded the body, an inflammatory response occurs. The affected tissues are surrounded by cells and fluids whose purpose it is to isolate, destroy, and remove the foreign substance and promote healing. The general effect is to increase circulation, the number of white blood cells, and the temperature of that immediate area. Therefore when an infection is localized, the area is swollen, reddened, warm or hot to the touch, and painful.

If the localized inflammatory response is unsuccessful, the body's next response is the cell-mediated immune response. This immune response involves formation of specific antibodies to identify specific antigens (foreign substances) and kill them. At this point the infection usually becomes systemic. During this process of forming antibodies, additional chemicals are released that stimulate the hypothalamus to reset the body's temperature at a higher point. This results in fever. The purpose of a fever is to increase the efficiency of the immune response while the increased temperature itself is damaging to most foreign invaders.

The type of organism and the organ system affected will often determine the signs and symptoms observed. Signs and symptoms can arise directly from the infecting organism or its products; however, the majority of signs and symptoms result from responses mounted by the body. Infectious diseases typically begin with general, nonspecific symptoms of fatigue, weakness, and loss of energy. Generalized aching and loss of appetite are additional common complaints. Further symptoms usually depend on the organ system affected. For example, if the lungs are the target organ, a dry cough progressing to a productive cough associated with chest pain may be common. An infection involving the gastrointestinal tract (gastroenteritis) may cause profuse diarrhea associated with spasmodic abdominal pain. The central nervous system is the target for meningitis, which may cause altered mental status with headache and photophobia associated with neck pain and stiffness. Each organ system, when affected, has its own particular type of complaint. The organ system affected can be deduced with an understanding of the anatomy, physiology, and pathophysiology of that system.

Fever

The hallmark of most infectious diseases is fever. Fever is body temperature regulated at a higher level than normal and is a beneficial protective mechanism. The interaction of the body's immune response with the agents of infection may excrete substances (pyrogens or endotoxins) that stimulate other chemicals (cytokinins such as interleukin, prostaglandins, etc.), which then cause the hypothalamus to reset body temperature to a higher level. Fever helps the body by killing many microorganisms; decreasing serum levels of iron, zinc, and copper needed for bacterial replication; stimulating destruction of cells; preventing viral replication; and increasing the efficiency of the body's immune system.

Presence of a fever has other effects too. Resetting of the body's temperature level causes the cells to increase their metabolic rate to maintain the fever. An increase in metabolic rate also increases nutrient and oxygen demand of the tissues and increases production of waste products. Heart rate and respiratory rate increase to help satisfy the demand for nutrients, oxygen, and waste removal. In general, children are better able to tolerate fevers than adults.

There are some effects of fever at the extremes of age that differ. The elderly may have a decreased or absent fever response to infection so the associated benefits are not present. As a result of the lack of fever response, the elderly have a higher morbidity and mortality. On the other hand, children develop higher temperatures than adults for relatively minor infections and, under the age of 5, have a greater tendency to precipitously raise body temperature. As a result of precipitous rising of temperatures, they are also more likely to develop febrile seizures. Febrile seizures usually occur with a rise to a temperature greater than 100.5° F (38° C) over a short period. In general, the faster the fever rises the more likely a seizure will occur. Febrile seizures in adults are not as common. At 106° F (41° C) nerve irritation and damage is more likely to produce a seizure in the adult.

Simple febrile seizures are generalized and brief, seldom lasting longer than 10 minutes. Complex febrile seizures are prolonged and may be focal. The most common cause of febrile seizures in children is ear infection. The most serious cause of febrile seizures is meningitis.

Rash

Another frequent finding, especially in childhood diseases, is the appearance of a rash. A rash is usually due to the body's reaction to chemicals, known as endotoxins, produced by the invading organism. Systemic infections such as chickenpox, measles, and roseola are all associated with characteristic skin eruptions. In chickenpox, the rash generally begins on the trunk as small red spots that become raised, fluid-filled blisters. The rash spreads to the face and throughout the body. After the blisters form scabs, the child begins to recover. Measles and roseola begin with high fevers, followed by a fine, red rash that begins on the face and spreads to the trunk and rest of the body. Many viral infections can cause a rash even though the origin of the exact virus is not known.

Another type of rash, a petechial rash, is indicative of meningitis. When found in the presence of a fever, it is highly suggestive of meningococcal meningitis, a contagious form of meningitis. This rash begins suddenly, usually in the skin folds, and spreads throughout the body. This may occur in adults, as well as children.

The presence of a rash does not always indicate an infection. A rash that itches may indicate an allergic reaction. A child with a fever who suffers an itching, raised rash that looks like hives is probably allergic to a medication such as an antibiotic or antipyretic (acetaminophen, ibuprofen, or aspirin). Scarlet fever, however, is an example of an allergic reaction to the toxins of an invading organism of strep throat. This condition is best treated with antibiotics to stop the production of the toxin.

Assessment

In general, an altered mental status in the presence of a communicable disease is always an indicator of the seriousness of the situation. Airway should be cleared of any foreign material, if present, and patency maintained. Abnormal sounds, such as stridor, suggest the possibility of impending airway obstruction and should be immediately reported to the receiving facility. Assessment of respiratory status includes the rate of respirations (noting presence of silent tachypnea in children) and presence and character of lung sounds. Assessment of the respiratory system is not complete without visualizing the chest wall and noting use of accessory muscles.

Assessing circulation includes evaluating pulses and the skin. Skin temperature (for presence/absence of fever), moisture (for hydration as well as diaphoresis) and color, as well as the presence of any rash, red streaks, or discoloration should be noted. The presence of any open wounds or sores should also be noted as potential sites for infection.

Baseline vital signs, as well as mental status, will help with evaluating perfusion. The potential for sepsis should be suspected in patients whose illness is extreme. Septic shock should be suspected in patients who have signs of decreased perfusion.

Treatment

Treatment is supportive. Airway and breathing should be maintained with suction used as appropriate. Oxygen should be administered both for increasing the supply but also to help manage fever. If wheezing is present, a bronchodilator, such as Alupent, can be helpful. The patient should be placed in the position of comfort to maintain perfusion of vital organs. When septic shock is suspected, oxygen, fluid replacement, and vasopressors such as dopamine are useful treatment options.

Treatment of fever is usually not encouraged unless the fever is excessive, such as >105° F (40.5° C) or if febrile seizures are present. Treatment of high fevers or febrile seizures is supportive, with management of the airway and measures to support heat loss. Removal of excess clothing, application of wet towels, and IV boluses are all useful measures to promote heat loss. Care should be taken to prevent shivering. Shivering indicates heat loss is occurring faster than the body's ability to adjust.

CASE 1

Dispatch: 16:00 hrs; 13 y/o male, difficulty breathing

On Arrival: You find 13 y/o Julio lying prone in bed. He appears pale and looks like he is sleeping. His chest is barely moving.

Initial Assessment Findings

Mental Status—He cries when you try to wake him, does not obey command, does not open his eyes

Airway—Open and clear

Breathing—R 26 and shallow; lung sounds clear bilaterally

Circulation—Skin pale, hot, and dry
        Radial pulse 166
        BP 112/78

Chief Complaint—According to mother he "turned blue"

Focused History

Events—Julio's mother tried to wake him to take him to the doctor's office. Julio became agitated, "shook all over and turned blue." That's when his mother called EMS.

Previous Illness—Julio has frequent upper respiratory infections, last one 6 months ago

Current Health Status—Last week, Julio came down with the worst "cold" he has ever had. Three days ago he began having a severe headache and yesterday could not get out of bed because it made his headache worse. Today he "wasn't making sense" so she made an appointment with the family physician. His mother first noticed a fever "sometime" last week.

Allergies—None known

Medications—Tylenol (acetaminophen) and aspirin for fever; last dose of Tylenol "maybe a few hours ago"

Focused Physical

Current Set of VS—P 166, R 26, BP 112/78, T 103.6° F (39.8° C)

Other Pertinent Findings—Julio weighs 112 lbs (51 kg); a fine petechial rash is present on Julio's trunk and seems to be spreading across his shoulders; his mother states the rash is new; Julio becomes agitated when you attempt to shine a light to evaluate pupil reaction; moving all extremities; pulse oximetry 99% on room air

ECG

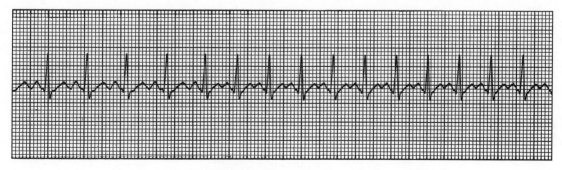

Figure 12-1

QUESTIONS

1. What is significant about Julio's history?

2. What body systems are affected?

3. What is the relationship between his tachycardia, tachypnea, and hot, dry skin?

4. Is there a relationship between his fever and his mother's description of headache, "not making sense," agitation when disturbed, and "shook all over and turned blue?"

5. What is significant about his petechial rash?

6. What is significant about Julio's agitation when you attempt to look at his pupils?

7. Is there any information from his history or physical examination that might be helpful?

8. How serious is Julio's current problem?

9. What is Julio at risk for?

10. What do you think is the cause of Julio's current condition?

11. How would you begin treatment?

12. What is the purpose of a fever?

13. When is a fever considered too high?

14. What special considerations does this case present for you and your partner in terms of BSI?

15. Would administration of antibiotics be an option for your system?

QUESTIONS AND ANSWERS

1. ***What is significant about Julio's history?***

Frequent URIs, severe headache followed by "not making sense," and agitation with "shaking all over and turned blue" in the presence of a fever and rash.

2. ***What body systems are affected?***

CNS—"not making sense," severe headache, suggestion of photophobia; GCS 9 (1 eye opening, 3 verbal response, 5 motor response)
Respiratory—tachypnea
Cardiovascular—tachycardia
Other—fever; hot, dry skin; rash

3. ***What is the relationship between his tachycardia, tachypnea, and fever?***

Tachycardia and tachypnea have a direct relationship to fever. As the set point in the hypothalamus is raised and fever begins, epinephrine is released to increase the metabolic rate to support the fever. With an increase in metabolic rate comes an increase in oxygen and nutrient demand. This increase in oxygen and nutrient demand is reflected in the resulting tachycardia and tachypnea.

4. ***Is there a relationship between his fever and his mother's description of headache, "not making sense," agitation when disturbed, and "shook all over and turned blue?"***

Headache is common when fever is present, "not making sense" suggests confusion or delirium, his agitation when disturbed and "shook all over and turned blue" suggests seizurelike activity or, at the least, heightened irritability of the brain. Together these signs and symptoms suggest significant brain irritation. A high fever may cause the confusion/delirium, as well as brain irritability.

5. ***What is significant about his petechial rash?***

A petechial rash in the presence of a high fever is highly suggestive of an infectious process. The process may be either bacterial or viral. A petechial rash in the presence of confusion in an ill patient suggests a meningococcus (a bacteria) infection. Although there are other viral causes of petechial rash that are more common, confusion is not usually present with those causes.

6. ***What is significant about Julio's agitation when you attempt to look at his pupils?***

This suggests photophobia. Photophobia is usually a result of irritation of the nerves supplying the eye. In nontrauma, an infection of the eye (such as inflammation of the anterior chamber, iritis, etc.), the brain itself or the meninges, along with tumors, high fever, or blood outside the vascular system may all result in photophobia.

7. ***Is there any information from his history or physical examination that might be helpful?***

Ask if he has been around anyone else in the family, friends, or people at school who have been ill and if so, do they know what the problem is. If any family members are also ill, do they have the same symptoms? Has this ever happened before?

8. ***How serious is Julio's current problem?***

Julio is seriously ill with evidence of CNS irritability probably resulting from an infectious process. This is a potential threat to life.

9. ***What is Julio at risk for?***

Grand mal seizures because of the high fever and history of an episode of "shook all over," respiratory compromise resulting from brain irritation and possibility of further seizures, and the possibility of increased intracranial pressure.

10. ***What do you think is the cause of Julio's current condition?***

An infection is the most likely cause. Because he has altered mental status in the presence of a high fever, meningitis or encephalitis are distinct possibilities.

11. ***How would you begin treatment?***

First, protect yourself. Wear a mask, as well as gloves, then continue with patient care. Remove any unnecessary clothing to promote heat loss. Apply oxygen by non-rebreather mask with a reservoir at 15 lpm. Try to start an IV of NS at a kvo rate.

12. What is the purpose of a fever?

A fever is a useful tool used by the body in response to an infection. Simple raising of body temperature kills many microorganisms and has adverse effects on the growth and replication of others. Higher body temperatures decrease serum levels of iron, zinc, and copper, all of which are needed for bacterial replication. Increased temperature also helps prevent viral replication in infected cells. Heat also increases the efficiency of the immune response. Although suppression of fever needs to be cautiously considered, fevers can become too high, resulting in serious side effects.

13. When is a fever considered too high?

Authorities disagree on a specific number or degree. However, they do agree that a fever is too high when it produces serious side effects, such as nerve damage or seizures. Children tend to cope with high fevers much better than adults.

14. What special considerations does this case present for you and your partner in terms of BSI?

Special considerations include the possibility of exposure or contamination to a potentially infectious process. The suspicion of meningitis or encephalitis is of concern. Organisms causing those diseases are primarily airborne. While gloves are routine and standard equipment on all runs, masks and goggles may not be. Both a mask and goggles should be worn when caring for this patient. Application of the non-rebreather mask as soon as an airborne organism is suspected is another part of patient care that helps protect the provider, as well as treat the patient. Other considerations include local policy and procedures regarding potential contamination, as well as exposures; and decontamination for airborne organisms, not only of equipment but also the patient compartment of your vehicle.

15. Would administration of antibiotics be an option for your system?

Paramedics who work in isolated areas or where transport time is >60 min would be most affected by such an option. Expanded scope of care in such isolated areas could greatly affect outcome in patients such as these. Elements that are imperative to ensure a successful program include specific training for paramedics, involving drawing blood for cultures before antibiotic use, accessing direct medical control, and on-line physician contact.

OUTCOME

Oxygen was applied with a mask non-rebreather and reservoir at 12 lpm. Medics started an IV of NS at kvo. En route to the hospital his clothing was removed and wet towels applied to his trunk and extremities. Just before arrival at the ED he suffered a grand mal seizure and pulled out his IV. He was rushed to the ED where another IV was started and lorazepam (Ativan) administered. Blood was drawn, labs ordered, blood cultures, and lumbar puncture done. Visual examination of the cloudy CSF (cerebrospinal fluid) was highly suggestive for meningitis. He was started on an IV antibiotic and admitted to the pediatric ICU. The CSF culture was positive for meningococcal pneumonia. He eventually recovered and was dismissed to home.

CASE 2

Dispatch: 15:30 hrs; 3 y/o male, seizure

On Arrival: You find 3 y/o Darin, in the bathtub, with about 3 inches of water. His mother is attempting to sponge him with the water. He is awake and crying vigorously.

Initial Assessment Findings

Mental Status—Awake and crying; obeys command; GCS 15
Airway—Open and clear
Breathing—R 12 with his crying; lung sounds clear on inhalation, unable to assess exhalation because of crying
Circulation—Skin appears flushed and hot
        Pulse rapid at 160
        BP not taken
Chief Complaint—Seizure

Focused History

Events—Mother went in to check on child and discovered him "shaking all over"
Previous Illness—Has an upper respiratory infection with a runny nose for last 2 days. Today began to run a fever of 101° F.
Current Health Status—Good
Allergies—None known
Medications—Tylenol (acetaminophen) for fever, last had 1 teaspoonful when he was put down for his nap at 1PM

Focused Physical

Current Set of VS—T 103.7° F (39.8° C), P 160, R crying, BP not taken
Other Pertinent Findings—The flush on his face appears to be a fine, red rash; the water in the tub is tepid; there are no other abnormalities noted
Diagnostic Tests—None done

ECG: Not done.

QUESTIONS

1. What is significant about Darin's history?

2. What body systems are affected?

3. Darin's pulse is high. What is the most likely reason for that?

4. Is there a relationship between his history of an upper respiratory infection, fever, and seizure?

5. Is there any information, from either his history or physical examination, that might be helpful?

6. How serious is Darin's current problem?

7. What is Darin at risk for?

8. What do you think is the cause of Darin's current condition?

9. How would you begin treatment?

10. Is a temperature of 103.7° F (39.8° C) high enough to cause a seizure?

11. If Darin was given Tylenol (acetaminophen) before his nap, why does he now have a fever of 103.7° F (39.8° C)?

12. What is significant about the fine, red rash noted on his face?

13. Are there any special precautions to take with Darin?

14. What is the most common cause of a febrile seizure in a child? Does that change your treatment?

15. What is the most serious cause of a febrile seizure in a child? What would you assess for that would suggest its presence?

16. How does Darin's signs and symptoms compare to Julio's signs and symptoms in Case 1?

QUESTIONS AND ANSWERS

1. What is significant about Darin's history?

Preexisting upper respiratory infection for last 2 days, onset of fever today, seizurelike activity in the presence of a fever

2. What body systems are affected?

Cardiovascular—tachycardia; hot skin

CNS—fever, seizure by history

3. Darin's pulse is high. What is the most likely reason for that?

There are two reasons for a high pulse. A fever causes the metabolic rate to be increased, which then increases the heart rate. The second is the history of a seizure, which will also cause the heart rate to increase. After time, the increased rate resulting from the seizure should decrease to the current "resting" rate.

4. Is there a relationship between his history of an upper respiratory infection, fever, and seizure?

Signs and symptoms of an upper respiratory infection in a child is a common first stage for many childhood diseases. The onset of fever should alert the medic to the fact that this is probably not a simple "cold." In young children, sudden fevers often cause seizurelike activity.

5. Is there any information, either from his history or physical examination, that might be helpful?

Has Darin ever suffered seizurelike activity before? If so, under what circumstances? Has Darin been rubbing or pulling at his ears? Has Darin had all his immunizations? Has he been exposed to any childhood disease?

6. How serious is Darin's current problem?

As long as Darin remains alert, it is relatively safe to consider him stable.

7. What is Darin at risk for?

Another seizure is unlikely; however, it is a possibility.

8. What do you think is the cause of Darin's current condition?

Sudden seizurelike activity in the presence of a fever suggests a febrile seizure.

9. How would you begin treatment?

Depending on your transport time and local protocols, you may choose to continue to sponge Darin down until his fever reaches 102° F (38.8° C). This process should not delay transport time. Ready Darin for transport by drying him off and loosely covering him until he is in the squad. Then uncover him and continue to try to cool him off according to your local protocol. Care must be taken to prevent shivering.

10. Is a temperature of 103.7° F (39.8° C) high enough to cause a seizure?

Yes. However, it is not the degree of the fever that is important, it is how suddenly it was reached. The faster a given temperature rises, the more likely a seizure will be triggered.

11. If Darin was given Tylenol (acetaminophen) before his nap, why does he now have a fever of 103.7°F (39.8° C)?

There are a few possibilities that could explain this. According to his mother, Darin was given acetaminophen at 1:00 PM or 13:00 hrs. You were dispatched at 15:30 hrs, which is approximately 2½ hrs later. It is possible the history is in error or he was given an inadequate dose of medication (a common cause of persistent fever). It is also possible that Darin's fever rose rapidly in spite of the medication. It is equally possible that his current fever could be much higher had he not received his medication. You probably will never know which it is.

12. What is significant about the fine, red rash noted on his face?

Because signs and symptoms of an upper respiratory infection is a common precursor to many childhood diseases, it is likely that this fine, red rash is an indicator of the disease process causing his fever. A fine, red rash is commonly viral in origin, though not always. The fact that this rash has started on his face suggests measles.

13. Are there any special precautions to take with Darin?

It is likely that Darin has a contagious, airborne disease. Appropriate personal protective equipment, such as masks, would be advisable.

14. What is the most common cause of a febrile seizure in a child? Does that change your treatment?

The most common cause of a febrile seizure in a child is an ear infection. That does not change treatment in the field.

15. What is the most serious cause of a febrile seizure in a child? What would you assess for that would suggest its presence?

The most serious cause of a febrile seizure in a child is meningitis. An altered mental status would be the earliest indicator. Another suggestive sign would be a fine petechial rash or the presence of large, purple blotches on the skin.

16. How does Darin's signs and symptoms compare to Julio's signs and symptoms in Case 1?

Darin is alert and obeys command; his rash is fine and red and started on his face. Julio has an altered mental status along with his fever and a petechial rash starting on his trunk.

OUTCOME

Darin was removed from the tub, dried off, and covered with a light blanket and carried to the squad. Once inside, he was undressed and allowed to sit on his mother's lap on the way to the hospital. En route, he calmed down and repeat VS were: P 120 and R 28. No BP was taken. On arrival in the ED, Darin's temperature was 102.4° F (39.1° C). An examination showed bulging, red eardrums, bilaterally. Further questioning of mother was done and it was discovered that Darin was never given his MMR (measles, mumps and rubella) immunization. A diagnosis of measles with bilateral otitis media was made. He was given amoxicillin, his mother given information on the MMR immunization, and Darin was dismissed to home.

CASE 3

Dispatch: 14:30 hrs; 58 y/o male with difficulty breathing

On Arrival: You find 58 y/o Memo lying in bed. He appears much older than his stated age. His skin is pale, he is awake, and he has a frequent cough.

Initial Assessment Findings

Mental Status—Awake, oriented, and obeys command; GCS 15

Airway—Open and clear

Breathing—R 22, speaks in phrases; lung sounds have rales and wheezes in the left posterior lower lobe

Circulation—Skin pale, warm, and dry with poor turgor

      Radial pulse regular at 98

      BP 100/78

Chief Complaint—"I'm just too tired . . . and out of breath . . . to get out of bed."

Focused History

Events—Today Memo was so tired and had such difficulty breathing that he just couldn't get out of bed.

Previous Illness—Relatives state he has had a cough for a year or more.

Current Health Status—Relatives note that he has had a gradual weight loss and been "feeling poorly" for about the last six months. He was urged to come visit relatives and has not been feeling well since he arrived. He has not seen a physician for 30 years.

Allergies—None known

Medications—OTC cough preparations

Focused Physical

Current Set of VS—P 98, R 22, BP 100/78, T 101.2° F (38.4° C)

Other Pertinent Findings—He has a wasted appearance and frequent, productive cough; sputum is yellow and blood streaked; complains of a dull ache in his chest on the left side; pulse oximetry is 86% on room air. Memo has been a hermit and lived in the hills for most of his life, does not abuse drugs, has an occasional whiskey (only if he makes it himself), and has a distrust of cities, banks, and the medical community in general.

Diagnostic Tests—BS 88; Tilt test positive, P 126 and BP 80/56

ECG

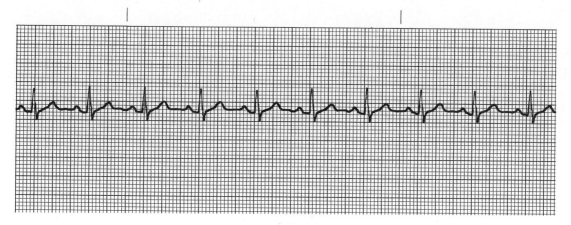

Figure 12-2

1. What is significant about Memo's history?

2. What body systems are affected?

3. What are possible causes of unilateral rales and wheezes?

4. What is the implication of unilateral rales and wheezes in the presence of a productive cough and fever?

5. What is Memo's complaint of fatigue most likely related to?

6. What could be the cause of his pulse oximetry value of 86% on room air?

7. How would you describe the ECG?

8. Is Memo's ECG related to his current problem?

9. What is the significance of a positive tilt test in this patient?

10. What is implied by a history of a cough for a "year," gradual weight loss, and "feeling poorly" for the last six months?

11. Is there any information, from either his history or physical examination, that might be helpful?

12. How serious is Memo's current problem?

13. What is Memo at risk for?

14. What do you think is the cause of Memo's current condition?

15. How would you begin treatment?

16. After initial treatment measures are completed, VS are: P 88, R 24, BP 106/80, lung sounds remain the same, and pulse oximetry is 88%. How would you continue treatment?

17 What is the significance of blood-streaked, yellow sputum?

18. What is the implication of his distrust of cities and the medical community in general?

QUESTIONS AND ANSWERS

1. What is significant about Memo's history?

Gradual weight loss and poor health for 6 months; hermit lifestyle with no medical contact for 30 years; fatigue with dyspnea, productive cough, and fever.

2. What body systems are affected?

Respiratory—unilateral rales and wheezes, productive cough, complains of ache in L chest
Cardiovascular—positive tilt test, pale skin with poor turgor
Other—wasted appearance, older than his stated age

3. What are possible causes of unilateral rales and wheezes?

Unilateral rales and wheezes, as long as there has not been prolonged immobility on one side, can be caused by an inhaled foreign body, an infection (such as pneumonia), a disease process (such as asbestosis), or long-term effects of a growth or tumor (pooling of fluid and secretions). Cardiac related fluid build up as a cause of rales and wheezes is usually bilateral.

4. What is the implication of unilateral rales and wheezes in the presence of a productive cough and fever?

This collection of signs and symptoms is consistent with an infection, the most common infection is pneumonia but also consider TB as a cause.

5. What is Memo's complaint of fatigue most likely related to?

In Memo's case, his fatigue could be related to several factors. Inadequate tidal volume (unable to talk in complete sentences) and thus inadequate oxygen supply, infection (productive cough with fever), and inadequate energy stores (wasted appearance) are all likely contributors to his fatigue.

6. What could be the cause of his pulse oximetry value of 86% on room air?

In the presence of normal blood pressure and perfusion, this value is inadequate. Whether the unilateral rales and wheezes are enough to explain this value is unclear. Regardless, whatever process is occurring in the lungs is significantly impacting his ability to adequately exchange.

7. How would you describe the ECG?

Regular sinus rhythm with no ectopy.

8. Is Memo's ECG related to his current problem?

There does not appear to be a relationship from this tracing.

9. What is the significance of a positive tilt test in this patient?

It suggests volume deficit. This is consistent with his poor turgor and indicates that the volume deficiency has exceeded his ability to compensate.

10. What is implied by a history of a cough for a "year," gradual weight loss, and "feeling poorly" for the last 6 months?

The implication is that this is a chronic problem that can't be corrected in the field. The fact that the chronic cough occurred before the weight loss and "feeling poorly" suggests that the origin of the problem is pulmonary but now has systemic effects.

11. Is there any information, from either his history or physical examination, that might be helpful?

How long has he been having a fever? Has he had any nausea, vomiting, or diarrhea? Has he been eating and drinking? How much weight has he lost? Has he noticed a regular pattern of sweating at night? Is there any pedal edema? What OTC medications has he been taking? How often and how much?

12. How serious is Memo's current problem?

This patient is losing his ability to compensate (extreme fatigue, pulse oximetry of 86%, and positive tilt test). At the moment he appears to be compensating. However, he may not stay that way long. He needs immediate transport to the hospital.

13. **What is Memo at risk for?**

   Respiratory failure, cardiac dysrhythmias from hypoxia, and rapid decompensation.

14. **What do you think is the cause of Memo's current condition?**

   Productive cough, unilateral wheezes and rales, and fever suggest pneumonia; those symptoms combined with a year long cough and weight loss suggests TB or cancer. His wasted appearance along with his hermit lifestyle suggests malnutrition.

15. **How would you begin treatment?**

   Oxygen by mask non-rebreather and reservoir at 15 lpm, an IV of normal saline with 250 to 500 ml bolus, reassess vital signs and pulse oximetry, apply a cardiac monitor, and keep the patient warm.

16. **After initial treatment measures are completed, VS are: P 88, R 24, BP 106/80, lung sounds remain the same, and pulse oximetry is 88%. How would you continue treatment?**

   If your transport time was especially short, you probably would go no further. If, however, your transport were longer, you might consider using a bronchodilator. His pulse oximetry is improved but still not very good. A bronchodilator, such as albuterol or metaproterenol, could be used to improve air movement and thus oxygenation. A second bolus of normal saline would also be a possibility. Signs of cardiac intolerance to increased preload, such as increased dyspnea, would need to be carefully monitored.

17. **What is the significance of blood-streaked, yellow sputum?**

   Yellow sputum suggests infection with pus in the sputum. Blood streaks suggests that capillaries have been broken. This may occur because of hard coughing or as a part of the infectious process.

18. **What is the implication of his distrust of cities and the medical community in general?**

   It may be difficult to get him to agree to transport. You may need to spend some time building a rapport to convince him to go with you. It is also possible that he finds it difficult to function in society, which you may not know. Depending on his responses, you may determine the possibility that he is a danger to himself or others. If so, there is the possibility of transport under the authority of local mental health laws.

OUTCOME

Memo was given oxygen by non-rebreather mask with a reservoir at 12 lpm. An IV of normal saline was started and, because of his orthostatic hypotension, a bolus of 300 ml was given immediately. A reassessment of his VS showed P 88, R 24, BP 106/80, lung sounds remained the same and the pulse oximetry was 88%. An inhalation treatment of albuterol was also given. Before arrival at the ED his pulse oximetry had improved to 95%. On arrival at the ED, VS were: P 84, R 22, BP 104/76 and pulse oximetry 94%. An additional bolus of 500 ml normal saline was delivered and blood work drawn. A chest x-ray revealed left-sided lobar pneumonia with multiple calcifications and a lesion highly suspicious for a tubercular cavitation. Cultures were done and IV antibiotics started. Memo was admitted to the ICU under respiratory isolation for active TB, pneumonia, septicemia, malnutrition, and dehydration. Shortly after admission he developed acute respiratory distress, was sedated, paralyzed, intubated, and placed on a ventilator. After a rocky course, Memo eventually recovered and was dismissed on INH (isoniazid), rifampin, and ethambutol.

CASE 4

Dispatch: 18:45 hrs; 30 y/o female complaining of dizziness and syncope

On Arrival: You find 30 y/o Debbie, lying on the couch in her robe. She is awake and appears very pale.

Initial Assessment Findings

Mental Status—Awake and oriented, obeys command, GCS 15

Airway—Open and clear

Breathing—R 28 and shallow, seems short of breath after talking; lung sounds faint, wheezes in bases

Circulation—Skin hot with bright red areas of peeling skin on palms of hands and extremities

Radial pulse rapid at 136

BP 92/54

Chief Complaint—Dizzy and lightheaded

Focused History

Events—When Debbie got up to go to the bathroom she got so dizzy she nearly passed out, so she crawled back to the couch and called EMS.

Previous Illness—Usually healthy

Current Health Status—About five days ago she came down with the worst case of the "flu" she has ever had. She complains of a sore throat and headache, which were followed by extreme muscle aches, fever, chills, vomiting, and diarrhea.

Allergies—Erythromycin

Medications—Advil (ibuprofen) for fever and Alka-Seltzer Plus Cold Medicine

Focused Physical

Current Set of VS—P 136, R 28, BP 92/54, T 103.2° F (39.6° C)

Other Pertinent Findings—Debbie's conjunctiva are extremely red, you note bright red blotches with peeling skin on both palms, as well as her extremities and trunk. Debbie states she noticed the red blotches the day she got sick. The peeling skin started yesterday. Pulse oximetry is 87%.

Diagnostic Tests—When raised to a sitting position she complained of feeling faint and her radial pulse disappeared; BS 150

ECG

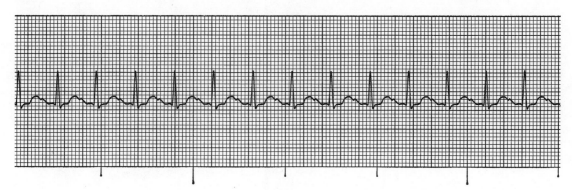

Figure 12-3

QUESTIONS

1. What is significant about Debbie's history?

2. What body systems are affected?

3. How would you describe Debbie's ECG?

4. What is the relationship between Debbie's respiratory rate, basilar wheezes, and pulse oximetry value?

5. Is Debbie perfusing adequately enough to have an accurate pulse oximetry value?

6. What are the main causes of bronchoconstriction, and which are most likely in this case?

7. What is the relationship between Debbie's pulse, blood pressure, and orthostatic hypotension?

8. What might explain Debbie's hypotension?

9. Is there a recognizable pattern of signs and symptoms with Debbie's illness?

10. Is there any information from her history or physical examination that might be helpful?

11. How serious is Debbie's current problem?

12. Debbie has bright red blotches and peeling skin. Is there a relationship between that and her other signs and symptoms?

13. What is Debbie at risk for?

14. What do you think is the cause of Debbie's current condition?

15. How would you begin treatment?

16. After administering oxygen and a fluid bolus there are no appreciable changes in her condition. However, upon moving her to your stretcher and then to the vehicle, she suddenly becomes acutely short of breath with audible wheezing. Repeat VS show the following: P 145, R 36, BP 70/46. How would you proceed?

17. What specific parts of her physical examination should you reassess?

18. In this situation, are there any special precautions you should take?

QUESTIONS AND ANSWERS

1. What is significant about Debbie's history?

Symptoms began about a week ago; describes it as the "worst case of the flu" she has ever had; red blotches began the day she became ill followed by peeling skin.

2. What body systems are affected?

Respiratory—tachypneic with basilar wheezes
Cardiovascular—tachycardia, hypotension
GI—vomiting and diarrhea
Other—fever; red, blotches with peeling skin

3. How would you describe Debbie's ECG?

Regular sinus tachycardia without ectopy.

4. What is the relationship between Debbie's respiratory rate, basilar wheezes, and pulse oximetry value?

Tachypnea can occur when tidal volume is limited or oxygen exchange is impaired. Basilar wheezes indicate that bronchoconstriction is present. Bronchoconstriction may limit tidal volume, as well as impair oxygen exchange. Pulse oximetry is an indicator of hemoglobin saturation, in other words, how well oxygen exchange is occurring at the alveolar level, provided there is adequate perfusion. In the presence of adequate perfusion, a low pulse oximetry value indicates incomplete hemoglobin saturation and may reflect inadequate tidal volume or impaired oxygen exchange or both.

5. Is Debbie perfusing adequately enough to have an accurate pulse oximetry value?

First assess your patient. As long as Debbie is lying flat, she has good mentation, which suggests that as long as she is supine, she is perfusing her brain adequately. Her shortness of breath after talking is an indicator of inadequate tidal volume at rest, which is abnormal. Your assessment indicates a problem exists, which is confirmed by pulse oximetry.

6. What are the main causes of bronchoconstriction, and which are most likely in this case?

The main causes of bronchoconstriction are irritation, allergy, infection, mucus, and presence of a foreign body. Irritation may be from an inhaled particulate matter (such as smoke) or from fluid, either on the outside of the terminal bronchiole or within the alveoli. Inhaled foreign proteins may cause an allergic reaction triggering a histamine response causing bronchoconstriction. Infections can also produce bronchoconstriction, as can mucus buildup. In this case, fluid or infection seem to be more likely causes of wheezing.

7. What is the relationship between Debbie's pulse, blood pressure, and orthostatic hypotension?

A BP of 92/54 suggests hypotension for which tachycardia is a compensatory mechanism. A tachycardia of 136 that can only generate a systolic pressure of 92 suggests a relatively serious problem with volume control. (In the case of sepsis, the patient may be vasodilated and/or have a fluid shift without suffering a true volume depletion; thus volume control becomes an issue.) Although it is true that Debbie has orthostatic hypotension when raised to a sitting position, thus confirming the suspicion of a volume-related problem, it is unnecessary to purposefully do so in the presence of these vital signs and history.

8. What might explain Debbie's hypotension?

There are several possibilities. Fever can result in a degree of dehydration. Debbie, by history, has had vomiting and diarrhea, which can also contribute to dehydration. Then there is the issue of infection. Septicemia can cause vasodilation with third spacing (shunting of fluid into the interstitial spaces), which will further contribute to relative hypovolemia.

9. Is there a recognizable pattern of signs and symptoms with Debbie's illness?

There is a pattern but not a common one. The onset of sore throat, headache, fever, chills, and extreme muscle aches with vomiting and diarrhea suggests a systemic infection and is common; her red blotches followed by peeling skin also are indicative of a systemic infection and are uncommon. Debbie is septic.

10. Is there any information from her history or physical examination that might be helpful?

Are her extremities swollen, especially her feet? Has this ever happened before? Is she having her menses? If so, is she using tampons? Does she have any open wounds or other potential sites of infection, such as a large pimple? Has she seen a physician?

11. How serious is Debbie's current problem?

This is a potential life threat. Her tachycardia cannot support a systolic pressure that will perfuse her brain when upright.

12. Debbie has bright red blotches and peeling skin. Is there a relationship between that and her other signs and symptoms?

This type of skin condition, red blotches followed by peeling, in the presence of a high fever, is sometimes referred to as "scalded skin" syndrome and is typical of a type of Staphylococcus aureus infection. Peeling skin could also represent toxic shock syndrome, which may be caused by streptococcus. In any case, a generalized infection could explain her broad variety of signs and symptoms highly suggestive of either staph or streptococcal infections.

13. What is Debbie at risk for?

Respiratory failure, cardiac dysrhythmias, and multiple organ failure.

14. What do you think is the cause of Debbie's current condition?

Debbie's collection of signs and symptoms, her skin color and peeling, presence of fever, tachycardia, and orthostatic hypotension, all suggest overwhelming infection.

15. How would you begin treatment?

Oxygen by non-rebreather mask with reservoir at 15 lpm, IV of normal saline followed by a 250 to 300 ml bolus and reassess lung sounds, respiratory effort, mental status, and ECG.

16. After administering oxygen and a fluid bolus there are no appreciable changes in her condition. However, upon moving her to your stretcher and then to the vehicle, she suddenly becomes acutely short of breath with audible wheezing. Repeat VS show the following: P 145, R 36, BP 70/46. How would you proceed?

She is in either septic shock or cardiogenic shock. The pharmacologic treatment is the same, start dopamine at 5 mcg/kg/min and titrate to effect. You may be using a premix solution or mix your own, regardless of which type of solution, care must be taken to adjust the drip rate to avoid delivering too much. The maximum dose is 20 mcg/kg/min. After the dopamine is on board, consider administering a second fluid bolus.

17. What specific parts of her physical examination should you reassess?

Systolic blood pressure and pulse rate, lung sounds or respiratory effort (accurate lung sounds are difficult to hear in the back of a moving vehicle), mental status, and ECG.

18. In this situation, are there any special precautions you should take?

The usual personal protective equipment, including masks and protective eyewear. Placing a non-rebreather mask on the patient is a fairly effective way to protect against airborne particles.

OUTCOME

Debbie was placed on oxygen with a non-rebreather mask and reservoir at 12 lpm and an IV of normal saline started. A bolus of 250 to 300 ml was delivered with no appreciable change in lung sounds but a systolic of 98. En route she suddenly became acutely short of breath and gray. VS were: P 145, R 36, BP 70/46. A dopamine drip was started at 5 mcg/kg/min and titrated to 8 mcg/kg/min to achieve a systolic of 94 and an improvement in skin color. On arrival at the ED blood work was done, a chest x-ray done, and cultures obtained. A second IV was started and an additional fluid bolus administered. On closer inspection, multiple small bug bites were noted on her lower legs with a small abscess on her lower left calf. IV antibiotics were begun, and she was admitted to the ICU with the diagnosis of acute toxic shock syndrome. After 6 weeks in the hospital and several surgical débridements of her abscess, she was dismissed to home.

BIBLIOGRAPHY

Aminoff, M. J., Greenberg, D. A., & Simon, R. P. (1996). *Clinical neurology,* (3rd ed.). Stamford, CT: Appleton & Lange.

Bartlett, J. G., Ciranowicz, M. M., & Meissner, J. E. (1995). *Infectious disorders.* New York: Springer Publishing.

Berkow, R. & Fletcher, A. J. (Eds.). (1992). *Merck manual of diagnosis and therapy.* Rahway, NJ: Merck Research Laboratories.

Bongard, F. S. & Sue, D.Y. (Eds.) (1994). *Current: Critical care, diagnosis and treatment.* Norwalk, CT: Appleton & Lange.

Cohen, F. L., Harriman, C. D., & Madsen, L. (1995). Symptoms and diagnosis of tuberculosis. In F. L. Cohen and J. D. Durham (Eds.). *Tuberculosis: A sourcebook for nursing practice.* New York: Springer Publishing.

Farley, J. A., Mooney, K. H., & Andrews, M. M. (1994). Alterations of neurologic function in children. In K. L. McCance and S. E. Huether (Eds.). *Pathophysiology: The biologic basis for disease in adults and children,* (2nd ed.). St. Louis, MO: Mosby.

Kelley, S. J. (1994). *Pediatric emergency nursing,* (2nd ed.). Norwalk, CT: Appleton & Lange.

Mandell, G. L. & Petri, W. A. (1996). Antimicrobial agents: Drugs used in the chemotherapy of tuberculosis and leprosy. In J. G. Hardman and L. E. Limbird (Eds.). *Goodman and Gillman's: The pharmacological basis of therapeutics,* (9th ed.). Philadelphia: McGraw-Hill.

Madsen, L. & Cohen, F. L. (1995). Medical treatment of tuberculosis. In F. L. Cohen and J. D. Durham (Eds.). *Tuberculosis: A sourcebook for nursing practice.* New York: Springer Publishing.

Nicol, N. H. & Huether, S. E. (1994). Alterations of the integument in children. In K. L. McCance and S. E. Huether (Eds.). *Pathophysiology: The biologic basis for disease in adults and children,* (2nd ed.). St. Louis, MO: Mosby.

Tierney, L. M., McPhee, S. J., & Papadakis, M. A. (Eds.). (1994). *Current: Medical diagnosis and treatment.* Norwalk, CT: Appleton & Lange.

13

Challenging Situations

OVERVIEW

Challenging situations for field providers often include the abuse and assault patient; the physically or mentally challenged patient; patients whose culture impacts their perception and/or willingness to seek help; the terminally ill; those whose religious beliefs preclude certain types of medical treatment; and the home care patient with tubes, shunts, ventilators, and other equipment with which providers are unfamiliar.

Abuse and Assault

The abuse and assault patient may be difficult to manage because of the situation. Frequently the use of alcohol is evident, as well as use of other recreational drugs. The patients may be abusive themselves toward caregivers. Because situations may be tense and volatile, care providers may feel at risk for violence themselves, and the presence of law enforcement personnel may be necessary. Although most services have protocols that prevent care providers from entering a scene until it is safe, it is not unusual to find care providers responding to a situation where violence does not become evident until they are well into the scene. Domestic altercations have one of the highest potentials of violence toward the caregivers. Recognizing when the scene has become unsafe is an experiential skill that is invaluable. Observational skills of the care providers are the key to this recognition. When in a residence, a person holding back in the doorway of another room or a person standing on the fringe of activity with one arm hidden or behind his or her back are both furtive actions that are highly suggestive for potential violence. When something does not seem right, it usually is not. Bystanders hiding behind trees or vehicles; crowds milling about; and people holding objects such as bats, poles, or chains are obvious signs of an unsafe scene. The more subtle scene signs are sometimes regionally dependent or characteristic of a city or location.

Some providers consider the most difficult abuse or assault scenes to be those that involve injury to a child. In such scenes, the emotions of the caregiver often conflict with the maintenance of a professional approach. Incidences of child abuse, rape, or incest are often emotionally difficult to handle. Debriefings may be necessary for the well-being of the caregiver(s).

Issues of evidence protection and collection are also important. Local law enforcement may be very helpful in educating personnel on proper procedure. Any clothing or personal items that are removed in the process of patient care should be placed in paper bags and then given to law enforcement. Plastic bags may cause degradation of some evidence, such as body fluids, and should not be used. Ropes with knots should not be untied; instead they should be cut well away from the knot, if possible.

Victims of assault may be very afraid, and their emotional support is also a concern. Documentation is always important, especially in a case of abuse. Take special care to document all body injuries found.

Physically or Mentally Challenged

The physically or mentally challenged patient presents a special challenge. Canes, braces, and splints come in various sizes and are designed to be worn both over and under clothing. It may be necessary to remove a brace for complete care. The patient is your best source to help you remove the appliance. Braces may be heavy and have straps that need to be undone carefully. Sometimes leg braces fit inside or onto a shoe. The shoe must be untied and either removed before taking off the brace or removed with the brace.

Torso braces or splints should not be removed unless absolutely necessary. However, you may encounter a torso brace that is not designed to accommodate the patient lying down with the brace on. Again, the patient is the best source of instruction. If the brace or splint must be removed, do it carefully, checking to make sure all of the necessary straps are undone before removing the apparatus. If a strap is well worn, that strap is usually the one to undo.

Remember that without the appliance, the patient may not be able to move or maintain his or her balance. Keep the appliance with the patient at all times. This is part of the patient's personal property and should be treated as you would a billfold or purse.

The mentally challenged patient may be particularly fearful, not only because something painful has happened to him or her but also because you are a stranger. Taking care to explain actions in simple terms, taking time to build a rapport, assuring that you will be with him or her all the way to the hospital and if necessary, including a parent or guardian in the care are all helpful actions.

Cultural Differences

Cultural differences can have a tremendous impact on not only whether a patient seeks help and how he or she reacts with the care provider but also in how the patient describes the nature of his or her problem. Effective care depends on recognizing and respecting the differences between cultures and recognizing how that difference will manifest itself, both in assessment and response to treatment.

Discussion of specifics regarding cultural differences can be found in textbooks with chapters on cultural diversity. Many organizations are recognizing the impact of culture to their service and are offering education on that subject to their personnel.

Terminally Ill

The terminally ill are a special population group that many care providers have difficulty dealing with. That difficulty may be in the training received. Death is somehow viewed as the "enemy" rather than another phase of life. Indeed, as care providers we strive to maintain the life of our patients as much as possible, so it is not hard to understand how death can be viewed in this manner. However, in the case of the terminally ill, a decision is usually made at some point not to have extraordinary means implemented to prolong life. When that decision is made, the patient is frequently sent home to be around those they love until the time of death. Care providers are usually not called to the home when that occurs. However, when the patient or family has not been able to make that decision, care providers may be called to a patient in extremis. In this case, most care providers will proceed to deliver the required treatment. In any such situation, care providers should follow their local protocols for dealing with such cases.

Religious Beliefs

Religious beliefs may complicate care delivered by providers. However, this is more common with definitive care providing blood products, immunizations, or other such invasive treatment.

Providers may encounter objections to intravenous fluids or to medications used in the field, but these instances are less common. In such cases, respecting the wishes of the patient is important. If any patient is an adult, of sound mind and alert, coherent, and oriented, he or she has the right to refuse any part of or all care. In the case of a minor, the issue is not as clear. Situations of child neglect are very real and may influence your actions. If at all possible, transport the child.

Home Care: Tubes, Shunts, and Machinery

As technology improves, more and more patients with chronic problems are being managed at home. Home care may involve a patient with tubes, such as gastric (through the nose) or gastrostomy tubes (through the stomach) for feeding or tracheostomy tubes. It may also involve those with central lines such as Groshong or Hickman catheters in the chest wall or venous access devices that are implanted just below the surface of the chest or abdominal wall. Other devices include shunts such as ventricular shunts (for hydrocephalus), dialysis access devices, Foley catheters, and colostomies. Technology may also be involved, including patients on home ventilators or on home IVs with pumps that are carried in a pocket or around the neck or in a backpack. More and more children with birth defects or chronic diseases are also being managed at home. This means that pumps, home ventilators, and additional tubes of all sorts may be encountered.

Most of these devices are not routinely found during patient calls. Since more and more people are being dismissed to home with such devices, it is increasingly likely that the care provider will encounter the patient with such a device. Each device has its own group of complications associated with it. The majority of the time when EMS is called in these situations it is to transport the patient to the hospital for an unrelated problem or for a complication that cannot be managed at home. The home caregivers will likely know more about the devices than anyone else on the scene and are your best resource. They will tell you how you can help them the most, what they need from you, and the best way to get the patient to the receiving hospital.

This chapter does not deal will all of the situations mentioned. Cases are presented that involve several of the more common situations or devices that may be encountered.

CASE 1

Dispatch: 21:30 hrs; Ill child, nature unknown

On Arrival: You find 8-month-old Sean in his crib. He is awake but has an intermittent weak cry. He appears pale, but his mother states that is his normal color.

Initial Assessment Findings

Mental Status—Eye opening to mother's voice, weak cry, no extremity movement

Airway—Open and clear

Breathing—R 24 with abdominal breathing; lung sounds clear and equal bilaterally

Circulation—Skin warm and dry

Brachial pulse regular at 100

BP not done

Chief Complaint—Mother states he isn't acting right.

Focused History

Events—Mother states Sean was acting normally earlier today, at dinner time he fell when he tried to climb out of his highchair but ate his dinner as usual, took his bottle, and went to bed about 8:00 PM. Sean began crying about 30 minutes ago. Mother noticed his cry and behavior wasn't normal so she called the doctor who recommended she call EMS.

Previous Illness—Ear infection diagnosed 2 days ago

Current Health Status—Since antibiotic started has been afebrile with normal activity

Allergies—None known

Medications—Amoxil (amoxicillin)

Focused Physical

Current Set of VS—P 100, R 24, no BP taken

Other Pertinent Findings—Eyes opening to voice and Sean focuses on the speaker; but no response to painful stimuli and extremities limp; continuous, intermittent, weak cry; no rashes, marks, or bruises noted; pulse oximetry 99%; aural temperature 98° F (37° C)

Diagnostic Tests—None done

ECG: Not performed

QUESTIONS

1. What is significant about Sean's history?

2. According to your assessment findings, what body systems are affected?

3. Is the presence of abdominal breathing in an 8 month old significant?

4. Does field treatment differ if Sean's problem was resulting from trauma or caused by a medical condition? Why or why not?

5. Is there any way to determine if trauma versus a medical condition is the cause of Sean's condition?

6. Is there any additional information, from either his history or physical examination, that might be helpful?

7. What is Sean at risk for?

8. How serious is Sean's condition?

9. What do you think is probably causing Sean's problem?

10. How would you begin treatment?

11. What would be necessary to tell his parents?

12. Does Sean's lack of fever indicate a lack of infection?

13. Would it be appropriate to check Sean's blood sugar?

14. How does a spinal cord injury in a young child differ from that in an adult?

15. Is it necessary to take a blood pressure on this child or would a capillary refill test be an adequate substitute?

QUESTIONS AND ANSWERS

1. ***What is significant about Sean's history?***

   There are two significant events. The first is his history of falling from his highchair, and the second is his history of an ear infection.

2. ***According to your assessment findings, what body systems are affected?***

   CNS—no extremity movement; eyes opening and focusing to mother's voice; weak, intermittent cry; mother states behavior not normal

3. ***Is the presence of abdominal breathing in an 8 month old significant?***

   The *absence* of it would be significant. It is normal for an 8 month old to have abdominal breathing. At this age the intercostal muscles have not developed enough to noticeably help with breathing.

4. ***Does field treatment differ if Sean's problem was resulting from trauma or caused by a medical condition? Why or why not?***

   Yes, if trauma were the cause, immobilization would be very important

5. ***Is there any way to determine if trauma versus a medical condition is the cause of Sean's condition?***

   At this point there really isn't. An argument can be made for trauma because of the apparent quadriplegia, but Sean continued to act normally and ate his dinner after the event. On the other hand, there are also disease processes that are specific for the CNS that could be involved. He has a history of an ear infection that could lead to encephalitis or meningitis but these conditions are usually associated with hard to manage fevers with altered mental status and don't cause quadriplegia. Polio is another disease but a history of progressive paralysis would be involved. Poisoning may have occurred but usually involves the entire CNS and not specifically the spinal cord. When quadriplegia is present the spinal cord is involved. The rule of thumb is to suspect trauma.

6. ***Is there any additional information, from either his history or physical examination, that might be helpful?***

   A thorough history including possibility of poisoning, known birth defects, any unusual or abnormal motor movement, palpate his fontanelle for any unusual or abnormal findings, are there any other children in the family ill.

7. ***What is Sean at risk for?***

   The obvious risk factor is respiratory arrest resulting from a suspected high cord injury causing quadriplegia. Seizure activity, cardiac arrest, and shock should also be considered.

8. ***How serious is Sean's condition?***

   Consider Sean's condition a potential threat to life.

9. ***What do you think is probably causing Sean's problem?***

   There could be a disease process that is specific for the central nervous system, or a metabolic genetic birth defect could be present, or this could be the result of a cord contusion. The most likely cause is cord contusion because of the quadriplegia. Child abuse may be a factor.

10. ***How would you begin treatment?***

    Carefully lift or log roll Sean and place him on a padded backboard. Apply oxygen by blow-by, keep him warm, and begin transport.

11. ***What would be necessary to tell his parents?***

    Depending on your system the parents may request a hospital or you may decide the most appropriate hospital. In either case it is important that the parents know to which hospital you are transporting. Your service program policy may allow you to have a parent up in front with the driver or in back with the baby. Because you don't know if a resuscitation will be necessary you might choose to have the parent ride up front or follow in their own vehicle. Ask for the child's favorite toy or blanket. If they ask what is wrong, be honest. Tell them you aren't sure but reassure them that his response to mom's voice and spontaneous breathing are good signs.

12. Does Sean's lack of fever indicate a lack of infection?

No, infection and sepsis can occur without fever. Because Sean has a history of an ear infection, there is the potential for an infectious process.

13. Would it be appropriate to check Sean's blood sugar?

Yes, because you don't know what is wrong. Abnormal blood sugar levels at this age would indicate a metabolic birth defect. These types of genetic problems usually become apparent during the first year of life.

14. How does a spinal cord injury in a young child differ from that in an adult?

A child's spine is hypermobile and has weak vertebral ligaments. This makes the cord susceptible to stretching without corresponding vertebral damage. The result can be spinal cord injury without radiographic abnormality. This is actually a syndrome called SCIWORA and is more common in unrestrained pediatric motor vehicle passengers, sports injuries, birth trauma, and pedestrians struck by motor vehicles. This type of injury usually occurs in the cervical cord (83% have cervical involvement), T_{12} and L_1.

15. Is it necessary to take a blood pressure on this child or would a capillary refill test be an adequate substitute?

A BP would be appropriate; however, a capillary refill test would tell you more about the actual state of perfusion. It is accurate in the presence of a normal body temperature and normal ambient air temperature. If Sean were hypovolemic a fluid bolus would be indicated, based on transport time.

OUTCOME

Sean's status did not change en route to the hospital. On arrival complete vital signs were P 104, R 22, BP 80/54, T 98°F (37° C) and an intraosseous IV was started. A CT scan showed a cervical cord contusion. Solu-Medrol was administered, and Sean was admitted to the pediatric ICU with the diagnosis of SCIWORA. A subsequent MRI revealed an extensive cervical cord contusion from C_5 to T_1. Why it took so long for neurodeficit to occur is unknown. It is possible that initial signs of neurodeficit were present but missed. Six months after the incident, Sean was learning how to walk again, with some residual weakness. Full outcome will not be completely determined for several years.

There are many occasions when paramedics will not have a clear idea of what the underlying problem is with a patient. In such cases it is more important to recognize body systems involved, support those body systems, and determine the significance of what is seen in terms of actual or potential life threat and to intervene accordingly. Knowing when to contact medical control is a significant part of this process.

CASE 2

Dispatch: 23:30 hrs; 18 y/o female; assault, police at the scene

On Arrival: On arrival you find 18 y/o Dorice, in an apartment, hunched over in the corner of the couch, clutching a blanket around her with blood smeared fingers. She is awake but her face is a mass of bruises, and she appears pale.

Initial Assessment Findings

Mental Status—Awake, alert, and oriented
Airway—Open and clear
Breathing—R 18 and regular; lung sounds present and equal bilaterally
Circulation—Skin pale, warm, and dry
         Pulse regular at 88
         BP 126/72
Chief Complaint—Abdominal pain

Focused History

Events—Police tell you that Dorice was assaulted and possibly raped by an unknown male who broke into her apartment. Apparently the assailant struck her face, chest, and abdomen with his fists. Neighbors called police when they saw someone run from the apartment and heard her crying.
Previous Illness—Asthma
Current Health Status—Good
Allergies—Pollen
Medications—Ventolin (albuterol) inhaler

Focused Physical

Current Set of VS—P 88, R 18, BP 126/72
Other Pertinent Findings—A small laceration above left eye, large contusion above her left eye and left cheek; abrasion on left temple; index and middle finger of right hand bruised with abrasions of right knuckles; she refuses to let go of her blanket, but is otherwise cooperative; she complains of pain when her abdomen and chest wall is palpated through the blanket; she denies loss of consciousness; she is very quiet; pulse oximetry is 99%
Diagnostic Tests—None performed

ECG

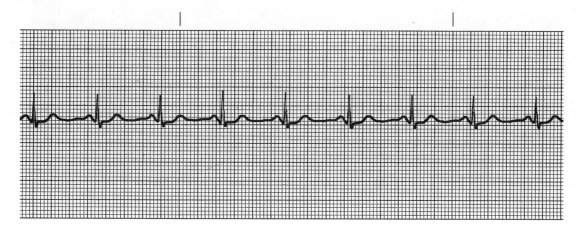

Figure 13-1

QUESTIONS

1. What is significant about Dorice's history?

2. According to your assessment findings and her behavior, what body systems are affected?

3. Is there any additional information from her history or physical examination that might be helpful?

4. How important is it to do a visual examination of her abdomen, chest, and extremities?

5. How serious is Dorice's condition?

6. How would you begin treatment?

7. You explain to Dorice that you need to take her to the hospital. She asks if you could wait a minute so she can clean up. How do you proceed?

8. What information is important to obtain?

9. What is an appropriate field impression to document?

10. En route to the hospital you notice tears on her face. When you ask if she is hurting anywhere, Dorice begins to sob. What do you do now?

QUESTIONS AND ANSWERS

1. *What is significant about Dorice's history?*

The police officer's statement of an assault, possible rape. This sets the stage for the rest of the call in terms of attention to potential injury, protection of potential evidence, awareness of legal aspects such as right to privacy and knowledge that any documentation will be closely scrutinized.

2. *According to your assessment findings and her behavior, what body systems are affected?*

Integumentary system (skin)—bruises and contusions
Abdominal/Reproductive—highly probable internal injuries
Psychologic—behavior suggests emotional trauma

3. *Is there any additional information from her history or physical examination that might be helpful?*

From the bruises on her face, she suffered significant blows to the head; assess her memory to determine if there is a gap suggesting a loss of consciousness. It is also important to find out if she has changed clothing. This clothing is evidence and should be given to the police or placed in a paper (NOT plastic) bag and taken to the hospital with the patient. Plastic holds in moisture and heat that may increase biodegradation, which may alter or destroy evidence.

4. *How important is it to do a visual examination of her abdomen, chest, and extremities?*

Although a visual examination is important, the emotional trauma this patient has suffered is also important. Do not force her. Close attention should be paid to her skin vitals, vital signs, and mental status. Try to find out where the blood on her fingers has come from. Ask her where she is bleeding. If you suspect that she has been stabbed, then ask her if that is so and proceed accordingly but do not force her, especially since she is stable. An important consideration is the presence of vaginal bleeding. With short transport times minor bleeding may not be an issue. With long transport times, it may become a major problem.

5. *How serious is Dorice's condition?*

Physically she is stable with no apparent threat to life.

6. *How would you begin treatment?*

Bring the gurney in to her, lay her down, and cover her with another blanket or sheet. If cold packs are available, cover with a washcloth or towel and apply to her face. Depending on your judgment and pulse oximetry values, you may apply oxygen.

7. *You explain to Dorice that you need to take her to the hospital. She asks if you could wait a minute so she can clean up. How do you proceed?*

Do NOT allow her to change clothing, go to the bathroom, brush her teeth, take a shower or change. This is to preserve evidence. These things need to be tactfully explained because she may be feeling "dirty" or "contaminated" and have an *extreme* need to wash.

8. *What information is important to obtain?*

It is not important for medics to know the details of the assault. However, it is important to know what she was struck by (fists, feet, any weapon, and so on), where she was hit, if she fell and what she may have hit (furniture, floor, and so on). It is also important to know physically where she hurts now.

9. *What is an appropriate field impression to document?*

The term "rape" is a legal term and not appropriate, "apparent assault victim" is one acceptable description. It is important to indicate specifically what the patient said and what EMS verified with direct observation.

10. **En route to the hospital you notice tears on her face. When you ask if she is hurting anywhere, Dorice begins to sob. What do you do now?**

This is a difficult situation. Emotions in a victim may range from anger and rage to terror and fright to emotionally shutting everyone out. The fact that she is openly crying is emotionally healthy but may be very disconcerting to care providers. Determining if she is physically hurting or if her pain has changed is necessary. Sometimes just reaching across and holding her hand or arm may help. To tell her that everything will be all right is NOT appropriate, nor is it correct. Handing her some Kleenex, assuring her that it's okay to cry, that she is safe now, and that you will be with her all the way to the hospital are supportive.

OUTCOME

En route to the hospital, Dorice remained stable but started to cry. She was reassured that she was safe now and that she could cry as much as she wanted. On arrival to the ED when she was transferred to the ED cart, she began to bleed vaginally. Physicians discovered a vaginal tear and she was sent to surgery where the examination was completed. Dorice suffered a vaginal tear that extended into the peritoneal cavity. She also sustained a fractured rib on the right and a bruised kidney. Two days after her surgical repair, she was dismissed to home.

Postscript: A few months later her assailant was shot and killed while trying to assault another woman.

CASE 3

Dispatch: 02:30; Assault victim, stabbing to the abdomen

On Arrival: You find 46 y/o Reggie, lying against a brick wall in an alley behind a shelter for the homeless. There are blood streaks and feces smeared over the front of Reggie's torn shirt. A strong odor of alcohol is present. Reggie is awake and yelling at the police.

Initial Assessment Findings

Mental Status—Awake, slurred speech, confused, obeys command
Airway—Open and clear
Breathing—R 18 and unlabored; lung sounds clear and equal bilaterally
Circulation—Skin warm, diaphoretic, color appears normal
        Radial pulse intact 108
        BP 136/72
Chief Complaint—"I can't get up"

Focused History

Events—Police tell you Reggie entered into an argument with another person in the shelter, both were told to go outside where the other party pulled a knife. Police suspect Reggie was stabbed in the abdomen.
Previous Illness—Unknown (Reggie refuses to answer)
Current Health Status—Unknown (Reggie refuses to answer)
Allergies—Unknown (Reggie refuses to answer)
Medications—Unknown (Reggie refuses to answer)

Focused Physical

Current Set of VS—P 108, R 18, BP 136/72
Other Pertinent Findings—Bruise with an abrasion over his right eye; old track marks on both arms; abdomen has old surgical scars (Reggie states from gunshot wound), is soft and diffusely tender; small opening with pink tissue oozing blood and feces at midabdomen just to the left of the umbilicus; abrasions noted on left knee and right shin; moving all extremities
Diagnostic Tests—Blood sugar 89; police at the scene state he blew a 0.35% alcohol level on the breathalyzer

ECG

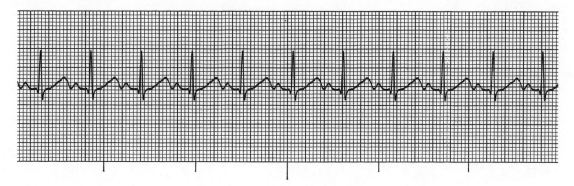

Figure 13-2

QUESTIONS

1. What is significant about Reggie's history?

2. What is significant about the mechanism of injury?

3. What body systems are affected?

4. What are the implications of such a high blood alcohol level in this patient?

5. When someone has suffered an evisceration, what are the characteristic physical signs that the peritoneum has been penetrated?

6. Is there any additional information from the physical examination or his history that might be helpful?

7. What do you think is wrong and why?

8. How serious is Reggie's current situation?

9. What is Reggie at risk for?

10. How would you begin treatment?

11. Why would a blood sugar test be appropriate in this situation?

12. Considering that Reggie doesn't look as bad as his mechanism suggests that he doesn't have all the signs of an evisceration, what might be another cause of the problem?

QUESTIONS AND ANSWERS

1. What is significant about Reggie's history?

The history of a knife-fight; presence of track marks on his arms suggest a history of drug abuse; abdominal scars caused by a previous gunshot wound; police determined an alcohol level around 0.35%.

2. What is significant about the mechanism of injury?

The amount of damage in a knife wound depends on the length of the blade and the location of the wound. The area of damage tends to be limited to the organs in the immediate vicinity of the wound. Because of Reggie's associated injuries (bruises and abrasions) it is also reasonable to assume that the mechanism included falling and/or fists.

3. What body systems are affected?

CNS—altered mental status, confused, and slurred speech
Cardiovascular—tachycardia
GI—presence of blood streaks and feces on shirt and abdomen along with wound

4. What are the implications of such a high blood alcohol level in this patient?

The absence of pain is unreliable; there are usually associated injuries that cannot be detected; mental status changes can rarely be discriminated between the effect of the alcohol and a head injury; and in general, information from the patient is unreliable.

5. When someone has suffered an evisceration, what are the characteristic physical signs that the peritoneum has been penetrated?

When the peritoneum has been penetrated, peritoneal fluid (a watery, serous fluid) may leak out, sometimes the omentum (fatty, yellow tissue) or bowel will protrude, but not always. If the bowel has been penetrated, feces may be present, but this is not always evident externally. The only reliable sign is the leaking of peritoneal fluid but even that is not always present.

6. Is there any additional information from the physical examination or his history that might be helpful?

It would be very helpful if Reggie were more cooperative with his history. If you could isolate what appears to be the wound and really examine it, that would be helpful. Ask Reggie what happened. It is just possible that Reggie did not get stabbed at all.

7. What do you think is wrong and why?

In the absence of more of a history and the lack of cooperation from Reggie, it is reasonable to assume the worst and assume that Reggie has a penetrating abdominal wound along with alcohol consumption.

8. How serious is Reggie's current situation?

Reggie appears to be stable at the moment.

9. What is Reggie at risk for?

Sudden deterioration, seizures from alcohol or head injury, and/or vomiting.

10. How would you begin treatment?

Apply pulse oximetry and try to clean up his abdomen as much as possible to look for other wound sites; cover the initial area with a trauma dressing (an occlusive dressing won't stay put—too much of a mess to seal edges) or sterile 4 × 4s. If pulse oximetry levels good, then apply oxygen by a nasal cannula. Depending on the amount of blood present, consider an IV of normal saline or lactated Ringer's.

11. Why would a blood sugar test be appropriate in this situation?

Such a high blood alcohol suggests that Reggie has been on a binge and probably hasn't eaten. Those who haven't eaten run the risk of hypoglycemia, especially over a prolonged period. Alcohol lowers blood sugar levels in those who have low glycogen stores, such as the malnourished.

12. *Considering that Reggie doesn't look as bad as his mechanism suggests that he doesn't have all the signs of an evisceration, what might be another cause of the problem?*

Reggie's history of a gunshot wound to the abdomen and no presence of peritoneal fluid but a small opening with pink tissue oozing blood and feces might be a colostomy, probably as a result of the previous gun shot wound. The amount of blood will certainly be a concern. But look at the scene carefully and especially inside his clothing. His colostomy bag might have been torn off in the scuffle.

OUTCOME

Reggie remained stable at the scene. A trauma dressing was applied to the wound, oxygen by nasal cannula was applied, and Reggie was transported to the trauma center. Once at the hospital, his wound was more closely examined and it was a colostomy. Reggie was asked what happened. Reggie said he was losing the fight so he ripped off the colostomy bag. The assailant ran away and "then lots of people came." Reggie was dismissed with a supply of colostomy bags.

CASE 4

Dispatch: 20:00 hrs; 58 y/o female, bleeding

On Arrival: You find 58 y/o Sally sitting on the edge of the tub in the bathroom. Her clothing is covered in blood. She is holding one end of a double catheter that is coming from her upper right chest wall. The catheter has a continuous flow of blood coming from the midportion of the catheter and one end.

Initial Assessment Findings

Mental Status—Alert and oriented, follows command
Airway—Open and clear
Breathing—R 24 and regular; lung sounds clear, bilaterally
Circulation—Skin pale, cool, and clammy
> Radial pulse weak at 124
> BP 80/56
Chief Complaint—Bleeding from central line

Focused History

Events—Sally had walked in the house from outside when she slipped and fell, striking her chest and shoulder against the metal rim of the kitchen table. Shortly after she got up, she noticed blood coming from a tear in her central line. She thought it would stop if she just sat for a minute. When her husband came to check on her and found the catheter still bleeding, he called EMS.
Previous Illness—Radical mastectomy for breast cancer, diagnosed 3 months ago
Current Health Status—"Not very good" since chemotherapy started; a central line (or venous access device) was surgically implanted 6 weeks ago for her chemotherapy
Allergies—None known
Medications—Rheumatrex (methotrexate) and Efudex (5-fluorouracil)

Focused Physical

Current Set of VS—P 124, R 24, BP 80/56
Other Pertinent Findings—An abrasion and contusion is noted on R shoulder extending onto R chest wall; a large swelling is noted between the catheter exit site and the shoulder incision site; the catheter has two branches with a tear in the catheter proximal to the branch, the main catheter has been jarred loose from the chest wall, blood is escaping around the exit site, through the tear and through one branch; there is a horizontal mastectomy scar on the L chest wall.
Diagnostic Tests—None done

ECG

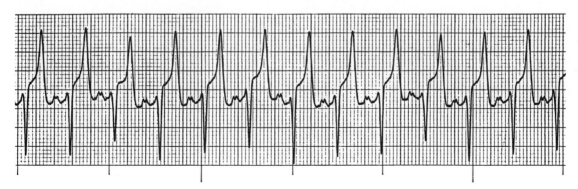

Figure 13-3

QUESTIONS

1. What is significant about Sally's history?

2. What is significant about the mechanism of injury and having a catheter in her chest?

3. What are the implications of Sally having this mechanism and being on chemotherapy?

4. What body systems are affected?

5. What is significant about the tear in the catheter?

6. What is significant about the swelling between the catheter exit site and the shoulder incision?

7. What is Sally at risk for?

8. How serious is Sally's current situation?

9. What is Sally's immediate problem?

10. How would you begin treatment?

11. Is there any other information from her history or physical examination that would help you?

12. What is important to reassess?

13. Sally was put on the monitor once she was taken to the squad. How would you describe her rhythm?

14. How would you know if Sally developed an air emboli?

15. People on chemotherapy are prone to several complications. What are the complications that you know about?

16. What should be included in further treatment?

QUESTIONS AND ANSWERS

1. What is significant about Sally's history?

Sally has a history of recent surgery for breast cancer, is currently undergoing chemotherapy, has a central line in place, and trauma is involved.

2. What is significant about the mechanism of injury and having a catheter in her chest?

Any patient who has a catheter inserted in the chest wall should be considered to have a central line or venous access device. It is called a central line because the catheter is inserted into a central vein, usually the subclavian or superior vena cava, to serve as a "line" for IV solutions, usually medications. Because the catheter is in a major vein, disruption by any means has the potential to cause significant bleeding.

3. What are the implications of Sally having this mechanism and being on chemotherapy?

Among other things, chemotherapy can lead to impaired clotting, which can worsen any bleeding; anemia, which can interfere with oxygen supply to the tissue; and fatigue, which impacts body reserves and may influence her ability to compensate.

4. What body systems are affected?

Cardiovascular—tachycardia; hypotension; and pale, cool, and clammy skin

5. What is significant about the tear in the catheter?

A tear in the catheter is not only a source of bleeding but also a source for air getting into the large vein. Although it is more of a threat to life for air to enter the arterial system, air in the venous system can also cause problems and is to be avoided.

6. What is significant about the swelling between the catheter exit site and the shoulder incision?

This may be evidence of internal bleeding at the site where the catheter was inserted into the subclavian vein. Suspect that the catheter has been pulled from the vein and bleeding is occurring at that site.

7. What is Sally at risk for?

Immediate problems include internal bleeding leading to exsanguination and an air embolus. Other problems include infection from contamination of a sterile body cavity, and injuries from her fall, such as bruising, skeletal injury, and the possibility of a cardiac contusion (from increased susceptibility to bruising).

8. How serious is Sally's current situation?

This is a threat to life; the greatest threat is from the excessive bleeding in the presence of a suspected clotting deficit. There is a lesser likelihood of development of an air embolus; but it is still a possibility.

9. What is Sally's immediate problem?

Hemorrhagic shock.

10. How would you begin treatment?

Direct pressure on the insertion site of the catheter, pinching the catheter closed. Cover the end of the catheter with a sterile dressing or tie a piece of umbilical tape around the catheter, between the exit site from the skin and the tear, to occlude the catheter. Administer oxygen by mask, nonrebreather with a reservoir at 15 lpm, lay her flat, feet elevated and start an IV in a peripheral line and bolus with 300 to 500 ml of crystalloid.

11. Is there any other information from her history or physical examination that would help you?

Why did Sally fall? Ask how she felt before the fall or if she knows why she fell.

12. What is important to reassess?

Her mental status, respiratory rate and effort, pulse rate, and blood pressure. It would also be important to reassess her contusions and the swelling in her shoulder. If she was having trouble with clotting, her bruises would be extending.

13. *Sally was put on the monitor once she was taken to the squad. How would you describe her rhythm?*

Sinus tachycardia. Sally has some interesting features in Lead II. There seems to be a notching of the P wave and an elevation of the T. Whether the notching of the P is an indicator of atrial enlargement or the elevation of the T is actually an indicator of elevation of the S-T segment is not only difficult to tell but does not change our care. However, this should heighten our awareness of the possibility of cardiac intolerance to increased preload and the development of congestive heart failure with large amounts of crystalloid administration.

14. *How would you know if Sally developed an air emboli?*

Sudden onset of difficulty breathing, anxiety, and air hunger, pleuritic chest pain, and increased pallor.

15. *People on chemotherapy are prone to several complications. What are the complications that you know about?*

Bleeding tendencies, anemia, infections (usually from the general public), pulmonary emboli, and stroke.

16. *What should be included in further treatment?*

Keep her warm, immobilize her right shoulder, and consider applying a cold pack to the swelling in the right upper chest. Because of the chance of air emboli, lie her on her left side. In this position, any air that has entered her vascular system will rise to the top or the right side of the heart, thus limiting or preventing air emboli from entering her lungs.

OUTCOME

Direct pressure was applied to the catheter exit site and Sally was placed on the gurney, supine with her feet elevated. Oxygen by mask, non-rebreather with a reservoir at 15 lpm was administered. Because of widespread venous collapse, an IV of normal saline was started in her left external jugular vein. A bolus of 500 ml was given en route to the hospital. Repeat VS showed a pulse of 116 and a systolic pressure of 92. On arrival at the hospital a chest x-ray was done, along with labs drawn, and a unit of blood started. Sally was taken to surgery where a torn subclavian vein was repaired. Sally developed pneumonia and had a rocky course but eventually recovered and was sent home. The rest of her chemotherapy treatment was much less eventful.

BIBLIOGRAPHY

Boum, M.K. (1997). Specialized adjuncts for therapy. In P. Pons & D. Cason (Eds.). *Paramedic field care: A complaint based approach.* St. Louis, MO: Mosby.

Braen, G.R. (1992). Sexual assault. In P. Rosen & R. M. Barkin (Eds.). *Emergency medicine.* (3rd ed.). St. Louis, MO: Mosby.

Pong, D. & Wilberger, J. E. (1982). Spinal cord injury without radiologic abnormalities in children. *Journal of Neurosurgery* 57:114.

Semonin-Holleran, R. (1994). Head, neck, and spinal cord trauma. In S. J. Kelley (Ed.). *Pediatric emergency nursing.* (2nd ed.). Norwalk, CT: Appleton & Lange.

Vanstralen, D & Goss, J.F. (1998). Damage control for pediatric spinal injuries. *Journal of Emergency Medical Services* March, pp. 114-125.

14

Trauma Emergencies

OVERVIEW

Trauma is the leading cause of death for persons between the ages of 1 and 40. Despite all efforts in prevention, trauma remains the fifth cause of death overall. There is a disparity between the genders, with male victims occurring about three times more frequently than female victims. For the caregiver, trauma continues to be an exciting response. Visual stimuli can be overwhelming. Impressive mechanisms may be present with dramatic physical injuries. Care is often fast-paced, involving transport considerations that include helicopters or light and sirens. Rapid recognition of significant injury usually determines the most appropriate facility to transport the patient. Other agencies such as law enforcement may be involved for a coordinated response.

One common problem is that the excitement of the scene and the frequent graphic injuries may leave the caregiver with tunnel vision. Maintaining an index of suspicion, attaining a knowledge of pattern recognition, and developing a concise approach that includes anticipating outcomes are all good characteristics that will help the caregiver avoid tunnel vision and deliver the best care possible.

The mechanism of injury is a valuable tool to help anticipate where the injury is most likely located. The age and physical condition of the victim is a guide to anticipating response and potential contributing factors. For instance, a 13 year old will have a very different response to a ground level fall than an 80 year old. The physical assessment findings of a 45-year-old insulin-dependent diabetic involved in a fender bender may dictate an additional assessment, that of checking a blood glucose level. The odor of alcohol or recreational drug use may alert the care provider to additional contributing factors that can be assessed for and managed appropriately. Use of seat belts, deployed air bags, penetrating injury, explosions, falls, and hangings all have their own significant patterns of injury to be assessed for and managed.

Anatomy, Physiology, and Pathophysiology

Suspicion of injury and potential for severity depends on a knowledge of organs, organ systems, and compensatory mechanisms. The type of mechanism involved usually predisposes to the type of direct or indirect organ injury such as soft tissue injury, fractures, bleeding, hollow organ spilling, swelling, irritation, organ rupture, and shock.

Critical body systems affected include the central nervous system (CNS), respiratory system, and the circulatory system (including the heart, vessels, and blood). The compensatory mechanisms include the epinephrine/norepinephrine system, the renin/aldosterone/angiotensin system,

281

and the biofeedback mechanisms of the brain to maintain perfusion to the CNS. Additional important pathophysiologic processes to understand include the concept of increased intracranial pressure and the pathophysiology of complete and incomplete spinal cord injuries.

Life threatening injuries or conditions include airway obstruction and hypoxia, tension pneumothorax, cardiac tamponade, uncontrolled bleeding (internal or external), multiple organ rupture or interrupted major vessels, increased intracranial pressure, multiple fractures of the pelvis, crush injuries of the chest or abdomen, and extensive burns including airway burns.

Potential threats to life include penetrating wounds to the cheek or neck, flail chest, multiple long bone fractures, and single organ rupture.

Assessment

Assessment of the trauma patient includes observation on approach. Scene safety is always a concern. Other observations include mechanism of injury, the number of patients, and deciding whether back-up is needed. Once the patient is identified many things happen simultaneously. Depending on the number of care providers, the initial survey may be done within seconds. The focused physical may occur very quickly with one provider conducting the physical and the second providing treatment. The assessment process involves recognition of patterns of signs and symptoms with treatment of threats to life begun on recognition of the problem.

Details such as patient positioning, presence of external blood, and skin color are all done on approach. Mental status, while immobilizing the head (c-spine), is the first to be assessed. Several threats to life have as their first sign an altered mental status. These include shock, hypoxia, and head injury. If the patient is talking, airway and breathing can also be assessed. Talking in 2 to 3 word sentences indicates inadequate minute volume. In the absence of exertion, this is abnormal. If the patient is not talking, opening the airway, ensuring its patency, and assessing for air exchange is next. Airway and breathing include assessing lung sounds and the chest wall, noting any abnormalities and treating as you go. Assessing the presence of the radial and/or carotid pulse, noting its rate and character along with skin temperature and moisture are next. Compensated shock often presents with sweat on the upper lip first. Internal bleeding may be indicated by pale, cool, clammy skin, and tachycardia with a low blood pressure. If signs and symptoms of shock are present but no external bleeding is noted, the patient is bleeding internally, either in the chest, abdomen, or multiple extremity fractures.

By the time the initial survey and focused physical is completed, threats to life should have been identified and treated. The following are patterns of signs and symptoms typical of injuries found in the multiple trauma patient.

Head Injuries. The major indicator of a head injury is altered mental status. However, there is also a typical pattern of assessment findings for increasing intracranial pressure. As the pressure inside the skull builds, headache and nausea/vomiting are common but unspecific. As the pressure builds and the brain stem is affected, altered mental status, pupil changes, alterations in respiratory rate, bradycardia, and hypertension occur. At about the time respiratory rate, bradycardia, and hypertension are occurring (Cushing's Triad), posturing also can be noted, either by flexion or extension. Posturing is a brain stem reflex.

Spinal Cord Injuries. Spinal cord injuries usually involve the sensation of pain, although this is not always true, especially if alcohol is involved. Careful assessment of extremity function and sensation will detect injury if there is nothing present to alter the patient's perception.

The presence of a low blood pressure and below normal heart rate in an unconscious trauma patient or a patient who cannot move should indicate high cervical cord interruption with neurogenic shock. If the patient can respond, the complaint is usually dyspnea. This is due to abdominal breathing. In complete cervical cord injury between C4 and C7, the diaphragm is the only muscle of respiration working. In cervical cord injury above C4, the diaphragm may not be able to work or is inefficient and assisted ventilations may be the only way the patient can breathe.

Injuries further down the cord involve the dermatomes. Useful reference points include T5 at the nipple line and T10 at the umbilicus. A sustained erection, or priapism, is another sign, usually of a low cord injury, in a trauma victim.

Partial cord injuries involve an unusual mixture of signs and symptoms. These can range from a complaint of numbness and tingling down one arm, in a completely mobile patient, to a feeling of water flowing down one leg. The rule of thumb is to suspect a spinal cord injury if weakness, paralysis, or altered sensation of any extremity occurs.

Chest Injuries. Life threatening chest injuries include tension pneumothorax and cardiac tamponade. The assessment pattern for a tension pneumothorax includes pallor, restlessness, distended veins (in the absence of blood loss), unequal lung sounds, tachycardia with a paradoxical pulse, and falling blood pressure. A deviated trachea is a very late sign. This is very similar to the pattern for cardiac tamponade: pallor, restlessness, distended veins (in the absence of blood loss), distant heart sounds, tachycardia with a paradoxical pulse, and falling blood pressure. The difference between the two is the presence or absence of unequal lung sounds.

A hemothorax may also be a threat to life, especially if bilateral, and may present as a tension pneumothorax.

Additional assessment findings that bear noting include those for flail segment. A flail segment may not be evident for the first 20 to 30 minutes after injury, depending on the number of ribs broken. Intercostal muscle spasm often splints the ribs in place requiring palpation of the chest wall to detect the presence of a flail. A flail segment interferes with air movement.

Abdominal Injury. There is a high correlation between the stated location of pain and an associated injury to the organ just under that area. Solid organs have pain associated with stretching of the organ capsule. Hollow organs, as well as solid organs, have pain with interruption of the organ wall. Radiating pain occurs in trauma most often with the liver and spleen. Stretched organ capsules irritate associated nerves radiating pain to the respective shoulders and neck area. The liver is associated with right sided shoulder and neck pain, whereas the spleen is associated with left sided shoulder and neck pain.

Interrupted organ walls are most often associated with bleeding. Solid organs will bleed extensively. Hollow organs will bleed minimally; however, it is the hollow organ contents that will predispose to peritonitis and sepsis hours later. This gives rise to the need for any patient with penetrating trauma of the trunk to be taken to a trauma center, regardless of presenting signs and symptoms.

The abdomen includes both the anterior peritoneal space and the retroperitoneal space. Because both areas have such a great capacity, suspect that a patient in shock with no visible bleeding site is bleeding either in the chest or abdomen until proven otherwise.

Extremity Injury. Over 50% of extremity injuries are missed in the multiple trauma patient. This is due to the concentration on managing the actual and potential threats to life. Because isolated extremity injuries are not considered a threat to life, this is considered an acceptable rate. Extremity injuries are identified by the following: the irregular contour of the limb involved and the presence of pain or crepitus on palpation. Distal circulation (pulse), sensation and movement should be assessed as appropriate. Multiple long bone fractures do have the potential to be a threat to life and should be assessed for and managed accordingly.

Shock. Of all assessment patterns, shock is probably the most talked about and the most frequently occurring syndrome in the trauma patient. The assessment findings for shock depend on how fast blood is lost, the previous state of health of the patient, and whether any preexisting conditions are present. Assessment findings can include such elements as recreational drug use, prescription medication that would interfere with compensatory mechanisms, or physical conditions, such as congestive heart failure, that would interfere with compensation.

Progressive and profound shock are easily recognized; compensated shock is not. A high index of suspicion and careful observation for subtle changes, such as increasing agitation or sudden drowsiness, may be the first indication of the presence of shock. Repeated assessments, especially serial vital signs, are most valuable. Regardless of the presence of any recognized injury, persistent anxiety in the presence of tachypnea or tachycardia should dictate rapid transport to the closest trauma facility.

Expose. Penetrating wounds, such as knife or gun shot/shot gun wounds, warrant removal of all clothing to find all the holes and penetrations.

Treatment

Treatment of the trauma patient is aimed toward supporting critical organs, organ systems, and the body's compensatory mechanisms. C-spine immobilization is performed on patient contact. Oxygen is administered by non-rebreather mask if the patient is awake and a good respiratory effort is noted. If unresponsive, an oral airway is placed and respirations assisted. If the patient accepts an oral airway without stimulating a gag reflex, intubation is indicated. The central nervous system, assessed by determining mental status, is supported by providing oxygen and ventilation. Adequate ventilation or tidal volume is at least 500 ml. This is determined by having good chest rise and fall.

The respiratory system is supported by oxygen, ventilation, and stabilization of the chest wall. This includes managing any open wounds to the chest wall or flail segments. Open wounds and flail segments are best managed by positive pressure ventilation. Covering an open wound to the chest with an occlusive dressing risks converting a simple pneumothorax to a tension pneumothorax. A tension pneumothorax is managed by reducing the tension. This is done by either loosening the occlusive dressing or by inserting a needle in the chest wall of the affected side.

A patient in profound shock that is unresponsive to treatment may have a tension pneumothorax or a cardiac tamponade. Cardiac tamponade is usually reduced as an in-hospital procedure.

The circulatory system is managed by gentle handling to help preserve any clots that may have formed, oxygen and ventilation, stopping bleeding, immobilizing the long bones (including the C-spine), limiting heat loss, and IV therapy with fluid boluses. Placing the patient on a backboard will help limit patient movement, thus preserving clot formation and immobilizing fracture sites. Appropriate oxygen therapy should be determined as soon as access to the patient is achieved. Heat loss can be limited by covering the patient with blankets after injury sites have been identified. IV therapy with fluid boluses is done on the way to the hospital.

Controversy exists regarding the total amount of fluid to be given. Current research suggests that systolic pressures above 100 disrupt clot formation and dilute clotting factors, thus increasing bleeding. Additional controversy exists regarding use of PASG. Those controversies are addressed in the appropriate cases cited in the chapter.

CASE 1

Dispatch: 22:00 hrs; personal injury accident, roll over, person pinned

On Arrival: You first see a sport utility vehicle, in the ditch, lying on its top. You find 31 y/o Cliff pinned under the roof at mid-chest. As you approach he opens his eyes and says, "I . . . can't . . . breathe." His lips are cyanotic. With the help of passers-by and a responding engine company, the vehicle is immediately lifted off Cliff.

Initial Assessment Findings

Mental Status—He opens his eyes to verbal stimuli, is verbally responsive but does not obey command, and is confused.

Airway—Open with bloody saliva

Breathing—R at 22 and shallow; lung sounds present but decreased bilaterally

Circulation—Skin pale and cool with cyanotic lips

Radial pulse absent, weak carotid at 116

BP none heard

Chief Complaint—Difficulty breathing

Focused History

Events—Another driver, who was behind Cliff, stated that Cliff was traveling at a high rate of speed when he swerved to miss a deer

Previous Illness—None known

Current Health Status—Not known

Allergies—None known

Medications—None known

Focused Physical

Current Set of VS—P 116, R 22, BP none heard

Other Pertinent Findings—Left side of chest tender to palpation; bruising noted across the sternum, chest, and upper abdomen; when the abdomen was palpated Cliff complained of pain and difficulty breathing; pelvis was stable; a large avulsion of the right knee noted; moving arms

Diagnostic Tests—None done

ECG

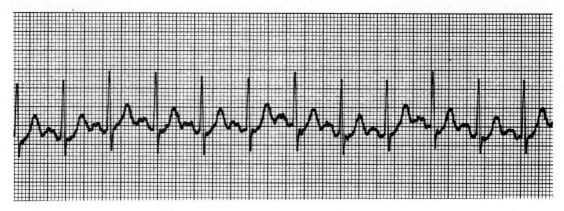

Figure 14-1

QUESTIONS

1. What is significant about Cliff's mechanism of injury?

2. From this mechanism, what type of injuries might you suspect?

3. What are your scene considerations?

4. After you have complete access to Cliff, what are your treatment priorities?

5. How would you accomplish your stated priorities?

6. What potential life threatening conditions is Cliff at risk for at the scene or en route?

7. How would you assess for each of them?

8. Of the signs and symptoms related to cardiac tamponade and tension pneumothorax, which one(s) would probably not be seen or not be accurate because of the situation?

9. Cliff complained of pain when his abdomen was palpated, but he also complained of difficulty breathing. What is significant about this associated complaint?

10. Is there any treatment for that condition?

11. Shortly after extrication and initial treatment with oxygen and IV fluids, you note that Cliff's cyanosis is increasing and he is complaining of increased difficulty breathing. What problems do you suspect, and how would you determine which problems were present?

12. Further assessment showed a weak, irregular carotid pulse of 166, in spite of a regular tachycardia by monitor; increasing respiratory distress; no detectable blood pressure; and unequal lung sounds (present on side but diminished or absent on the other side). Cliff's skin is cold and clammy with a gray color. There is a recognizable pattern of signs and symptoms described. What does it indicate?

13. What is the treatment for this condition?

14. How would you know if you were successful?

15. If you should suspect cardiac tamponade, what is the problem with trying to listen to heart sounds in the field?

16. How would you continue treatment?

17. Assuming fluid replacement is successful and the systolic pressure rises, what is Cliff at risk for developing as a result of increased pressure?

18. What must you continually reassess and why?

QUESTIONS AND ANSWERS

1. What is significant about Cliff's mechanism of injury?

Because Cliff was found pinned under the vehicle, he was ejected. Ejection greatly increases the likelihood of head and spinal injury. Because he was *under* the vehicle the phenomenon of traumatic asphyxia must also be considered.

2. From this mechanism, what type of injuries might you suspect?

Suspected injuries include head injuries, spinal cord injuries, flail chest with lower airway injury (pulmonary contusions, ruptured bronchi or vessels, and pneumothoraces), mediastinal injuries (contused heart, major vessel injury, and traumatic aortic aneurysm or rupture), broken pelvis and femurs, solid organ rupture (liver, spleen, and pancreas), ruptured diaphragm, hollow organ rupture (stomach, intestines and bladder), an evisceration, major vessel rupture/traumatic aneurysm, and extremity fractures. Immediate exsanguination is a possibility once the vehicle is off the patient.

3. What are your scene considerations?

A big consideration is how to prevent the overturned car, which has just been lifted off Cliff, from being a safety hazard. Because there is an engine company present that can handle the physical aspects of moving the vehicle, your concern is to move Cliff, as soon as possible, to an area of safety. You are also in a ditch. Although that might not present a hazard in itself, it may present problems getting out of the ditch, and it is a difficult place to be when you need light.

4. After you have complete access to Cliff, what are your treatment priorities?

Airway and breathing with oxygen and ventilation; circulation with fluid resuscitation and hemorrhage control, and immobilization of the skeletal system.

5. How would you accomplish your stated priorities?

It would be helpful if you could move Cliff to a backboard, either with a scoop stretcher or manually lift (or logroll). Airway management is a priority along with management of hemorrhage and C-spine immobilization. The biggest risk to lifting the car off is immediate exsanguination. Therefore some systems would advocate use of the PASG device, placing them on the backboard and then immediately inflating them while the airway was being managed. Of course, use of the PASG is controversial and is up to your local medical control.

Airway management would include immediate clearing of the oral cavity (suctioning) and use of the bag-valve-mask. This could be done while a C-collar was applied. If you are trying to get out of the ditch, you may be placing a mask non-rebreather with a reservoir at 15 lpm on him until you can get to a place where you can further manage the airway.

Once you have Cliff in a place where you can further treat, then start an IV of crystalloid, normal saline or Ringer's lactate, and start with a 500-ml bolus and repeat.

6. What potential life threatening conditions is Cliff at risk for at the scene or en route?

As soon as the vehicle is lifted off Cliff, exsanguination (bleeding out) is the immediate risk. From that point on Cliff is at risk for developing profound shock from excessive and uncontrollable bleeding, airway obstruction from lower airway crushing injury, cardiac tamponade, tension pneumothorax, and developing increased intracranial pressure from a head injury.

7. How would you assess for each of them?

Exsanguination as the immediate risk could be observed for and should be assumed to be occurring internally. Observation of visible blood and the abdominal size and presence of rigidity would confirm internal bleeding. The presence of tachycardia and low blood pressure would confirm the presence of shock.

Airway obstruction from lower airway crushing injury would be confirmed by the presence of bloody sputum, difficulty breathing, and inadequate tidal volume.

Cardiac tamponade and tension pneumothorax have very similar presentations with distended veins and a paradoxical pulse. Cardiac tamponade has distant heart sounds, whereas a tension pneumothorax has absent or unequal lung sounds on the affected side and eventually a deviated trachea occurs.

Increasing intracranial pressure from a head injury would be suspected with deterioration in mental status, posturing, and developing unequal/unreactive pupils.

8. *Of the signs and symptoms related to cardiac tamponade and tension pneumothorax, which one(s) would probably not be seen or not be accurate because of the situation?*

Both conditions have distended veins as a characteristic sign. In a patient who is also suffering blood loss, distended veins will usually not be seen.

In cardiac tamponade, distant heart sounds is also a sign. Listening to heart sounds in an uncontrolled and noisy environment is very difficult and inaccurate.

A tension pneumothorax can produce a deviated trachea. In reality this is a late sign. The trachea does, indeed shift, and it shifts very quickly. However, we can only see the trachea above the sternal notch. The trachea extends about 3 to 4 inches below the sternal notch and that is where it starts deviating first. By the time tracheal deviation has extended up to the sternal notch the patient is either dead or close to it.

9. *Cliff complained of pain when his abdomen was palpated, but he also complained of difficulty breathing. What is significant about this associated complaint?*

Because of the location of the crush injury, suspect a ruptured diaphragm.

10. *Is there any treatment for that condition?*

No field treatment; however, it would negate the use of the PASG, if that were an option.

11. *Shortly after extrication and initial treatment with oxygen and IV fluids, you note that Cliff's cyanosis is increasing and he is complaining of increased difficulty breathing. What problems do you suspect, and how would you determine which problems were present?*

An increase in cyanosis implies either a respiratory or a circulatory problem. His complaint seems to indicate a respiratory problem; however, if hypoxia is worsening due to impaired circulation, a sense of dyspnea is common. Problems to suspect include lower airway obstruction (most likely from blood), a tension pneumothorax, cardiac tamponade, extreme cardiac contusion, or an increasing state of shock.

12. *Further assessment showed a weak, irregular carotid pulse of 166, in spite of a regular tachycardia by monitor; increasing respiratory distress; no detectable blood pressure and unequal lung sounds (present on one side but diminished or absent on the other side). Cliff's skin is cold and clammy with a gray color. There is a recognizable pattern of signs and symptoms described. What does it indicate?*

This collection of signs and symptoms indicates a tension pneumothorax. The unequal lung sounds along with the irregular carotid pulse are the tip-off. Unequal lung sounds indicate a problem with ventilation in one side of the chest. An irregular pulse in the presence of a regular cardiac rhythm is a paradoxical pulse. Unequal lung sounds in the presence of a paradoxical pulse are signs of a tension pneumothorax. On the other hand, *equal* lung sounds in the presence of a paradoxical pulse in a chest trauma patient, are usually signs of cardiac tamponade.

13. *What is the treatment for this condition?*

Chest decompression with a large bore needle (14 or 16 gauge), using either the anterior approach, (in the intercostal space between the third and fourth rib, midclavicular line, up and over the rib) or the midaxillary approach (between the fourth and fifth rib).

14. *How would you know if you were successful?*

There should be an immediate release of air and a noticeable improvement in skin color, as well as a noticeable ease of ventilating. The pulse, in this case the carotid pulse, should lose its irregularity.

15. *If you should suspect cardiac tamponade, what is the problem with trying to listen to heart sounds in the field?*

An accurate auscultation of heart sounds is best done in a quiet environment to be most accurate. Determining if heart sounds are distant or not, requires the experience of regular listening of heart sounds, which most field medics do not have.

16. *How would you continue treatment?*

After chest decompression, stabilize the large bore needle and continue to assist ventilations. Monitor fluid replacement and continue fluid boluses until the return of a blood pressure that supports perfusion or until you reach local maximum for fluid replacement.

17. *Assuming fluid replacement is successful and the systolic pressure rises, what is Cliff at risk for developing as a result of increased pressure?*

Cardiac tamponade, recurring or increased bleeding, signs and symptoms of increased intracranial pressure, development of a traumatic aneurysm or rupture of same.

18. *What must you continually reassess and why?*

Mental status for evidence of increased intracranial pressure; respiratory status for recurrence of the tension pneumothorax; pulse and BP for signs of increased bleeding or improvement.

OUTCOME

After the vehicle was lifted off Cliff, a scoop stretcher was used to place him on a backboard. A C-collar and mask, non-rebreather with a reservoir at 12 lpm, was placed and Cliff was immediately removed from the ditch to the squad. There he was ventilated with a bag-valve-mask while two large bore IVs were started and turned wide open. En route to the hospital Cliff became difficult to ventilate and became more agitated and cyanotic. His left chest seemed to be larger than his right chest. Lung sounds on the left were absent. An anterior chest decompression, with a 14-gauge IV needle was performed with immediate improvement. A second set of VS were: P 120, R 24, BP still not heard or felt. On arrival at the trauma center, hemoglobin/hematocrit levels were obtained while chest x-rays, cross-table C-spine, and pelvic films were completed. A rapid infuser began O negative blood and he was taken to surgery within 20 minutes. His full extent of injury included bilateral pneumothoraces, ruptured spleen (requiring removal), lacerated liver, and ruptured diaphragm. He also suffered 5 fractured ribs on the left and 3 on the right with bilateral pulmonary contusions. The avulsion of his right knee was repaired. Cliff suffered adult respiratory distress syndrome (ARDS), kidney failure, and became septic. He eventually recovered.

CASE 2

Dispatch: 14:40 hrs; motorcycle personal injury accident, one victim

On Arrival: As you round the corner you see a motorcycle imbedded in the front of a late model compact car. There is a dent in the top of the roof and the windshield is broken, from an outside impact. Approximately 30 feet beyond the vehicle is 20 y/o Hirohoto. He is lying flat on his back. A full-face helmet is in place along with a leather jacket and leather trousers. As you kneel beside him he gasps, "I . . . can't . . . breathe . . . can't . . . feel . . . any . . . thing."

Initial Assessment Findings

Mental Status—Alert, verbally responsive, oriented

Airway—Open and clear

Breathing—R labored at 24, with accessory muscle use noted in his neck, talking in one-word sentences; lung sounds clear on the right, coarse sounds on left, in midsternal area

Circulation—Skin pale, warm, and dry

Radial pulse 60

BP 86/64

Chief Complaint—Complaining of difficulty breathing and inability to feel

Focused History

Events—Hirohoto had just received the motorcycle for his birthday and was taking it out for a ride when he entered the intersection and ran head-on into the automobile at a high rate of speed.

Previous Illness—Unknown

Current Health Status—Unknown

Allergies—None known

Medications—Unknown

Focused Physical

Current Set of VS—P 60, R 24, BP 86/64

Other Pertinent Findings—His full-face helmet is intact with extensive scuffing on the left side and top; a midsternal bruise about the size of a grapefruit is noted. No chest wall movement is noted, but regular, rhythmic movement of the diaphragm synchronized with his respirations is present. Bilateral lower leg anterior gouges extending down to the tibia, approximately 10 cm in length are also noted but are not bleeding; a laceration on the left lateral hip, extending posteriorly to the left buttock is bleeding profusely.

Diagnostic Tests—Administration of 300 ml normal saline bolus resulted in VS of: P 58, R20, BP 100/72

ECG

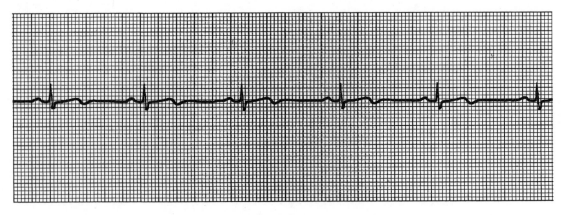

Figure 14-2

QUESTIONS

1. What is significant about Hirohoto's mechanism of injury?

2. From this mechanism, what type of injuries might you suspect?

3. What is significant about the scuff marks on Hirohoto's helmet?

4. What was the benefit of Hirohoto's helmet and leather jacket and trousers?

5. What are your scene considerations?

6. What is the significance of Hirohoto's complaint of difficulty breathing and inability to feel?

7. What are your treatment priorities?

8. What will you do with the helmet?

9. What would be your initial treatment?

10. What is the significance of Hirohoto's abdominal movement?

11. What is the significance of the midsternal bruise?

12. What might be the cause of the coarse lung sounds heard?

13. Is there any treatment for these conditions?

14. What is the relationship among Hirohoto's pulse, skin vitals, and BP?

15. Are Hirohoto's vital signs consistent with any other signs or symptoms?

16. Hirohoto has a recognizable pattern of signs and symptoms. What are the signs and symptoms of that pattern, and what do they indicate?

17. Is there any field treatment for this condition?

18. What is Hirohoto at risk for and why?

19. How would you assess for each of them?

20. How would you describe Hirohoto's ECG?

21. Is Hirohoto's rhythm related to his signs, symptoms, or chief complaint?

22. After your initial treatment was completed and you were en route to the hospital, Hirohoto tells you he is an insulin dependent diabetic. How would you continue treatment?

23. Based on this information, how would you revise your impression of what he was at risk for in the field?

24. Earlier you noted that the laceration on Hirohoto's left hip and buttock was bleeding profusely but the deep gouges on the anterior surface of his shins were not. What is the most likely explanation for that?

25. You also noted that Hirohoto's chest wall was not moving. What is the most likely explanation for that?

26. Given Hirohoto's signs, symptoms, and complaints, where do you think his cord injury is located?

QUESTIONS AND ANSWERS

1. What is significant about Hirohoto's mechanism of injury?

The significance is in the ejection and number and velocity of impacts. When impacting the car, Hirohoto first struck either or both the handles of his motorcycle and/or the hood of the vehicle, then the roof of the vehicle was impacted and finally the ground. Each time the outside of the body impacts the organs inside the body also impact. The total number of impacts could have been around five or six. Each time an impact occurs the body risks injury. The velocity of the impact is also significant in terms of the amount of kinetic energy reaching the body. In most cases the velocity is more important than the weight of the object.

2. From this mechanism, what type of injuries might you suspect?

Head injury, spinal cord injury, multiple fractures (especially extremity), pulmonary contusions, pneumothoraces, solid organ rupture (liver, spleen, kidney), fractured pelvis, and soft tissue injury (abrasions, avulsions). Hollow organ rupture is not as likely, neither are facial injuries.

3. What is significant about the scuff marks on Hirohoto's helmet?

There was a significant impact to his head. Inspect the helmet carefully; it may have cracked.

4. What was the benefit of Hirohoto's helmet and leather jacket and trousers?

The helmet is designed to protect the head but does not mean that a head injury has not occurred, it just minimized the potential for death resulting from head injury. The "leathers" protect the skin from extreme friction if contact with pavement occurs. Again it minimized the potential for extreme abrasions and avulsions in case of "laying the bike down" or other such impacts where friction may occur.

5. What are your scene considerations?

Primarily scene safety (which in this case was safe) and determining the number of patients. Someone was driving the car. That person needs to be identified and checked.

6. What is the significance of Hirohoto's complaint of difficulty breathing and inability to feel?

The inability to feel implies a central nervous system problem and possible cord injury. The complaint of difficulty breathing given this mechanism may have many causes, but when occurring at the same time as an inability to feel it implies a high cord problem.

7. What are your treatment priorities?

Gaining access to and securing an airway; Immobilization is a high priority; maintaining adequate perfusion and preserving body heat are also priorities.

8. What will you do with the helmet?

A full-face helmet does not allow access to the airway and must be removed. Although it is true that Hirohoto currently appears to have an open airway, he is in respiratory distress. There is nothing to guarantee that his airway will stay clear, and there is reason to believe that he has a high potential to vomit. You do not want to get caught with a full-face helmet on a patient who is vomiting.

9. What would be your initial treatment?

With manual stabilization and using a two-man technique, the helmet should be removed. Once the helmet is removed oxygen should be applied; you might try a mask non-rebreather first, but if not successful, then assist with a bag-valve-mask and time to the movement of his abdomen. Then move the patient to a backboard, either with a scoop stretcher or by logrolling. Apply dressings to the bleeding areas if they are accessible. Cover with blankets and move to the back of the squad.

10. What is the significance of Hirohoto's abdominal movement?

This is a description of belly or abdominal breathing. Sometimes it is missed when the abdomen is not bared and directly observed. When it occurs in the presence of a mechanism of injury, no chest wall movement, complaints of dyspnea, and an inability to feel, it indicates a high cord injury.

11. *What is the significance of the midsternal bruise?*

    Bruises occur where impacts to the body have happened. In a young, healthy person it usually takes a significant impact to cause bruising, especially one that can be observed at the scene. The vital organs in this location are especially important to survival. Evaluation of the cardiac rhythm is important, as are lung sounds, and close attention to ventilatory status.

12. *What might be the cause of the coarse lung sounds heard?*

    Since they seem to be unilateral and in close proximity to the bruise, the cause might be air escaping from a torn bronchus, blood collecting in the bronchioles, a pneumomediastinum, or an inhaled foreign body. Ask if he had been eating something just before the crash.

13. *Is there any treatment for these conditions?*

    There is no treatment for air escaping from a torn bronchus or a pneumomediastinum. A foreign body down that low in the bronchiolar tree cannot be removed in the field. The only other treatment is to closely monitor ventilations and assist when necessary.

14. *What is the relationship among Hirohoto's pulse, skin vitals, and BP?*

    His pulse is 60, which is the bottom end of normal. For someone involved in a traumatic incident this is lower than expected, especially in the presence of hypotension. His skin is pale, warm, and dry. Pale skin in the presence of skin warmth and dry texture does not fit the expected results of a normal epinephrine/norepinephrine response. The BP is hypotensive but not too low. While it is possible that this patient may normally have a low pressure, that cannot be assumed in an obviously injured patient. The rate is not slow enough to produce hypotension without another problem. The pale, warm, dry skin may be the result of vasodilation. (The reason the skin is not flushed is because after the initial flushing, blood has a tendency to settle in the most dependent parts.) The presence of vasodilation with a pulse of 60 could, however, cause hypotension.

15. *Are Hirohoto's vital signs consistent with any other signs or symptoms?*

    Yes, they are consistent with his abdominal breathing and complaint of lack of feeling.

16. *Hirohoto has a recognizable pattern of signs and symptoms. What are the signs and symptoms of that pattern, and what do they indicate?*

    The pattern consists of a mechanism of injury in the presence of abdominal breathing, lack of feeling, bradycardia, and low blood pressure. These indicate spinal cord injury or neurogenic shock.

17. *Is there any field treatment for this condition?*

    Standard treatment consists of immobilization, oxygenation with assistance as needed, a fluid bolus (usually 200 to 300 ml) and preservation of body heat. Usually the fluid bolus is enough to increase the blood pressure as long as there is no blood loss. If the heart rate is extremely slow, atropine 1mg may help.

18. *What is Hirohoto at risk for and why?*

    Internal bleeding because of the mechanism; increasing intracranial pressure (ICP) because of the mechanism, a head injury is still possible and a small bleed could take time to develop signs; vomiting because high cord injuries usually affect the GI tract; loss of body heat resulting from the vasodilation that occurs; and respiratory arrest as a result of swelling of the cord after injury.

19. *How would you assess for each of them?*

    Internal bleeding could be detected by continued fall in BP; increasing ICP by changes in mental status, especially in the presence of unequal or unresponsive pupils (posturing and grand mal seizure activity will most likely not be seen because of the cord damage); vomiting by close attention to the airway and presence of reverse swallowing; respiratory arrest by weak or irregular respiratory effort or a decrease in spontaneous rate; loss of body heat cannot be detected easily and is a danger that should be presumed.

20. *How would you describe Hirohoto's ECG?*

    Regular sinus rhythm without ectopy.

21. *Is Hirohoto's rhythm related to his signs, symptoms or chief complaint?*

    His rhythm is not the cause of any obvious sign, symptom, or complaint.

22. *After your initial treatment was completed and you were en route to the hospital, Hirohoto tells you he is an insulin dependent diabetic. How would you continue treatment?*

   A blood sugar level should be checked to establish a baseline. It is unlikely that his level is too low since he is oriented and seems alert. However, in a state of stress, blood sugar levels can change very quickly. The implication is that if he should have a change in mental status, check his blood sugar.

23. *Based on this information, how would you revise your impression of what he was at risk for in the field?*

   It would be revised to include hypoglycemia, as well as hyperglycemia and ketoacidosis.

24. *Earlier you noted that the laceration on Hirohoto's left hip and buttock was bleeding profusely but the deep gouges on the anterior surface of his shins were not. What is the most likely explanation for that?*

   In neurogenic shock, vasodilation occurs, which expands the container. Vasodilation in the absence of a compensatory increase in rate causes an initial settling effect where blood settles to the most dependent parts. If the patient is supine, blood will settle to the back and buttocks, away from the anterior surface. Thus breaks in the skin on the anterior surface have a tendency not to bleed, whereas those in the dependent surfaces will bleed profusely.

25. *You also noted that Hirohoto's chest wall was not moving. What is the most likely explanation for that?*

   No chest wall movement in a patient with a cord injury indicates the injury has occurred above the site where the intercostal nerves exit the spinal cord.

26. *Given Hirohoto's signs, symptoms, and complaints, where do you think his cord injury is located?*

   The phrenic nerve that supplies the diaphragm is still working so the injury is below that point (C2-C4). The chest wall has no movement so the injury is above that point (T1-T5). Therefore the injury is somewhere between C4 and T1-T2. However, permanent damage cannot be determined in the field, neither can additional lower vertebral or cord injury be ruled out.

OUTCOME

At the scene Hirohoto's helmet was immediately removed using a two-man technique. Once access to the airway was obtained a bag-valve-mask was used to assist ventilations and timed to his respiratory effort. He was exposed and abdominal breathing noted. At that point he was logrolled onto a backboard and dressings applied to his hip and buttock. He was covered with blankets and placed inside the squad. En route to the ED the cardiac monitor was applied, an IV of normal saline was started, and a fluid bolus of 200 ml was administered. Repeat VS showed: P 58, R 20, BP 100/72. On arrival at the ED, he notified personnel of his diabetic status. X-rays of his C-spine showed a crushed C6 and subluxated C7, fractured T5-T6, and a small fracture of the left ilium (pelvic wing). The laceration was superficial. Hirohoto was admitted to the ICU and had a rough few days with bradycardia and a labile blood pressure. His diabetes became very difficult to manage. Insulin resistance developed with repeated episodes of hypoglycemia, hyperglycemia, and ketoacidosis. He developed pneumonia, became septic, and expired 2 weeks after admission.

CASE 3

Dispatch: 00:45; personal injury, pedestrian hit by train

On Arrival: You find 45 y/o Dan, face down on the train tracks with body parallel to the tracks. He is dressed in old, tattered clothing with blood staining the left side of his shirt at waist level. Deformities of both extremities are apparent but no obvious amputations or extremity bleeding is noted. There is a strong odor of alcohol.

Initial Assessment Findings

Mental Status—Moaning on approach, no intelligible speech, does not obey command but thrashes arms when disturbed, eye opening only to painful response

Airway—Open and clear

Breathing—R 24, chest rise equal; lung sounds diminished on left, right clear in upper lobes, crackles in lower right lobe

Circulation—Skin normal color, warm, and dry

        Radial pulse 106

        BP unable to take because of thrashing of arms

Chief Complaint—Multiple trauma

Focused History

Events—It is unknown how this man was injured. It was speculated that Dave was attempting to either jump off a boxcar or jump on a boxcar when he was apparently hit by the train. Dave was found by a lineman. The last train passed by about 15 minutes ago.

Previous Illness—Unknown

Current Health Status—Unknown

Allergies—Unknown

Medications—Unknown

Focused Physical:

Current Set of VS—P 106, R 24, BP unable to take

Other Pertinent Findings—Subcutaneous emphysema with crepitus noted on palpation of right lower, lateral chest wall; abrasions noted to left lateral abdomen and flank with a quarter size open wound located at hip level of left lateral abdomen; pelvis has crepitus to palpation, obvious deformities to both femurs, lower legs, and right ankle.

Diagnostic Tests—None done

ECG

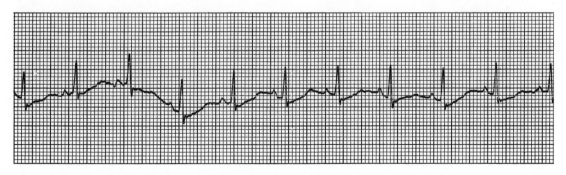

Figure 14-3

QUESTIONS

1. What is significant about Dave's mechanism?

2. From this mechanism, what type of injuries might you suspect?

3. What are your scene considerations?

4. What conclusions can you make regarding Dave's mental status?

5. What are your treatment priorities?

6. What would be your initial treatment?

7. With lung sounds diminished on the left, crackles in the right lower lobe, and presence of subcutaneous emphysema with crepitus on palpation of the right lower chest wall, what must you suspect and check for?

8. Is there any immediate field treatment for those conditions?

9. How does the presence of alcohol complicate the assessment, or does it?

10. What is Dave at risk for developing?

11. How does the presence of alcohol alter those risk factors, or does it?

12. How would you continue treatment?

13. What are the pros and cons to using the PASG (pneumatic antishock garment)?

QUESTIONS AND ANSWERS

1. *What is significant about Dave's mechanism?*

   His initial appearance does not suggest that he was run over by the train, giving more weight to the supposition that he may have been hit by the train. There is a significant mechanism by virtue of the sheer weight and speed (even if relatively slow) of the force. Crush and shear injury would be suspected.

2. *From this mechanism, what type of injuries might you suspect?*

   Amputation would be a reasonable suspicion though not apparent, head injury, pneumothorax with multiple rib fracture and pulmonary contusions, multiple extremity fractures, and fractured pelvis. If he was actually hit by the train (versus wheels running over him), it is possible that solid organ injury (liver, spleen, kidney) and/or hollow organ injury has occurred. From his first appearance and history he is lucky to still be alive.

3. *What are your scene considerations?*

   Scene safety—when is the next train scheduled to come by. Dave must be removed from the tracks and taken to a safe area.

4. *What conclusions can you make regarding Dave's mental status?*

   Dave has a GCS of 9 (eye opening to painful stimulus, localizes pain, unintelligible noises), but this is complicated by the possibility of alcohol. About the only conclusion that can accurately be made is that his mental status is impaired and a head injury must be suspected.

5. *What are your treatment priorities?*

   Stabilization of the spine; airway is currently clear but oxygenation is necessary; circulatory support with finding the site of bleeding and starting bleeding control; and rapid transport.

6. *What would be your initial treatment?*

   Logroll onto a backboard and apply oxygen by a mask non-rebreather with a reservoir at 15 lpm; move to the back of the unit and expose to find bleeding sites and injuries; control bleeding; and start an IV of normal saline.

7. *With lung sounds diminished on the left, crackles in the right lower lobe, and presence of subcutaneous emphysema with crepitus on palpation of the right lower chest wall, what must you suspect and check for?*

   Suspect multiple rib fractures bilaterally and a flail segment on the right; also suspect a developing pneumothorax on the left. Check for a possible tension pneumothorax on the left.

8. *Is there any immediate field treatment for those conditions?*

   Multiple rib fractures and a flail are best treated in the field with oxygen and positive pressure ventilation (harder to do than to say). There is no field treatment for a pneumothorax (other than supportive oxygen therapy) unless it becomes a tension pneumothorax; then a chest decompression is the treatment.

9. *How does the presence of alcohol complicate the assessment, or does it?*

   Alcohol does complicate assessments because of the effect on mental status and pain perception, among other things. Altered mental status caused by the effect of high levels of alcohol cannot be discriminated from altered mental status as a result of brain injury. Additionally, high levels of alcohol dull pain receptors so the ability of the patient to perceive pain is impaired. This implies that even on palpation, the absence of pain does not imply absence of serious injury at the point of palpation. Perhaps the greatest danger is the tendency by the care provider to assume the patient is "just a drunk" and not perform a complete assessment.

10. *What is Dave at risk for developing?*

    Shock, increased intracranial pressure, a tension pneumothorax, and loss of body heat.

11. How does the presence of alcohol alter those risk factors, or does it?

The affect of alcohol on the development of hemorrhagic shock is probably slight at best. Alcohol's effect in intracranial pressure is again negligible; however, there is some research that suggests the effect of alcohol on patients with head injuries is more on the outcome (it's worse). Alcohol has no effect on the development of a tension pneumothorax. Alcohol does, however, have an effect on the loss of body heat. Alcohol is a general body vasodilator so there is an increased risk of losing body heat.

12. How would you continue treatment?

After Dave was moved to the transport vehicle and clothing removed to find all areas of injury, a dressing would be applied to the bleeding areas. Because he has pelvic crepitus and multiple long bone fractures, the PASG might be useful. If your protocol allows for its use in such a situation, all three compartments would be inflated, starting with the legs first, then the abdomen. A close watch on the respiratory system would also be required, especially since multiple rib fractures are suspected.

13. What are the pros and cons to using the PASG (pneumatic antishock garment)?

The PASG is a device that is useful as a splint for multiple long bone fractures and pelvic fractures. Because it exerts pressure on the abdomen, the diaphragm may also be affected, requiring more work from the patient to breathe. When a ruptured diaphragm is suspected or when penetrating trauma above the navel has occurred, application of the PASG may aggravate a ruptured diaphragm and increase intrathoracic bleeding. In some systems, medical directors would rather not use the device at all, in other systems, medical directors authorize the PASG for situations like this one.

OUTCOME

At the scene a dressing was placed over the penetrating wound of the abdomen; PASG was applied and all three compartments were inflated. A monitor was applied and sinus tachycardia was noted. Two large bore IVs of normal saline were started with 1000 ml infused by arrival. Mental status did not change en route, Dave continued to thrash about with any stimulus. A second set of VS: P 110, R 24, BP unable to gain cooperation to obtain. On arrival at the ED, VS: P114, R 22, BP 108/44. A GCS was obtained then he was sedated, paralyzed, and intubated. He then had portable x-rays done, which revealed multiple rib fractures and a left sided flail segment with bilateral pneumothorax. Bilateral chest tubes were placed in the trauma room. ABGs showed a pH 7.19, pO_2 155, pCO_2 37.9, HCO_3^- 19.7, blood alcohol 348, hemoglobin/hematocrit 14.8/44.4. X-ray revealed multiple fractures of the pelvis. CT showed no brain injury, no obvious abdominal organ injury, but seven pelvic fractures with one communicating with the open abdominal wound. He was taken directly to the OR where the PASG was slowly deflated and surgical repair began. He was admitted to the ICU. His recovery was complicated with infection and kidney failure. He was dismissed to a rehabilitation unit 6 weeks after admission.

CASE 4

Dispatch: 01:30; personal injury accident, person pinned

On Arrival: You see a compact car up on the sidewalk lying on its driver's side. It is wedged between a cement retaining wall and a pole. The car door of the passenger side has been opened and a person is standing in the inside of the car, looking out the opened door and yelling to you to hurry because his friend is bleeding. An engine company has arrived at the same time you have and is starting to secure the scene. You find out that your patient is the driver, 16 y/o Muhallah, who lost control of his vehicle and it jumped the curb. He and his passenger, the person standing in the car on your arrival, were unrestrained. After about 15 minutes, firefighters extricate Muhallah from the vehicle and he helps himself crawl out. He is bloody from his left neck to his fingertips and a neck wound is bleeding profusely. He is awake and appears anxious.

Initial Assessment Findings

Mental Status—Alert, anxious, obeys command
Airway—Open and clear
Breathing—R 18 and normal; lung sounds present and clear bilaterally
Circulation—Skin pale, cool, and clammy
        Radial pulse regular at 120
        BP 106/86
Chief Complaint—Pain in left arm

Focused History

Events—He and his friend were on the way home from a party when he lost control on a curve.
Previous Illness—None known
Current Health Status—Good
Allergies—Artichokes
Medications—None

Focused Physical

Current Set of VS—P 120, R 18, BP 106/86
Other Pertinent Findings—There is a laceration that begins on the left side of his neck just above the juncture of his neck and shoulder that extends to his left axilla. The clavicle is broken and bone ends are exposed. There is an extensive degloving injury that begins on the posterior side of his left upper arm at the shoulder and extends to mid-forearm. Bone, muscle tissue, tendons, and ligaments are exposed. There is profuse bleeding from his neck, clavicular area, and axilla. Chest wall palpates intact with the exception of his left clavicle. No other abnormalities are noted.
Diagnostic Tests—None done

ECG: None done

1. What is significant about Muhalla's mechanism?

2. From this mechanism, what type of injuries might you suspect?

3. What are your scene considerations?

4. What are your treatment priorities?

5. What special considerations must be taken when dealing with lacerations to the neck, and why?

6. How do the special considerations affect treatment?

7. What anatomic structures are located under the clavicle?

8. How does that knowledge affect field treatment?

9. What is the relationship between Muhalla's pale, cool, clammy skin and his vital signs?

10. What would be your initial treatment?

11. What is Muhalla at risk for?

12. What anatomic structures are located in the axilla?

13. Does that knowledge affect field treatment?

14. How would the degloving injury be managed?

15. How would you continue your treatment?

QUESTIONS AND ANSWERS

1. What is significant about Muhalla's mechanism?

With a vehicle being turned on its side and no restraints used, there is considerable tossing of the occupants. Every object inside the vehicle then becomes a potential impact point for the occupant.

2. From this mechanism, what type of injuries might you suspect?

Head injuries, fractured ribs, pneumothorax, multiple fractures, solid organ rupture, (hollow organ rupture is possible but not as likely), and spinal fractures.

3. What are your scene considerations?

Scene safety in terms of stabilization of the vehicle. On approach it seems that the vehicle is wedged pretty securely but stability of the vehicle should be evaluated very carefully. With people moving about (in and out of the open door) it may not remain stable. The other concern regards the pole. Consideration must be given to the potential for the pole to fall. If this is a power pole, are the lines secure or are there any lines down?

4. What are your treatment priorities?

Treatment priorities in terms of immobilization, airway and oxygenation, breathing, and circulation don't change. However, since he helped himself crawl out and he appears alert and oriented, the assumption is that for the moment he is exchanging and cord function is intact. Because of the copious amounts of bleeding you will probably be applying pressure to the bleeding sites, then directing immobilization, oxygenation, and so forth from that point.

5. What special considerations must be taken when dealing with lacerations to the neck, and why?

The neck contains vital structures such as the spinal cord, major vessels, and the trachea. If lacerations to the neck involved the spinal cord, paralysis might also be involved, with respiratory effects a common result. If major vessels are involved bleeding may be extensive and the patient may exsanguinate. If arteries are involved, the interruption of arterial pressure may cause a vacuum effect and air may gain entry into the arterial system. Air emboli in the cerebral circulation can lead to a stroke. If the trachea is involved then patency of the airway is a concern and must be immediately managed.

6. How do the special considerations affect treatment?

If the spine is involved, then immobilization is needed; if the trachea is involved, then inserting an endotracheal tube in the tracheal wound and inflating the cuff may be the effective way to secure the airway; if arterial bleeding is involved, then place an occlusive dressing over the wound with direct pressure to control bleeding and place the patient on his left side in a slight Trendelenburg position. This position will theoretically keep any air in the system floating to the top which is now the right side (venous side of the heart) and toward the feet (away from the brain).

7. What anatomic structures are located under the clavicle?

The clavicle protects major vessels, the subclavian artery, subclavian vein, and the brachial plexus (C5-T1), all of which lie close together just under the clavicle.

8. How does that knowledge affect field treatment?

Because of the presence of a major artery and a major vein, direct pressure to control massive bleeding is necessary. If direct pressure is applied, it would not be unusual for the patient to complain of numbness, tingling, or burning pain resulting from the irritation of the nerve by the pressure. The other problem is the presence of broken bone ends. Broken bone ends are very sharp. Care must be taken to avoid direct pressure on a bone end to prevent lacerating through gloves. It is also possible that bone ends may lacerate the brachial plexus, resulting in nerve damage. The priority in the field is bleeding control, which is direct pressure. Keep in mind that monitoring and assessing extremity feeling and function is also an assessment task and should be done throughout transport.

9. *What is the relationship between Muhalla's pale, cool, clammy skin and his vital signs?*

His pale, cool, clammy skin indicates an epinephrine/norepinephrine response and vasoconstriction are present. This is also consistent with his tachycardia. With a normal blood volume a heart rate of 120 would significantly increase the blood pressure, but his is low normal, suggesting that a significant blood loss has probably already occurred.

10. *What would be your initial treatment?*

Start direct pressure to the bleeding site(s) as soon as you have access to the patient, then direct spinal immobilization while someone is applying an oxygen mask. Because most paramedics do not work alone, the assumption is that you will have one or more people to help you.

11. *What is Muhalla at risk for?*

The initial risk is exsanguination or airway occlusion. The biggest risk is missing another serious injury such as an internal bleed or head injury due to the distraction of the massive degloving injury.

12. *What anatomic structures are located in the axilla?*

Major nerves (brachial nerve) supplying the arm and vessels (brachial artery), as well as the lymph nodes. This area does not have large muscle bodies so the ribs and intercostal muscles are very close to the surface.

13. *Does that knowledge affect field treatment?*

With direct pressure, complaints of numbness and tingling may occur if the brachial nerve is irritated by the pressure. If the radial pulse is weak or absent you may not know if it is due to your direct pressure on the brachial artery or if it is because there is an occlusion further down the "line."

Check for frothy blood in the axilla or subcutaneous emphysema down the lateral side of the chest wall. A pneumothorax could be present and missed.

14. *How would the degloving injury be managed?*

The exposed tissue should have moist dressings applied with dry dressings over that. That, however, is a perfect world and may not be possible. The goal is to cover the exposed tissue as much as possible. The problem will be the bleeding sites. Dressings should be applied to bleeding sites with direct pressure maintained over the dressings. Do the best you can. Do *not* use hemostats or clamps of any sort. If these instruments are used when tissue is not adequately visualized, vital structures can be permanently damaged. In the field, direct pressure is the best method for bleeding control. There are some exceptions such as excessive transport time and limited help.

15. *How would you continue your treatment?*

If possible, start an IV in the opposite extremity. The priority is bleeding control so the majority of your time will be concentrated with that task.

OUTCOME

Muhalla crawled out of the vehicle with help from the firefighters. He has no complaints other than extreme pain in his left arm. He is very anxious. Direct pressure was immediately applied to the neck and shoulder area. A standing backboard was placed next to him, and the "standing board" procedure was utilized to maintain spinal immobilization. Since there was plenty of help, he was rapidly placed on the gurney and taken to the medic unit. Because of his wounds, manual cervical immobilization was maintained. Once inside, dry dressings were placed to the clavicular bleeding site and axilla and manual pressure applied. An occlusive dressing was applied to the neck area along with manual pressure. The laceration did not extend around to the trachea or to the spine. Oxygen by mask, non-rebreather with a reservoir at 15 lpm was also applied and an IV of normal saline started and a bolus of 500 ml was given. His left arm was placed on a sterile burn pad with dry dressings placed on the exposed tissue, sterile saline was used to moisten the dressings, and the pad was wrapped around the arm and tissue. A second set of vital signs showed: P 102, R 20, BP 112/80.

On arrival at the ED, rapid exploration of the wounds revealed major vessel transection and he was taken to surgery. A punctured subclavian artery was repaired along with a lacerated external jugular vein, lacerated brachial vein, and severely contused brachial plexus. The degloved tissue was débrided and reattached. After 3 weeks and many débridement sessions, Muhalla was dismissed to an outpatient treatment center. He underwent physical therapy for 6 months and now has almost full function.

CASE 5

Dispatch: 08:00 hrs; construction site electrical accident, 32 y/o male burn victim

On Arrival: You find 32 y/o Dale inside a newly constructed office building. He is sitting in a chair just outside a room where the floor and walls are covered in soot except for footprints in the floor near an electrical panel. Dale is awake but his face is gray. His face appears abnormally wrinkled and is sagging downward, as if his skin were melting. His hands have the same effect up to his wrists. He has no eyebrows and the hair at his hairline is singed off. His shirt is scorched at the neckline and cuffs but otherwise intact. He tells you, "Man, this really hurts!"

Initial Assessment Findings

Mental Status—Awake, oriented, and obeys command

Airway—Open and clear, tongue and mucous membranes appear normal color

Breathing—R regular at 20; lung sounds present, clear, and equal bilaterally

Circulation—Skin of arms is normal color, warm, and dry

> Brachial pulse 88
>
> BP 146/86

Chief Complaint—Pain around wrists and lower neck area

Focused History

Events—Dale is an electrician and was working at the electrical panel when a flash occurred.

Previous Illness—Hypertension

Current Health Status—Good

Allergies—None known

Medications—Lotensin (benazepril)

Focused Physical

Current Set of VS—P 88, R 20, BP 146/86

Other Pertinent Findings—Both ears are reddened and have blisters; his eyes are clear but all lashes are gone. The skin on his face is a gray color and appears to be sliding downward, as if it is melting. The top button of his work shirt had been open so the area of his lower neck that is burned is a V-shaped area ending just below the sternal notch. That area is also reddened and blistered. Both hands are fully involved with the same appearance as his face, gray in color with the appearance of melting skin. Both wrists have circumferential red, blistered skin that extends about 2 to 3 inches above the base of his thumbs. There are no other apparent injuries.

Diagnostic Tests—Blood sugar level 94

ECG

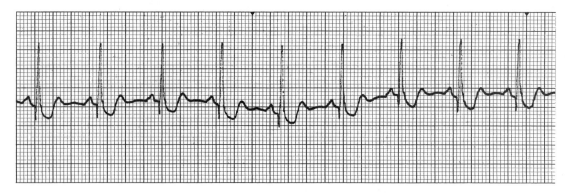

Figure 14-4

QUESTIONS

1. What is significant about Dale's mechanism of injury?

2. From this mechanism, what type of injuries might you suspect?

3. What are your scene considerations?

4. What are your treatment priorities?

5. Dale states his face and hands really don't hurt that much, but his neck and wrists really hurt. What is the most probable reason for the lack of pain in his face or hands?

6. What is the estimated percent of body burn for Dale?

7. Does Dale meet the criteria for a burn center?

8. What would be your initial treatment?

9. What makes electrical flash burns different from a flame burn?

10. What is Dale at risk for?

11. In Dale's case, what specific body functions must be continually reassessed?

12. What is Lotensin (benazepril)?

13. How could the presence of Lotensin (benazepril) affect Dale's assessment findings?

14. Does Dale's history of hypertension or taking Lotensin (benazepril) alter his treatment?

15. How would you continue treatment?

16. How could Dale's pain be managed, or can it?

17. A special challenge in this case is how to deliver oxygen when the face is burned. How would you do it for Dale?

QUESTIONS AND ANSWERS

1. *What is significant about Dale's mechanism of injury?*

This is a burn from an electrical source and occurred in an enclosed space.

2. *From this mechanism, what type of injuries might you suspect?*

Electrical contract burns follow the nerve and blood vessel tracts in the body and can cause violent muscle contractions that will literally throw a person. Cardiac dysrhythmias, respiratory arrest, internal burns that are "hidden," and traumatic injuries (usually involving joints and long bone fractures) from being thrown are all common with electrical burns. Electrical sources of ignition can also cause flame burns. In an enclosed space, flame burns can also cause heat related injuries to the respiratory system. Electrical sources can also cause flash burns, which are caused by arching of electrical current. In this type of burn, clothing may be intact but exposed skin may be severely burned. Inhalation burns are rare.

3. *What are your scene considerations?*

Scene safety from the source of electricity. Other electricians or members of the public power district should be available to help secure the scene. Until that occurs designate a person to keep others away from the scene and remove the patient to a safe area. In this case the scene is safe. There was another electrician and a member of the public power district present when the event occurred.

4. *What are your treatment priorities?*

Ensuring an open airway with adequate oxygenation and ventilation; determining adequacy of circulation and perfusion to vital organs, and determining if immobilization is needed.

5. *Dale states his face and hands really don't hurt that much, but his neck and wrists really hurt. What is the most probable reason for the lack of pain in his face or hands?*

Considering that his face and hands have been noticeably burned suggests the most likely reason there is no pain is that they have suffered a third degree or full thickness burn.

6. *What is the estimated percent of body burn for Dale?*

The areas burned are the front of his face, a small area at the lower neck-upper sternum, and both hands extending up his wrists about 2 to 3 inches. Using the rule of 9s he has suffered about 4.5% to his head, 3% to each hand/wrist, and 1% to the lower neck. This amounts to about an 8% to 9% body surface area of partial and full thickness burn.

7. *Does Dale meet the criteria for a burn center?*

Yes, not because of the percent burned, but because of the critical areas involved—his face, hands, and circumferential nature of the burns on his wrists.

8. *What would be your initial treatment?*

Oxygenate, cover burned areas with dry dressings, start an IV, and transport.

9. *What makes electrical flash burns different from a flame burn?*

Flash burns are seen when a victim is too close to an open electrical source. This results in thermal burns, usually to skin unprotected by clothing on the side next to the flash. Because there is no direct contact with electricity, there is no associated violent muscle contraction throwing the victim, neither is there an entrance nor exit point.

10. *What is Dale at risk for?*

Immediate prehospital risks include airway compromise, either upper airway or lower airway; and cardiac dysrhythmias, even though that has a low probability. In field care can also contribute to such in-hospital risks as hypothermia and infection.

11. *In Dale's case, what specific body functions must be continually reassessed?*

Respiratory and cardiac function must continually be reassessed.

12. What is Lotensin (benazepril)?

Lotensin or benazepril is an ACE (angiotensin converting enzyme) inhibitor. Angiotensin is a substance produced by an enzyme in the kidney that can cause peripheral vasoconstriction, which then contributes to hypertension. ACE inhibitors interfere with the enzyme that creates angiotensin, thus preventing vasoconstriction and resulting hypertension.

13. How could the presence of Lotensin (benazepril) affect Dale's assessment findings?

The presence of an ACE inhibitor may have little effect other than preventing the BP from elevating as much as it might.

14. Does Dale's history of hypertension or taking Lotensin (benazepril) alter his treatment?

No, not in the prehospital environment.

15. How would you continue treatment?

Put Dale on a cardiac monitor and consider pain management. Since Dale's BP is within normal limits, regulate the IV flow so he gets approximately 150 ml/hr.

16. How could Dale's pain be managed, or can it?

One of the biggest problems in the prehospital treatment of any patient is the management of pain. Pain from burns is excruciating, but unfortunately, there is very little that can be done effectively. Use of cold on the burn has been advocated in the past. However, resultant hypothermia and vasoconstriction has a severe negative impact on patient outcome. Cool, moist dressings applied to burn areas that are less than 9% BSA usually do not produce the hypothermia that cold dressings applied to larger burn areas produce. Use of cool, moist dressings rather than cold also limits the amount of vasoconstriction. In general, for major burns, use of moist dressings is not advocated.

Morphine, 5 mg IV push and repeated, may take the edge off, but patients will most likely suffer a respiratory arrest before enough can be given to really relieve the pain. In cases where associated injury or inhalation burns are involved, morphine may be contraindicated.

Nitrous oxide has been used in the prehospital environment and may be useful for isolated extremity burns, but for larger burns it can cause the phenomenon of diffusional hypoxia if used in amounts greater than 50%.

Diazepam (Valium) 5 to 10 mg IV can be useful for eliminating memory for the time it is used but can cause respiratory depression when given rapidly or in large amounts.

If and when pharmacologic agents are used will be up to local medical control.

17. A special challenge in this case is how to deliver oxygen when the face is burned. How would you do it for Dale?

In this case a mask, non-rebreather with a reservoir at 15 lpm was chosen. Sterile 4 × 4s were used to line the elastic headband and the plastic mask where it touched facial tissue.

OUTCOME

As soon as it was determined that Dale was not thrown and a flash burn was the mechanism, oxygen by mask, non-rebreather with a reservoir at 15 lpm was started. Sterile 4 × 4s were used to line the elastic and the plastic portion that touched the skin. He was then taken to the medic unit and his shirt removed. Sterile burn dressings were used to wrap his hands and wrists. Vital signs were taken, a cardiac monitor applied, and an IV of normal saline running at 100 ml/hr was started. En route to the hospital he developed frequent PVCs. At the local hospital he developed runs of PVCs that affected his BP (106/78). He was given 150 mg lidocaine IV push; PVCs were then reduced and a lidocaine drip started. Based on the areas of burn and the presence of full-thickness burn, ground transport transferred to the burn center. Dale eventually recovered 90% of hand function with minimal scarring of his face.

CASE 6

Dispatch: 17:30 hrs; 27 y/o pregnant female, personal injury collision

On Arrival: You find 27 y/o Cassie, lap and shoulder belt in place, behind the wheel of a small compact car. She is awake, appears pale, and is obviously pregnant. She is anxiously asking, "Is my baby going to be okay?"

Initial Assessment Findings

Mental Status—Awake, repeatedly asking the same question, does not obey command
Airway—Open and clear
Breathing—R 24 and regular; speaking in complete sentences but seems out of breath. Lung sounds clear and equal bilaterally
Circulation—Skin pale, warm, and dry
        Pulse regular at 100
        BP 110/72
Chief Complaint—"Is my baby going to be okay?"

Focused History

Events—Cassie's car was hit broadside on the passenger side front door, at an intersection by another vehicle whose driver ran a red light.
Previous Illness—Unknown, repeatedly asking same question
Current Health Status—Unknown, repeatedly asking same question
Allergies—Unknown
Medications—Unknown

Focused Physical

Current Set of VS—P 100, R 24, BP 110/72
Other Pertinent Findings—Fundal height midway between xiphoid and umbilicus; small glass cuts to left hand; small hematoma with abrasion on left temple; no other injuries noted; unable to hear fetal heart tones; she moves all extremities and movement is purposeful.
Diagnostic Tests—None done

ECG

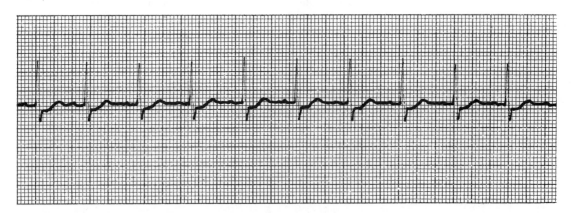

Figure 14-5

QUESTIONS

1. What is significant about Cassie's mechanism of injury?

2. From this mechanism, what type of injuries might you suspect?

3. What are your scene considerations?

4. What are your treatment priorities?

5. What is significant about Cassie's repeated question?

6. Cassie's fundal height is midway between the xiphoid and umbilicus. What trimester is she most likely in?

7. What are the special treatment considerations that must be taken into account when the patient is in the second or third trimester?

8. What would be your initial treatment?

9. Regarding her pregnancy, what is Cassie at risk for?

10. Why should fetal heart tones be assessed in the field?

11. What is the significance of the absence of fetal heart tones?

12. How would the onset of premature labor be detected in the field?

13. How do signs of internal bleeding differ in a pregnant woman in her second or third trimester?

14. If Cassie is bleeding internally, how would you know?

15. How would you continue treatment?

QUESTIONS AND ANSWERS

1. *What is significant about Cassie's mechanism of injury?*

   The mechanism is a vehicular crash where her vehicle was impacted on the passenger side. She was belted in, so seat belt injuries are possible.

2. *From this mechanism, what type of injuries might you suspect?*

   Head injury (hitting the side of the head versus the front of the head), clavicular injury, rib fracture, pulmonary contusion or pneumothorax, neck injury, hip injury, and abdominal injury including fetal injury, bruised uterus, and/or ruptured bladder.

3. *What are your scene considerations?*

   Determining the number of patients (other occupants of Cassie's car, the other driver and possible occupants of that car) and scene safety (traffic control, leaking fuel).

4. *What are your treatment priorities?*

   Ensuring an open airway and adequate ventilation, ensuring perfusion to vital organs including the fetus.

5. *What is significant about Cassie's repeated question?*

   Cassie's repeated question suggests the presence of a head injury. Together with her inability to obey command, purposeful movement, and spontaneous eye opening, she has a GCS of 13.

6. *Cassie's fundal height is midway between the xiphoid and umbilicus. What trimester is she most likely in?*

   The fundus is at the level of the umbilicus at 5 months and the xiphoid at 9 months. If the fundus is located somewhere in between, the assumption is approximately 7 months.

7. *What are the special treatment considerations that must be taken into account when the patient is in the second or third trimester?*

   Treatment should include positioning on the left side or displacing the uterus to the left to avoid supine hypotensive syndrome.

8. *What would be your initial treatment?*

   Immobilize and extricate from the vehicle, apply oxygen by mask, non-rebreather with a reservoir at 15 lpm and start an IV of normal saline at kvo rate

9. *Regarding her pregnancy, what is Cassie at risk for?*

   Premature labor, abruptio placentae, a "silent" abdominal bleed, and/or shock

10. *Why should fetal heart tones be assessed in the field?*

    Fetal heart tones can be an indicator of the seriousness of a pregnant woman's condition or condition of the fetus.

11. *What is the significance of the absence of fetal heart tones?*

    In a quiet environment, absent fetal heart tones indicate the fetus is either dying or dead. In the field it is very hard to hear fetal heart tones without a Doppler or similar device. It may be more accurate to ask the mother if she can feel the baby move or when she last felt the baby move. If a Doppler or similar device is available, and medics are trained in its use and are comfortable using it, the absence of fetal heart tones is an indicator of extreme fetal distress.

12. *How would the onset of premature labor be detected in the field?*

    The mother may complain of vague, diffuse abdominal pain, or low back pain; gentle palpation of the abdomen may reveal a periodic tensing and relaxation of the uterus, which may or may not be detected by the mother; or presence of bloody vaginal drainage. Sometimes premature labor is occurring but cannot be detected in the field.

13. ***How do signs of internal bleeding differ in a pregnant woman in her second or third trimester?***

When the peritoneum stretches from the enlarging uterus, normal peritoneal pain perception is dulled. Complaints of abdominal pain that would normally occur when the peritoneum is irritated by chemicals released by ruptured organs and capsules are diminished or absent. When internal bleeding occurs the body considers the fetus and uterus to be an extremity. Because there are no valves in the uterus or placenta, blood is shunted from the pregnant uterus to the rest of the body. This cannot be observed. If the bleeding is occurring within the uterus, the uterus will enlarge so periodic measurements of fundal height can be a valuable tool. Blood pressure is normally a bit low because pregnancy is a vasodilatory state and the heart rate normally in the 80s or 90s. Repeated observations of heart rate and skin vitals are valuable for noting trends.

14. ***If Cassie is bleeding internally, how would you know?***

The first sign is altered mental status. In this case when altered mental status may be caused by a head injury (she has a hematoma with abrasion on the left temple), close attention to pulse rate, skin vitals, response to a fluid challenge, and measurement of fundal height can all be indicators of internal bleeding.

15. ***How would you continue treatment?***

Shift Cassie to her left side by putting a towel roll under the right side of the backboard. Continue to orient Cassie to what happened and where she is and monitor for any change in her mental status. If you have a long transport, you might choose to administer a fluid bolus of 250 to 300 ml of normal saline and repeat vital signs. If there is no change, there is a high probability of internal bleeding.

OUTCOME

Cassie was immobilized on a backboard and quick extrication performed. Oxygen by mask, non-rebreather with a reservoir at 15 lpm was applied. In the back of the medic unit, the backboard was tipped on its left side and an IV of normal saline was started at kvo rate. Vital signs remained the same. En route to the hospital Cassie became more oriented and obeyed command. She stated her due date was in 6 weeks. On arrival at the hospital fetal heart tones were detected at a rate of 160, a contraction monitor was applied, which showed regular contractions every 90 seconds to 2 minutes lasting for 20 to 30 seconds. An ultrasound detected no damage to the placenta or fetus. A mild bruise was noted to the uterine wall. During her time in the ED, Cassie was alert, oriented, and obeyed command. She was admitted to the OB unit with premature labor. Approximately 5 weeks later, Cassie delivered a healthy baby girl.

CASE 7

Dispatch: 19:45 hrs; personal injury collision, 81 y/o male injured

On Arrival: You see two vehicles at odd angles to each other in an intersection and a truck that has apparently run head-on into a tree. The truck appears to have also been impacted on the driver's side door and the rear bumper is torn off. Your patient is in the truck. You find 81 y/o Karl, unrestrained, lying across the front seat of his truck. The steering wheel is bent.

Initial Assessment Findings

Mental Status—Opens eyes to voice, is disoriented to where he is and what happened, inconsistently obeys command

Airway—Open and clear

Breathing—R regular at 22; lung sounds faint wheezes in both bases, clear in upper lobes

Circulation—Skin pale, cool, and dry

Radial pulse irregular at 70

BP 112/82

Chief Complaint—No complaints of pain

Focused History

Events—Bystanders state he ran a red light, was hit in the driver's side door, which knocked him into another lane where he was rear-ended and then jumped the curb and hit the tree.

Previous Illness—Hypertension, "heart problems"

Current Health Status—Good

Allergies—Sulfa

Medications—Lasix (furosemide), Lanoxin (digitalis), hydrochlorothiazide, K-chlor (potassium supplement), Theo-Dur (theophylline), and Micronase (glyburide)

Focused Physical

Current Set of VS—P 70 and irregular, R 22, BP 112/82

Other Pertinent Findings—Bruise noted on sternum, complains of pain when left chest wall palpated, no crepitus noted; abdomen soft and nontender; pelvis intact; bilateral bruising with contusions on knees; deformity of right ankle noted; pulse oximetry is 80%

Diagnostic Tests—Blood sugar 40

ECG

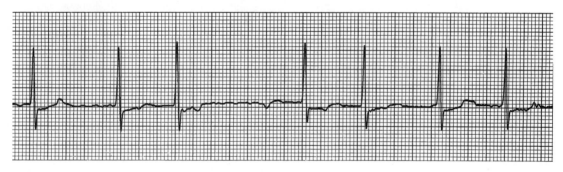

Figure 14-6

QUESTIONS

1. What is significant about Karl's mechanism of injury?

2. Given this mechanism, what type of injuries might you suspect and do those differ with age?

3. What are your scene considerations?

4. What are your treatment priorities?

5. According to your assessment findings, what body systems are affected?

6. How do normal changes of aging regarding the CNS affect your assessment?

7. How do normal changes of aging affect your assessment of Karl's skin?

8. Considering the medications Karl is taking, what preexisting problems does Karl have?

9. Would a pulse oximetry value of 80% on room air be considered normal for Karl?

10. How would you describe Karl's ECG?

11. Is Karl's ECG a result of the chest trauma he sustained, or is it caused by a preexisting condition?

12. How do Karl's preexisting problems affect your assessment?

13. What specific treatment considerations do Karl's preexisting cardiovascular problems require?

14. Karl has a midsternal bruise. How would a cardiac contusion be recognized?

15. What is Karl at risk for?

16. What is your initial treatment of Karl?

17. What other considerations, related to Karl's age and preexisting medical problems, must you take into account when assessing and treating Karl?

18. When you try to ask Karl what happened, he seems easily distracted and inattentive. When he does respond he asks questions of his own but doesn't answer your questions. What additional assessment should be done?

19. How does aging change the picture of the patient in shock?

20. How would you know if Karl were in shock?

21. During your time with Karl you have determined that he is hard of hearing but can lip read. Answers to your questions are inconsistent, and his response to command is also inconsistent. His pupils are equal; he moves all extremities but his left side is noticeably weaker. Karl's blood sugar is 40. How would you continue treatment?

1. What is significant about Karl's mechanism of injury?

Multiple collisions with at least two other vehicles and a tree. There were multiple body impacts with each vehicular impact because no restraints were used.

2. Given this mechanism, what type of injuries might you suspect and do those differ with age?

Suspected injuries include: head injury, spinal fractures, rib and sternal fractures with pulmonary contusion, cardiac contusion, aortic injury, liver and spleen lacerations, hip and pelvic fractures, and multiple long bone fractures.

Yes, injury patterns differ with age. The elderly are more likely to become injured on impact. Among other things, bones are more prone to breaking, subdural bleeds are more common, aortic injury is more likely (because of arteriosclerosis the arteries become more rigid and fixed, making the aorta more prone to a "shear" injury), the skin is more likely to tear rather than lacerate, and bruising tends to be more extensive.

3. What are your scene considerations?

Determining how many patients you have, if back up is needed, traffic control and scene safety (fuel leaks, etc) are important.

4. What are your treatment priorities?

Ensure airway patency and spinal immobilization along with adequate oxygenation, ventilation, and perfusion of vital organs.

5. According to your assessment findings, what body systems are affected?

CNS—disorientation and inconsistent response to command
Respiratory—basilar wheezing
Cardiovascular—pale, cool, dry skin with an irregular pulse
Musculoskeletal—bruise midsternum and deformed right ankle

6. How do normal changes of aging regarding the CNS affect your assessment?

Normal changes of aging of the CNS involve the size of the brain, which gradually shrinks over the years, slower reaction time, and susceptibility to medical incidents, such as stroke. Shrinking of the brain leads to increased incidence of subdural bleeds from relatively minor trauma to the head. Slower reaction time requires that, when trying to communicate with the elderly, you should allow time for a response. Hearing deficits can also contribute to a confusing picture of mental status. Look for the presence of a hearing aid. Sometimes getting jostled will dislodge a hearing aid, resulting in a confused elder whose confusion has nothing to do with a head injury. Taking a minute to really look around, the immediate environment may reveal the missing hearing aid.

Susceptibility to medical incidents, such as stroke, can precipitate traumatic events, as well as result in altered mental status. Assessment of mental status needs to be done repeatedly. Access to the patient's wallet where a record of preexisting conditions, such as stroke, diabetes, or other information, may be listed will be particularly valuable.

7. How do normal changes of aging affect your assessment of Karl's skin?

Normal changes of aging result in less subcutaneous support for the skin and blood vessels. This leaves the skin more fragile and prone to bruising and tearing rather than lacerating. Skin tears occur under clothing and may be easily missed.

8. Considering the medications Karl is taking, what preexisting problems does Karl have?

Preexisting problems include: congestive heart failure (with a high likelihood of atrial fibrillation), emphysema, and type II diabetes.

Furosemide and digitalis along with an antihypertensive (in this case, hydrochlorothiazide) are typical medications for a patient with atrial fibrillation and congestive heart failure. K-chlor is a potassium supplement that is consistent with a patient on furosemide and hydrochlorothiazide.

Theophylline (Theo-Dur) is a bronchodilator commonly prescribed for patients with chronic obstructive pulmonary disease, usually emphysema or asthma.

Glyburide (Micronase) is an oral hypoglycemic agent usually prescribed for patients with adult onset or type II diabetes.

9. *Would a pulse oximetry value of 80% on room air be considered normal for Karl?*

No, even patients with a known history of chronic obstructive pulmonary disease would not be considered normal if a pulse oximetry value were this low. There are some patients who have such extreme disease process where values of 88% may be considered the low end of acceptable normal. However, such values cannot be assumed and must be taken into account with the rest of the assessment findings.

10. *How would you describe Karl's ECG?*

Atrial fibrillation (QRS narrow, no P wave, irregular rate).

11. *Is Karl's ECG a result of the chest trauma he sustained, or is it caused by a preexisting condition?*

You can't tell in the field. His medications might lead you to believe that preexisting atrial fibrillation was highly probable. What you don't know is if the chest trauma affected his ventricular rate. Neither do you know if a more serious dysrhythmia will develop later.

12. *How do Karl's preexisting problems affect your assessment?*

If a cardiac monitor wasn't considered before, it is now. Checking a blood sugar level is also a necessary assessment step. Assuming that atrial fibrillation was a "normal" rhythm for this patient is not wise. The important factor is to determine adequacy of perfusion of vital organs, especially the CNS, and to detect changes or trends in vital signs.

13. *What specific treatment considerations do Karl's preexisting cardiovascular problems require?*

Karl's heart may not be able to tolerate an increase in preload, therefore fluid replacement must be done carefully and judiciously. Because of his history of hypertension, a BP of 112 systolic may be too low for adequate perfusion. A fluid bolus may be a diagnostic tool. Preventing hypothermia is another treatment consideration.

14. *Karl has a midsternal bruise. How would a cardiac contusion be recognized?*

Cardiac contusions are not common, but if they are present, field recognition is limited to rhythm changes on the cardiac monitor. The most common are premature ventricular contractions (PVCs) and AV blocks. ST and T wave changes can also occur.

15. *What is Karl at risk for?*

Sudden decompensation and shock; cardiac dysrhythmia and v-fib; respiratory distress and ruptured bleb if positive pressure is used to ventilate; hypothermia; missed injuries (from assuming signs of injury are because of preexisting medical problems); and missed medical problems (from assuming signs of a medical problem are caused by an injury) resulting in inappropriate treatment.

16. *What is your initial treatment of Karl?*

Immobilize and quickly extricate to a sheltered environment. Apply oxygen. You might start with a nasal cannula, frequently reassessing or with a mask, non-rebreather and a reservoir at 12 lpm, and monitor the effect by pulse oximetry and mental status. Start an IV of normal saline.

17. *What other consideration(s), related to Karl's age and preexisting medical problems, must you take into account when assessing and treating Karl?*

Karl has a history of type II diabetes as evidenced by his glyburide (Micronase). Hypoglycemia may be a major factor in this incident. Testing his blood sugar level is a critical part of his assessment and may be a major factor in treatment.

18. *When you try to ask Karl what happened, he seems easily distracted and inattentive. When he does respond he asks questions of his own but doesn't answer your questions. What additional assessment should be done?*

It is possible that Karl cannot hear you. It is also possible that Karl has suffered either a head injury or a stroke. The additional assessment should be to determine which problem may be present. If Karl is hearing impaired, many hearing impaired people have learned to lip read. Get his attention, either with your hand on his shoulder while you talk, or your hand on his face. Speak clearly and distinctly asking a simple question, such as his name. You may ask if he has a hearing aid and gesture to your ear.

If Karl has a head injury or has suffered a stroke, there should be other signs of neurologic deficit that a neuro assessment should be able to detect. Hypoglycemia may also present in this manner. Checking his blood sugar is necessary.

19. **How does aging change the picture of the patient in shock?**

    Compensatory mechanisms are delayed and may be inefficient. The ability to vasoconstrict is affected by the presence of aortosclerosis, as well as the number and efficiency (both are reduced) of alpha-receptors. The ability of the heart to function, both in its ability to tolerate an increased preload (from peripheral vasoconstriction), as well as an increase in rate and oxygen demand, is another factor. The ability to mount a compensatory response may be complicated by medications such as beta-blockers, calcium channel blockers, ACE inhibitors, or diuretics. The heart may not be able to tolerate the increase in preload or the increase in oxygen demand. Shock may actually worsen with normal supportive treatment, such as fluid replacement.

20. **How would you know if Karl were in shock?**

    The first sign would be a change in mental status. Because Karl already has an abnormal mental status, look for a change in his current state, either to becoming quiet and sleepy or restless and combative. The skin and pulse rate will be the next most likely places to show a change.

21. **During your time with Karl you have determined that Karl is hard of hearing but he can lip read. Answers to your questions are inconsistent, and his response to command is also inconsistent. His pupils are equal; he moves all extremities, but his left side is noticeably weaker. Karl's blood sugar is 40. How would you continue treatment?**

    Hypoglycemia is considered a life threat. However, giving 50% dextrose IV to a patient with a head injury may worsen his prognosis if hemorrhage is involved. Although Karl is not unconscious, he does have neurological deficit that may be consistent with a stroke or head injury. With a history of diabetes, most protocols allow use of 50% dextrose if other signs of increased intracranial pressure are not present, such as unequal/unreactive pupils and/or posturing. Karl has neither.

OUTCOME

Karl was immobilized and quickly extricated. Oxygen by nasal cannula raised his pulse oximetry level to 90%. A card in his wallet listed his hearing impairment, medications, allergies, and physician. He also had a BP card in his wallet. His BP a week before this incident was 144/86. He was placed on a monitor and an IV started. Dextrose 50% slow IV push was administered. Karl became alert and his left sided weakness corrected itself after 10 g. Vital signs were reassessed. A fluid bolus of 100 ml was given with a resulting BP 126/80. On arrival at the ED Karl was switched to a mask, non-rebreather with a reservoir at 12 lpm, which raised his pulse oximetry level to 95%. Blood work was drawn and x-rays taken. Karl had suffered 5 fractured ribs on the right and 3 on the left. There was no flail segment but significant pulmonary contusion. During examination, a 5 cm abdominal aortic aneurysm was also discovered. There was no cardiac effect noted from his midsternal bruise. After a rocky course involving pneumonia, Karl eventually recovered and was sent home after 10 days in the hospital and 1 week in a rehab unit. His abdominal aortic aneurysm was considered stable.

CASE 8

Dispatch: 14:30 hrs; injured child

On Arrival: You find your patient, 5 y/o Yurba, sitting on her mother's lap on the porch. She is awake, has a tear-stained face, and appears alert. Her color seems normal. Her tee shirt is grass stained.

Initial Assessment Findings

Mental Status—Awake, alert, and oriented
Airway—Open and clear
Breathing—R 22 without distress; lung sounds clear in all lobes
Circulation—Skin normal color, warm, and dry
        Pulse 120 and regular
        BP 82/56
Chief Complaint—"My tummy hurts"

Focused History

Events—Yurba was playing around the car in the driveway when suddenly she cried out. When the mother turned around she saw Yurba get up and run toward her. The car had rolled down a slight incline, to the end of the driveway. No one saw exactly what happened.
Previous Illness—None
Current Health Status—Good
Allergies—None known
Medications—None

Focused Physical

Current Set of VS—P 120, R 22, BP 82/56
Other Pertinent Findings—An 8 cm wide abrasion began on her right chest wall at the nipple line and extended across her chest and abdomen to the left side at about the level of her waist. She moves all extremities on command; pulse oximetry 99%; Yurba weighs about 50 lbs.
Diagnostic Tests—None done

ECG: Not done

1. What is significant about Yurba's injury pattern, and what mechanism is suggested?

2. Given this mechanism, what type of injuries might you suspect?

3. How do these injuries differ from those an adult might suffer with the same mechanism?

4. What are your scene considerations?

5. What are your treatment priorities?

6. Given Yurba's vital signs, are they within a normal range or is she in shock?

7. How could you rapidly calculate what value would indicate hypotension in a young child?

8. How do early signs and symptoms of shock differ in a child from those in an adult?

9. How would you recognize shock in Yurba?

10. What is Yurba at risk for?

11. Does Yurba require immobilization?

12. How would you begin treatment?

13. If you needed to start an IV on a child, what sites would you use?

14. If fluid resuscitation is required for a child, how much should be given? Is there a limit?

15. Is a fluid bolus appropriate for this situation? Why or why not?

16. En route to the hospital Yurba becomes quiet and sleepy. Repeat vital signs show: P 126, R 26, BP 80/64. What does this change suggest and what should be assessed?

17. How would you continue treatment?

18. What must be reassessed?

19. How would you identify early respiratory distress in a child Yurba's age?

20. What is the danger of using positive pressure to ventilate a child?

21. If a child Yurba's size would need to have ventilatory assistance, how could you ensure a good tidal volume?

QUESTIONS AND ANSWERS

1. What is significant about Yurba's injury pattern, and what mechanism is suggested?

Yurba's injury pattern of the abrasion that is approximately 8 cm wide and extends from the upper right chest to the lower left abdomen suggests that the tire of the car rolled over her. What is significant is that the major organs of the chest and abdomen are both involved.

2. Given this mechanism, what type of injuries might you suspect?

Fractures, pulmonary contusion, diaphragmatic rupture, solid organ rupture (liver, spleen and pancreas), hollow organ rupture (stomach, intestine, colon, bladder), pelvic fracture, and spinal cord injury.

3. How do these injuries differ from those an adult might suffer with the same mechanism?

Yurba is not as likely to suffer from skeletal fractures as an adult. She is more likely to sustain internal organ damage that is not readily visible. She is also more likely to suffer a spinal cord contusion than a vertebral fracture.

4. What are your scene considerations?

Check out the stability of the car.

5. What are your treatment priorities?

Ensure a patent airway, oxygenation, ventilation, and perfusion to vital organs.

6. Given Yurba's vital signs, are they within a normal range or is she in shock?

Yurba's vital signs are: P 120, R 22, BP 82/56. Her pulse rate is within normal limits as is her respiratory rate and BP. However, her BP is at the low end of normal even with a tachycardia of 120. This is suggestive of compensated shock, even though no single vital sign is clearly outside "normal" limits.

7. How could you rapidly calculate what value would indicate hypotension in a young child?

Hypotension in children is defined as a systolic blood pressure less than 70 mm Hg $+ 2 \times$ the age in years. For Yurba that would be a systolic less than 80 mm Hg (70 mm Hg $+ 2 \times 5$).

8. How do early signs and symptoms of shock differ in a child from those in an adult?

A child will compensate more efficiently than an adult, probably because of a much more resilient cardiovascular system (they haven't abused their bodies as much). Young children, however, do not have the benefit of an increase in contractility of heart muscle. Therefore a sustained tachycardia in a quiet child is one of the best indicators of early shock. Other signs include a change in mental status and decreased activity, as well as presence of pallor or delayed capillary return in a central area. Skin color is a valuable assessment sign. Because peripheral vasoconstriction is so effective, increased preload can often compensate for small volume losses very effectively. If pallor is ignored because the heart rate "isn't fast enough" or because the child is quiet and "good," the child will deteriorate before any problem is suspected.

9. How would you recognize shock in Yurba?

Yurba's assessment findings already suggest that she is compensating. If shock would become progressive, there would be a change in her mental status, an increase in heart rate, and an increase in pallor.

10. What is Yurba at risk for?

Progressive shock resulting from continued or unrecognized internal bleeding, respiratory distress from pulmonary contusions, pneumothorax or tension pneumothorax, or sudden collapse from an unrecognized spinal cord contusion.

11. Does Yurba require immobilization?

Because Yurba's history includes an episode of getting up, running to her mother, and sitting upright on her mother's lap, the prospect of immobilization may seem unnecessary. However, to rely only on this history to determine presence or absence of cord injury is very risky. Acute stress reaction can effect children, as well as adults, therefore more of an assessment needs to be done to determine probability of cord injury. If you are in a system where the need for field immobilization is based on assessment of spine pain or tenderness, motor function (finger abduction/adduction, finger/hand extension, foot/great toe flexion/dorsiflexion), and sensory examination (abnormal sensation/pain), then this will be done before moving the child. If your system is such that the need for immobilization is based on mechanism, then full immobilization will probably be done.

12. How would you begin treatment?

Immobilization based on your protocols, oxygen by nasal cannula or mask, non-rebreather with a reservoir (based on which one is tolerated by Yurba), keep her warm and begin transport. Depending on your transport time, an IV may or may not be started.

13. If you needed to start an IV on a child, what sites would you use?

First look to the obvious sites, antecubital space or back of hand. In children the age of 6 or under, sites include the top of the foot or interosseous route. An additional site in infants includes the forehead.

14. If fluid resuscitation is required for a child, how much should be given? Is there a limit?

Fluid resuscitation in children is done by bolus, 20 ml/kg, repeated up to 3 times for a total of 60 ml/kg.

15. Is a fluid bolus appropriate for this situation? Why or why not?

Yes, Yurba has assessment findings consistent with compensated shock. To wait until her blood pressure drops would be to wait until she is in late shock, which is too long. A child loses approximately 25% of blood volume before BP falls.

16. En route to the hospital Yurba becomes quiet and sleepy. Repeat vital signs show: P 126, R 26, BP 80/64. What does this change suggest and what should be assessed?

This suggests that shock is progressing. Rapidly assess skin vitals and lung sounds.

17. How would you continue treatment?

If a nasal cannula was used initially, switch to a mask, non-rebreather with a reservoir at 12 to 15 lpm. Based on her response, you may need to assist her ventilations. If an IV was not started before, an IV is needed now. Use a crystalloid such as normal saline or Ringer's lactate and administer a bolus of fluid at 20 ml/kg (450 ml). If possible, warm the fluid. Turn up the heater in the patient compartment to help keep Yurba warm.

18. What must be reassessed?

A repeat set of vital signs, especially respiratory rate and effort and heart rate. Monitor closely for respiratory distress.

19. How would you identify early respiratory distress in a child Yurba's age?

Look for nasal flaring, intercostal retractions and an increase in respiratory rate.

20. What is the danger of using positive pressure to ventilate a child?

If too much pressure is used, gastric distention can occur (stimulating vomiting and limiting tidal volume) and/or resulting pulmonary trauma can cause a pneumothorax.

21. If a child Yurba's size would need to have ventilatory assistance, how could you ensure a good tidal volume?

Prevent or minimize gastric distention by good positioning and inflate just enough to have her chest rise.

OUTCOME

After a thorough assessment, Yurba was placed on the gurney and a mask, non-rebreather with a reservoir at 15 lpm applied with mother's help. She was kept warm and transported. En route she became sleepy with a rise in heart rate and change in pallor. There were no veins readily seen and an IV was not started in the field. At the ED an IV was started in her left antecubital space and 500 ml of normal saline was rapidly infused. A CT scan showed bilateral pulmonary contusions with extensive lacerations to her liver. Because the liver capsule was intact, the decision was made to allow the liver to heal itself. No other internal injuries were identified. One unit of packed cells was started in the ED and she was admitted to the ICU on strict bed rest with close monitoring of her hemodynamic status. After 3 days a significant pleural effusion was identified and a chest tube was inserted on the right. The rest of her hospital course was uneventful. She was dismissed after 6 weeks to home and after another 6 weeks was permitted to restart preschool.

BIBLIOGRAPHY

Campbell, J. E., & Alabama Chapter of the American College of Emergency Physicians (Eds.). (1998). *Basic trauma life support: For paramedics and advanced EMS providers* (3rd ed.). Englewood Cliffs, NJ: Prentice-Hall.

Caroline, N. L. (1995). *Emergency care in the streets,* (5th ed.). Boston: Little, Brown.

Eichelberger, M. R., Ball, J. W., Pratsch, G. L., & Clark, J. R. (1998). *Pediatric emergencies* (2nd ed.). Upper Saddle River, NJ: Brady, A Prentice-Hall Division.

Harrahill, M. (1997). Maternal trauma care: A brief review. *J Emer Nurs* 23 (6):649.

Kelley, S. J. (1994). *Pediatric emergency nursing* (2nd ed.). Norwalk, CT: Appleton & Lange.

Pre-Hospital Trauma Life Support Committee. (1994). *PHTLS basic and advanced: Pre-hospital trauma life support* (3rd ed.). St Louis, MO: Mosby.

Troiano, N. H. (1991). Trauma during pregnancy. In C. J. Harvey (Ed.). *Critical care obstetrical nursing.* Gaithersburg, MD: Aspen.

15

Cardiac Emergencies

OVERVIEW

The heart, along with the vascular network and blood, has the job of maintaining perfusion to the body cells. When there is a problem with the heart, or any other part of this system, complex compensatory mechanisms are stimulated to help maintain perfusion. Assessment findings often reveal which part or parts of the compensatory mechanisms is/are working. This helps direct treatment. The goal of all treatment of cardiovascular problems is to maintain perfusion.

Anatomy, Physiology, and Pathophysiology

The heart functions to pump blood to the cells of the body. Blood functions as the medium that carries oxygen, nutrients, and other substances needed by the cells. Blood also functions in the role of waste removal, carrying substances such as dissolved gases to the lungs for exhalation and other substances to the kidneys for excretion. As such, the heart maintains perfusion to the cells of the body. There are a number of characteristics of cardiac muscle that help with the efficiency of cardiac function. There is also the Frank-Starling law that, within limits, helps the heart keep up with almost any energy demand the body may require. Cardiac muscle itself is very sensitive to chemicals known as catecholamines, otherwise known as epinephrine, norepinephrine, and dopamine. While epinephrine and norepinephrine exist within the sympathetic nervous system, their release along with dopamine, into the blood stream is a function of the adrenal glands above the kidneys. The presence of these catecholamines serves to enhance the efficiency of cardiac function by stimulation of receptors sites in cardiac muscle and conduction tissue.

The conduction system of the heart functions independently of the rest of the body, and has a system of back-up pacemakers. There is one outside nerve that influences heart rate. That is the vagal nerve, which comes from the brain stem and only innervates the SA and AV node of the heart. When stimulated, this nerve slows the heart rate.

Normally the heart functions as a master pump, maintaining a certain cardiac output to satisfy perfusion needs. Through a system of biofeedback mechanisms, the cardiovascular system is extremely sensitive to adjusting to the perfusion needs of the body. The majority of perfusion needs are satisfied by the vascular system by use of vasoconstriction, vasodilation, and/or capillary sphincter actions at the cellular level, in response to tissue needs for oxygen, nutrients, or waste removal. When the need is extreme or cardiac output cannot keep up with the demand, the biofeedback mechanisms may trigger stimulation of the sympathetic nervous system, causing the release of epinephrine/norepinephrine from the adrenal glands and/or stimulate the renin/aldosterone/angiotensin pathway in the kidneys.

Those events that interfere with perfusion can be roughly divided into those that interfere with volume, rate, or cardiac muscle failure. Loss of volume may be directly related to loss of blood, such as hemorrhage or other cause of anemia, or loss of body water, such as dehydration or third spacing of body fluid. Cardiac emergencies that also involve a degree of body water loss or dehydration are very common. However, cardiac emergencies resulting from the loss of whole blood are not common and, when they do occur, usually occur in the elderly.

Rates that interfere with perfusion include those that are too slow, such as the bradycardias; those that are too fast, such as supraventricular tachycardia (SVT); or those that are inefficient because of their site of origin, such as ventricular tachycardia. The numbers sometimes associated with bradycardia (rates < 60 bpm) and SVT (rates > 150 bpm) are somewhat arbitrary, and do not substitute for a thorough patient assessment. Cardiac muscle failure relates to actual muscle damage, such as that which results from a myocardial infarction or chronic hypertension, insufficient valve function, or obstructive conditions such as pulmonary emboli, cardiac tamponade or tension pneumothorax.

Of the obstructive causes of cardiac emergencies, pulmonary emboli are more frequent. History is the key to detecting the problem. Patients on birth control pills, those who have been immobile for a length of time, those with fractured long bones, or those with a history of smoking in conjunction with any of the previously mentioned conditions are at greatest risk. Emboli usually are fragments of a distal thrombus, commonly located in the lower legs, which break off and lodge in the pulmonary arteries. Large saddle emboli frequently cause death within a short time. Multiple smaller emboli may break off causing "clot showers". They usually do not cause immediate death but death may occur over a period of time (days to weeks). These clot showers cause a localized inflammatory reaction that can cause pleuritic chest pain, tachycardia, shortness of breath, sudden syncope, a sensation of impending doom, a persistent cough, and other symptoms that may be vague and non-specific.

A tension pneumothorax in a medical patient is usually due to a ruptured bleb. Patients who are susceptible to blebs include those with a history of COPD. The bleb may act as a one-way valve, trapping air in the pleural space. The history may involve an activity such as heavy lifting, laughing, or coughing with a sudden onset of sharp, localized chest pain associated with an immediate onset of difficulty breathing that rapidly worsens. Lung sounds are clear with significantly diminished or absent sounds on the affected side.

Cardiac tamponade in a medical patient is not common. Pericarditis, chronic conditions such as cancer of the mediastinum or systemic lupus, may cause cardiac tamponade. The onset in a medical patient is usually gradual with vague, diffuse chest pain, gradually increasing in intensity as the chief complaint. As the fluid builds up in the pericardial sac, the ventricles are prevented from fully expanding, thus dropping cardiac output. As a result, tachycardia, the sensation of dyspnea, and hypotension result.

With the exception of obstructive causes, pulmonary edema is often one of the first signs associated with inefficient cardiac function and may begin insidiously. As cardiac muscle becomes inefficient, cardiac output falls. This triggers the compensatory mechanisms through the biofeedback mechanisms. When cardiac output drops, epinephrine and norepinephrine are released in an attempt to maintain cardiac output by increasing the strength of myocardial contractions, thereby increasing heart rate and stimulating peripheral vasoconstriction causing an increase in preload. This also increases the workload and oxygen demand of the heart. As long as the heart can compensate by maintaining a balance between the increase in preload and the increase in workload, cardiac output will be maintained. However, the increased workload further contributes to left ventricular inefficiency causing the body to gradually decompensate. Eventually, what is termed *cardiac* or *congestive failure* becomes pronounced. In the meantime, a delicate balance is maintained. If there is any disturbance in this balance, such as a rise in blood pressure, rapid signs of failure will occur and frank pulmonary edema is a common result.

Because of the build up of pressure and the back-flow that is caused from the left ventricle to the left atria, the mitral or bicuspid valve becomes inefficient. A murmur develops that can be heard with a stethoscope. It is easiest to hear the murmur in a relatively quiet environment. Because of the pressure in the atria, the atria will enlarge. As the pressure in the system is transmitted to the right atria, the SA node is eventually affected. Atrial fibrillation is a common result, although other dysrhythmias may also occur. Atrial fibrillation also contributes to inefficient cardiac function.

The disease process known as congestive heart failure is not a simple condition and has many consequences. How many are present depends on the length of time, the extent of the precipitating process, and the efficiency of the compensatory mechanisms.

When approximately 40% of cardiac muscle is no longer able to function, cardiogenic shock results. Frank pulmonary edema along with hypotension are the hallmarks of cardiogenic shock.

Not all patients with an underlying cardiac problem will have pulmonary edema and not all patients with pulmonary edema have cardiac problems. Whether or not pulmonary edema occurs is dependent on several factors. It is important to remember that it takes approximately 1 liter of fluid to cause crackles or rales with wheezing often occurring first. Therefore the absence of crackles does not rule out a cardiac problem. The medication that a patient is already on and the history related to the current problem will often indicate the source of the problem. Common home medications for congestive failure includes a digitalis preparation (digoxin or Lanoxin), a diuretic (commonly furosemide or Lasix), and an antihypertensive. A potassium supplement may also be prescribed.

Those who have a history of sudden onset tachycardia may be on a beta-blocker, a calcium channel blocker or an alpha-blocker.

Because of the close association between the cardiovascular system and the respiratory system, a thorough assessment of the respiratory system is wise in all patients with a cardiac complaint, as is a thorough assessment of the cardiovascular system in all adults with a respiratory complaint.

Assessment

Common complaints of patients with cardiac related problems include chest pain and/or difficulty breathing. Patients with an excessively fast heart rate may complain of a "fluttering" in their chest. A thorough history will often indicate the origin of the problem.

Assessment begins with the ABCs. If the patient is talking, the airway is intact. The ability to talk in complete sentences suggests adequate minute volume. Respiratory rate is usually rapid in the patient with hypoxia or hypoxemia. Lung sounds are related to the amount of fluid back-up, if any. The absence of lung sounds on one side suggests the presence of a tension pneumothorax. In cardiac tamponade the lung sounds are clear and equal. The sensation of shortness of breath is present before any detectable pulmonary problem. If pulmonary edema is involved, wheezing followed by crackles (or rales) eventually occurs.

Skin color, temperature, and moisture are related to the amount of vasoconstriction and hypoxia (from a drop in cardiac output and/or pulmonary edema) that is present. Skin may range from pale, cool, and dry to cold, clammy, and dusky (gray/blue in color). If volume loss is a factor, skin turgor is another important assessment sign.

In many patients the back-up of body water creates a back pressure within the system that is slow and gradual. After a prolonged time, usually weeks, peripheral edema may be evident. Check for pitting edema in the dependent parts, such as the feet and lower legs. Distended neck veins may also be present.

The cardiac monitor will be a valuable diagnostic tool. The heart rate may help determine the cause of the cardiac failure. Rates generally faster than 150 or slower than 50 are too slow to maintain cardiac output in most adults. Heart rates between 100 and 150 generally are in response to a volume deficit or epinephrine/norepinephrine response.

Pay particular attention to the pulse and check it with the ECG monitor. A paradoxical pulse may indicate the presence of a tension pneumothorax or cardiac tamponade, or may occasionally occur in congestive heart failure.

Bradycardia may be associated with a second or third degree block, which will dictate treatment options as will the presence of an SVT or VT.

Blood pressure is an indication of the adequacy of perfusion. High blood pressure in the presence of congestive heart failure may be the stressor that triggered the pulmonary edema.

Treatment

Oxygen is the initial treatment option for any patient with a cardiac emergency. Further treatment options are directly related to the cause of the cardiac emergency. A lack of fluid or volume dictates an IV with a fluid bolus, usually 250 to 500 ml for the adult. Obstructive causes include a needle chest decompression for the tension pneumothorax, a pericardiocentesis for the cardiac tamponade (usually a physician procedure); and symptomatic treatment for a patient suffering a pulmonary emboli.

For the patient with pulmonary edema, treatment depends on the cardiac rhythm and the blood pressure. If the rhythm cannot support perfusion, correct the rhythm. Oxygen atropine and pacing with appropriate sedation are the options for bradycardia. Adenosine, verapamil and cardioversion with appropriate sedation are options for supraventricular tachycardia. Lidocaine and cardioversion with appropriate sedation are options for ventricular tachycardia.

If the cardiac rhythm can support perfusion and the blood pressure is high or normal, offloading the cardiovascular system is the usual treatment of choice. Nitroglycerin, furosemide, and morphine consist of the pharmacologic choices.

If the cardiac rhythm can support perfusion but hypotension exists in the presence of pulmonary edema, cardiogenic shock is present. The drug of choice is dopamine.

CASE 1

Dispatch: 68 y/o with difficulty breathing

On Arrival: 68 y/o Fred is sitting in a recliner, with family members present. He is awake but looks pale and diaphoretic. He also looks very tired.

Initial Assessment Findings

Mental Status—Awake, alert, and oriented, GCS 15
Airway—Open and clear
Breathing—RR 24 and labored, talking in 3 to 4 word sentences, faint wheezes are audible; lung sounds are absent in bases, wheezes and rales in upper lobes, bilaterally
Circulation—Skin pale, cool, and clammy; nail beds and lips are dusky
      Radial pulse strong, irregular at 116
      BP 194/110
Chief Complaint—"Can't breathe"

Focused History

Events—Onset occurred shortly after watching Super Bowl
Previous Illness—Hypertension, previous MI 4 years ago
Current Health Status—Felt fine this morning before watching the game; has had similar problems several times a year, usually when he doesn't follow his diet or take meds regularly
Allergies—None known
Medications—Furosemide (Lasix), digitalis (Lanoxin), spironolactone with hydrochlorothiazide (Aldactazide), potassium chloride (K-Dur), salt restricted diet; forgot to take his meds yesterday and today, has been eating potato chips, pretzels, carbonated beverages, etc.

Focused Physical

Current Set of VS—BP 194/110, P 116 and irregular, R 24
Other Physical Findings—Pitting edema bilaterally to midshin; denies pain
Diagnostic Tests—Pulse oximetry 87%

ECG

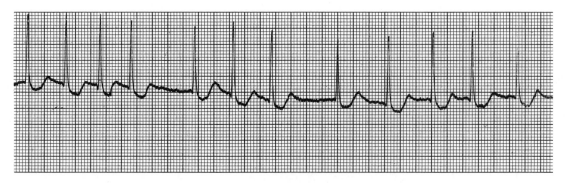

Figure 15-1

QUESTIONS

1. What is significant about Fred's history?

2. What body systems are affected?

3. What is the significance of the combination of medications that Fred is on?

4. How does Fred's history relate to his current problem?

5. What is Fred's cardiac rhythm?

6. Is there a relationship between Fred's rhythm and his difficulty breathing?

7. Would you treat Fred's rhythm?

8. What is the significance of the pulse oximetry value of 87%?

9. How do Fred's dusky lips and nail beds relate to his pulse oximetry value?

10. What is the significance of Fred's inability to talk in complete sentences?

11. What is the pathophysiology behind Fred's skin color, temperature, and moisture?

12. Fred has absent lung sounds in the bases with wheezes and rales in the upper lobes. Explain the physiology behind these signs.

13. How serious is Fred's situation, and how do you know?

14. What is the significance of Fred's pitting edema?

15. What is the first thing you would do for Fred before any pharmacologic therapy?

16. Is there a recognizable pattern to Fred's signs and symptoms?

17. Explain the pathophysiology behind congestive heart failure.

18. Is there any other problem that might be present?

19. What is Fred at risk for?

20. What pharmacologic agents do you have available that could help Fred, and how do they work?

QUESTIONS AND ANSWERS

1. What is significant about Fred's history?

Previous history of being on digitalis, diuretics, and antihypertensives; noncompliant with meds and diet; has been eating high salt content foods

2. What body systems are affected?

Cardiovascular—pitting edema, tachycardia, hypertension

Respiratory—R 24, wheezing and rales, nail beds and lips dusky; pulse ox 87%

3. What is the significance of the combination of medications that Fred is on?

The combination of Lasix (furosemide) and Lanoxin (digitalis) is very common for patients with atrial fibrillation and congestive heart failure. The addition of another antihypertensive (Aldactazide) is a common practice for additional hypertension control. K-Dur (potassium supplement) or a similar supplement is needed due to the diuretic effects of Lasix and Aldactazide "wasting" potassium.

4. How does Fred's history relate to his current problem?

His history of eating foods high in salt, combined with failure to take medication may affect his blood pressure by causing retention of body water leading to high blood pressure and exacerbate inefficient cardiac function, resulting in pulmonary edema.

5. What is Fred's cardiac rhythm?

Atrial fibrillation. No discernible P wave, QRS < 0.10 sec, and an irregular ventricular response meets the criteria for atrial fibrillation.

6. Is there a relationship between Fred's rhythm and his difficulty breathing?

Fred's difficulty breathing is caused by his pulmonary edema. Fred's pulmonary edema is exacerbated by fluid overload from failure to take his medication and high salt diet. Atrial fibrillation for Fred is a chronic problem (you know that from his medications). When the atria are fibrillating the left ventricle becomes less efficient. The combination of less efficient ventricular function and fluid overload has a high probability of precipitating pulmonary edema.

7. Would you treat Fred's rhythm?

No, it is not going fast enough to interfere with perfusion. Medications used to treat atrial fibrillation (digitalis preparations) are not routinely carried in the field.

8. What is the significance of the pulse oximetry value of 87%?

An 87% saturation is too low. This is most likely an indication of how much his pulmonary edema is interfering with oxygen-carbon dioxide exchange, preventing full saturation of RBCs at the alveolar level.

9. How do Fred's dusky lips and nail beds relate to his pulse oximetry value?

Dusky lips and nail beds are signs of desaturation of hemoglobin. Usually at least 5% of hemoglobin must be desaturated before cyanosis occurs.

10. What is the significance of Fred's inability to talk in complete sentences?

Adequate minute volume (RR × tidal volume) is required to speak in complete sentences. Since Fred's respiratory rate is within normal limits, the tidal volume must be impaired. This is an indicator of how much his pulmonary edema is interfering with his ventilations.

11. What is the pathophysiology behind Fred's skin color, temperature, and moisture?

Fred is having an epinephrine/norepinephrine release and is pale and cool because of vasoconstriction. There are two possibilities for his diaphoresis. First, it is work for Fred to breathe. Hard work causes an increase in metabolic rate and sweat may be a result of the body's effort to cool off. However, in this case, Fred is also hypoxic. Hypoxia is the most likely cause of his epinephrine/norepinephrine release, a side effect of which is diaphoresis. Thus Fred has two likely causes for his diaphoresis, the work it takes to breathe and his hypoxia.

12. ***Fred has absent lung sounds in the bases with wheezes and rales in the upper lobes. Explain the physiology behind these signs.***

    Pulmonary edema is caused by body fluid collecting in the air passages of the lungs. Because body water follows gravity and the patient is sitting up, the type of sound heard on auscultation depends on the amount of fluid present at that level. There are no lung sounds in the bases because there is so much fluid in the alveoli that no air is entering at that level. At the next level, rales are heard because the alveoli are only partially filled with fluid. Wheezes are caused by fluid in the interstitial spaces and within the alveoli, causing enough irritation to the bronchi to cause constriction. Wheezes are often heard in conjunction with rales.

13. ***How serious is Fred's situation, and how do you know?***

    Fred is in acute respiratory distress and needs treatment immediately. The first signs are his skin color and his diaphoresis. Combine that with his dusky lips, talking in 3 to 4 word sentences, lung sounds, and vital signs and you have a pretty good idea of the degree of respiratory distress. His history tells you the most likely cause of the problem.

14. ***What is the significance of Fred's pitting edema?***

    Since it takes time (days to weeks) for enough fluid to build up enough for "pitting" to occur, its presence is an indication of a chronic problem. Fred may live with some degree of pitting edema, but his noncompliance doesn't help.

15. ***What is the first thing you would do for Fred before any pharmacologic therapy?***

    Ensure that he is sitting upright and give him high flow oxygen.

16. ***Is there a recognizable pattern to Fred's signs and symptoms?***

    Yes, hypertension, tachycardia, atrial fibrillation, and pulmonary edema are part of the pattern of congestive heart failure. The pattern is confirmed by his history.

17. ***Explain the pathophysiology behind congestive heart failure.***

    When left ventricular function is inefficient for whatever the reason (e.g., muscle damage, atrial fibrillation), cardiac output (CO) drops. When CO drops, epinephrine and norepinephrine are released in an attempt to maintain CO by increasing the strength of myocardial contraction, increasing heart rate, and stimulating peripheral vasoconstriction (PVC) causing an increase in preload. But unfortunately, all these actions also increase the workload (and oxygen demand) of a heart that already is being strained. The increased workload further contributes to left ventricular inefficiency, or failure. In addition to causing a drop in CO and more epi/norepi release, ventricular failure also causes fluid to back up into the pulmonary capillary beds, disturbing the hydrostatic pressure gradient, causing fluid to cross the capillary membrane and collect in the interstitial spaces around the alveoli and terminal bronchioles. This increases the distance O_2 and CO_2 must cross leading to hypoxia. If the pressure gradient is changed enough, fluid will cross into the alveoli (pulmonary congestion) further increasing the hypoxia. Hypoxia itself stimulates an epi/norepi release, thus perpetuating the cycle, making the resultant congestive heart failure worse. This is typical of left sided heart failure.

18. ***Is there any other problem that might be present?***

    Yes, Fred may be having a silent MI.

19. ***What is Fred at risk for?***

    Sudden decompensation and cardiogenic shock.

20. ***What pharmacologic agents do you have available that could help Fred, and how do they work?***

    The pharmacologic agents are: nitroglycerine, furosemide (Lasix), and morphine. *Nitroglycerine* works as a general body vasodilator with special emphasis on dilating the coronary arteries and the pulmonary capillary bed. By dilating the coronary arteries, more oxygenated blood can reach cardiac muscle. By dilating the pulmonary capillary bed, fluid in the alveoli and interstitial spaces is pulled back into the vessels. By dilating the peripheral blood vessels, preload and afterload are decreased (BP is decreased) thus decreasing the workload on the heart. Nitro is short acting, can be given sublingually by pill or spray, and can be repeated up to three times in the field. A side effect is decreased BP requiring the BP to be monitored closely.

Furosemide, or Lasix, works as a diuretic. It has another, less well known effect that can help improve pulmonary edema relatively quickly. That effect is localized vasodilation, not only in the kidneys but also in the lungs. This effect typically works within 3 to 5 minutes, pulling fluid from the alveoli and interstitial spaces back into the vascular bed. Patients will start to feel better before the diuretic effect is noticed. The diuresis off loads excess body fluid and decreases preload, decreasing the workload on the heart, thus decreasing the oxygen demand. Because the fluid is also decreasing in the alveoli and interstitial spaces, better exchange of O_2 and CO_2 (resulting in better O_2 saturation) is available to cardiac muscle, increasing efficiency of function. The dose of furosemide is 40 to 120 mg IVP (depending on the patient's history). A side effect is dehydration with decreased BP. With short transport times this may not be problem for field providers.

Morphine Sulfate works in several ways. First it functions as a venous vasodilator, decreasing preload and thus decreasing the workload on the heart. Morphine is also an analgesic, binding with pain receptors and increasing the comfort level of the patient. In binding with pain receptors, morphine also provides a sedative effect that further decreases myocardial oxygen demand. Morphine is a very valuable drug for its hemodynamic effects. The dose is 2 to 10 mg slow IVP. However, a side effect is the significant respiratory depression that may occur, primarily at the higher doses. For this reason, Narcan (naloxone) must be readily available. In cases of pulmonary edema, 2 to 3 mg increments, repeated as needed, are recommended.

OUTCOME

Fred was put on a non-rebreather mask, which raised his pulse ox to 89%. An IV was started, kvo and nitro was given sublingually and repeated once. His breathing improved, pulse ox was up to 92%, and his resultant BP was 190/100. Furosemide 80 mg was then given with steady improvement. On arrival at the hospital Fred was talking in complete sentences, his lips and nail beds were normal color, and his skin was dry. Fred's pulse ox was up to 97%, heart rate 88, and BP 180/94. Another 40 mg of furosemide was given, a Foley catheter inserted, and chest x-ray and labs were done. After a total output of 2,000 ml, Fred's pulse ox was 99%, heart rate 74, and BP 166/88. He was admitted for congestive heart failure and regulation of medication.

CASE 2

Dispatch: A 56 y/o male with medical problem, nature unknown

On Arrival: 56 y/o Michael is sitting at his desk in his office. He is awake but has a gray color to his face and is diaphoretic. His secretary is with him.

Initial Assessment Findings

Mental Status—Alert and oriented, obeys command; GCS 15
Airway—Open and clear
Breathing—RR 18, talking in complete sentences; lung sounds very faint in bases, clear in upper lobes
Circulation—Skin ashen, cold, very diaphoretic
　　　　　　Radial pulse none present, carotid faint and hard to feel
　　　　　　BP 74/40
Chief Complaint—"Very dizzy"

Focused History

Events—Michael was working at his desk when he suddenly broke out in a cold sweat, became faint, and nauseated. Michael called for his secretary. She took one look and called for an ambulance.
Previous Illness—Michael was diagnosed with adult onset diabetes 6 months ago, as well as hypertension, ulcers
Current Health Status—He has not been feeling well for several days with flu-like symptoms: achy, indigestion, no energy, and no appetite. He denies a fever. He needed to complete some contracts so came into work today.
Allergies—None known
Medications—Glipizide (Glucotrol), cimetidine (Zantac), atenolol (Tenormin); takes meds regularly

Focused Physical

Current Set of VS—P 66 irregular, R 18, BP 74/40
Other Pertinent Findings—Denies any pain, denies vomiting, denies diarrhea or loose stools, no edema noted, no abnormalities noted
Diagnostic Tests—BS by glucometer "high"

ECG

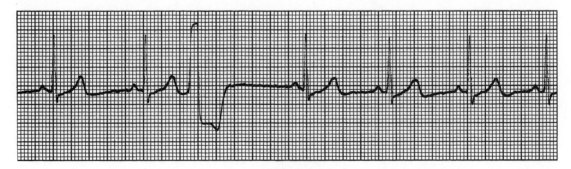

Figure 15-2

QUESTIONS

1. What is significant about Michael's history?

2. What body systems are affected?

3. How would you describe Michael's rhythm?

4. Would you treat Michael's rhythm? Why or why not?

5. Is there a relationship between Michael's rhythm and his blood pressure?

6. Is there anything that could interfere with normal compensatory mechanisms?

7. What is the significance of Michael's diabetes to his current complaint?

8. What is the significance of a blood sugar reading that is "high"?

9. How serious is Michael's situation?

10. What is Michael at risk for?

11. Is there a recognizable pattern to Michael's signs and symptoms? What are all the possibilities?

12. What is the first priority of care?

13. Which body systems are the ones to specifically reassess to help you tell where or what the origin of the problem is?

14. What is your impression?

15. How would you continue treatment?

16. In patients who present with this type of problem, why would fluid boluses be useful?

17. Would a fluid bolus of 200 to 500 ml make the cardiogenic shock patient worse?

18. Dopamine is the drug of choice for cardiogenic shock in the field. What is the dose and how does it work?

19. If the problem with Michael was sepsis, could treatment for cardiogenic shock be harmful?

QUESTIONS AND ANSWERS

1. What is significant about Michael's history?

Michael is a diabetic with a history of ulcers and hypertension. His problem has been developing over the last several days with an acute episode today.

2. What body systems are affected?

Cardiovascular—hypotension and inadequate perfusion with ashen, cold, sweaty skin

3. How would you describe Michael's rhythm?

Sinus rhythm with one PVC. Underlying rhythm is regular, PRI within normal limits, QRS < 0.10, one extra beat with wide QRS and R opposite the T.

4. Would you treat Michael's rhythm? Why or why not?

No, this rhythm is capable of sustaining cardiac output and perfusion. The single PVC is not pathologic by itself. Treatment is aimed toward oxygenation and restoring adequate perfusion.

5. Is there a relationship between Michael's rhythm and his blood pressure?

His rhythm does not explain his hypotension, nor does it exhibit normal compensatory mechanisms (normally a low BP would stimulate a tachycardia). A single PVC in the presence of inadequate perfusion may indicate developing irritability of cardiac muscle.

6. Is there anything that could interfere with normal compensatory mechanisms?

His antihypertensive medication is a beta blocker that prevents abnormally fast rates and suppresses strength of contractions. Usually, even with a beta blocker on board, sufficient stimulation of compensatory mechanisms over-rides the effect of normal doses of beta blockers to cause an increase in heart rate. In Michael's case, the lack of an increase of heart rate in the presence of hypotension is significant and most likely is a reflection of his cardiac status.

7. What is the significance of Michael's diabetes to his current complaint?

Diabetics are prone to accelerated cardiovascular disease and peripheral neuropathy. Peripheral neuropathy might explain why Michael has no complaint of chest pain.

8. What is the significance of a blood sugar reading that is "high"?

There are several factors that are significant. First, this makes hypoglycemia unlikely; second, acute stressors can cause release of emergency stores of sugar resulting in high blood sugar levels that are not related to diabetic ketoacidosis.

9. How serious is Michael's situation?

Michael is in shock and decompensating rapidly.

10. What is Michael at risk for?

Further decompensation and arrest within a short period of time.

11. Is there a recognizable pattern to Michael's signs and symptoms? What are all the possibilities?

Yes, he is in shock. The problem is determining what type of shock it is. Michael's signs and symptoms are *too* general. In the absence of pain or specific discomfort, Michael's signs and symptoms are not specific enough to clearly pinpoint the origin of the problem. There are, however, distinct possibilities. With a history of hypertension and his age, an acute myocardial infarction and cardiogenic shock are likely. Considering his history of ulcers, an internal bleed is also likely. Septic shock is also a strong possibility given a history of diabetes, vague illness, and the time period involved. A diabetic reaction (hypoglycemia, ketoacidosis, or severe dehydration) is unlikely. Anaphylaxis and neurogenic shock are also highly unlikely.

12. What is the first priority of care?

High flow oxygen.

13. Which body systems are the ones to specifically reassess to help you tell where or what the origin of the problem is?

The respiratory system, particularly reassessing lung sounds, is probably the one system that will tell you the most in the shortest amount of time. Other body systems and reassessments include cardiovascular (skin vitals, pulse, ECG, blood pressure) and central nervous system (mental status).

14. What is your impression?

Michael is predisposed to a "silent" myocardial infarction because of his diabetes. His condition is highly suggestive for cardiogenic shock with an acute MI as the precipitating cause. Even though he has a history of ulcers, a bleeding ulcer usually presents with a tachycardia, as does sepsis. Using a fluid bolus to guide treatment would be very useful in this case.

15. How would you continue treatment?

After administering high flow oxygen by non-rebreather mask at 15 lpm with a reservoir, start an IV of normal saline at a kvo rate. Consider a fluid bolus and after reassessment repeat or consider dopamine.

16. In patients who present with this type of problem, why would a fluid bolus be useful?

Given a normal heart rate, a fluid bolus ensures adequate volume and may help determine if the problem is cardiac in nature. Initially a fluid bolus of 200 to 500 ml is followed by reassessment of lung sounds, blood pressure, pulse, and ECG. If lung sounds remain clear then repeated fluid boluses can be given. If, however, lung sounds begin to change to wheezes or rales, then the problem is cardiac in nature and dopamine can be instituted.

17. Would a fluid bolus of 200 to 500 ml make the cardiogenic shock patient worse?

At first impression, this may seem to be true because it is the intolerance to the fluid addition (change in lung sounds or increased difficulty breathing) that points the caregiver in the direction of correct treatment. However, the general consensus is that a *small* bolus probably doesn't hurt and may actually help. There are two reasons for this. First, most patients (not all) are also on diuretics for BP control and enter into the problem slightly dehydrated. The second reason is that a small fluid bolus appears to increase the effectiveness of the dopamine.

18. Dopamine is the drug of choice for cardiogenic shock in the field. What is the dose and how does it work?

Dopamine is a naturally occurring catecholamine in the sympathetic nervous system and in the adrenal glands. As a catecholamine, it has effects on both alpha and beta receptor sites, as well as dopaminergic receptors. Which type of receptor is affected depends on the dose. Dopamine is a powerful medication so relatively low doses (mcg/kg/min) can be very potent. One to 2 mcg/kg/min primarily has a beta effect (renal and mesenteric artery vasodilation occurs). Five to 10 mcg/kg/min have the best beta effect on cardiac muscle. Increased contractility and dilated coronary arteries are the desired effects typical for this dose. At 10 mcg/kg/min and above, increased rate begins to be seen along with vasoconstriction and increased oxygen demand. At 15 to 20 mcg/kg/min almost the entire effect is alpha with peripheral vasoconstriction, increased preload, increased rate, and increased oxygen demand. In most systems, dopamine is started at 5 mcg/kg/min (a 180 pound man [82 kg] would start at 410 mcg/min) and increased to maintain perfusion, roughly measured in the field by BP. Dopamine must be closely regulated so the drip rate doesn't exceed the need.

19. If the problem with Michael was sepsis, could treatment for cardiogenic shock be harmful?

No, fluid boluses with dopamine is also the treatment of choice in the field for septic shock.

OUTCOME

A non-rebreather mask was applied, an IV of normal saline started and, after a fluid bolus of 300 ml, his BP improved slightly. After the bolus was repeated, Michael complained of having difficulty breathing and his BP started to fall. Dopamine was immediately begun at 5 mcg/kg/min. His BP slowly improved en route. VS were BP 96/68, P 82, R 16. On arrival at the hospital, Michael stated he felt better and his skin was dry but his color did not improve. The dopamine was stopped and dobutamine and IV nitro were started. During the 12-lead ECG, Michael complained of increased difficulty breathing. PVCs became frequent, dopamine was restarted, and lidocaine given. Ventricular tachycardia rapidly degenerated into v-fib, which could not be converted. Cause of death was cardiogenic shock resulting from an AMI.

CASE 3

Dispatch: A 76 y/o male with difficulty breathing.

On Arrival: You find Howard, sitting at the kitchen table. He is awake, appears pale, and his son is with him.

Initial Assessment Findings

Mental Status—Alert and oriented, obeys command; GCS 15

Airway—Open and clear

Breathing—RR 32 and labored, talking in complete sentences but seems out of breath; lung sounds are wheezes in bases bilaterally

Circulation—Skin is pale with pronounced circumoral pallor, cool but dry

Radial pulse faint, hard to feel; carotid 150

BP 90/62

Chief Complaint—Difficulty breathing

Focused History

Events—Howard started to have an ache in his chest and dyspnea when working in his yard. He came in the house to rest, the ache in his chest went away, but the dyspnea remained and seemed to get worse. He did not take any meds. His son called the squad.

Previous Illness—Hypertension, "heart problems," denies history of a heart attack

Current Health Status—Considers it relatively good, woke up feeling fine

Allergies—Penicillin

Medications—Hydrochlorothiazide, Lopressor, Nitro-Bid; takes pills regularly

Focused Physical

Current Set of VS—98/64, P 150, R 32 and labored

Other Physical Findings—No pitting edema, nail beds dusky

Diagnostic Tests—Pulse oximetry 86%

ECG

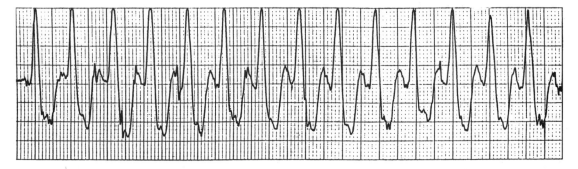

Figure 15-3

QUESTIONS

1. What is significant about Howard's history?

2. What body systems are affected?

3. What is the relationship between Howard's cardiovascular signs and symptoms and his respiratory signs and symptoms?

4. What is significant about Howard's pulse ox value?

5. How would you describe Howard's cardiac rhythm?

6. Is there a relationship between Howard's rhythm and his BP? Dyspnea?

7. How bad is Howard's condition?

8. What is Howard at risk for?

9. Is there a recognizable pattern to Howard's signs and symptoms? What are the possibilities?

10. Would you treat Howard's rhythm and when?

11. What is your first priority of care and why?

12. After your first priority is taken care of, what are your choices for treatment?

13. What is your field impression?

14. How would you treat?

15. In this case, lidocaine was chosen to treat Howard. What is the most likely explanation?

16. Would there have been any harm in trying adenosine first?

17. When a lidocaine bolus is successful, a lidocaine drip is often started but not always. Why?

18. Is the potential for side effects of lidocaine increased when repeat boluses are used?

19. How does this patient compare to the patient in Case 1?

QUESTIONS AND ANSWERS

1. *What is significant about Howard's history?*

   History of cardiac problems, type of meds suggests coronary artery disease. Onset of symptoms with exertion. Anginal type pain relieved with rest, dyspnea not relieved.

2. *What body systems are affected?*

   Cardiovascular—angina, tachycardia, hypotension, pallor
   Respiratory—complaint of difficulty breathing, wheezes, pulse ox 86%

3. *What is the relationship between Howard's cardiovascular signs and symptoms and his respiratory signs and symptoms?*

   Yes, tachycardia can result in lowered cardiac output, hypotension, and decreased perfusion. Tachycardia also causes increased oxygen demand. Decreased perfusion and increased oxygen demand both lead to angina. Tachycardia in an overburdened heart can also result in a backup of blood to the left atria, correspondingly disrupting hydrostatic pressure in the pulmonary capillary beds and leading to pulmonary edema and wheezing.

4. *What is significant about Howard's pulse ox value?*

   The value of 86% may indicate the degree to which his pulmonary edema is interfering with his ability to oxygenate his blood. However, pulse oximetry is inaccurate when a person is in shock with vasoconstriction. Even though the value seems appropriate, there is the chance it is inaccurate. Depend on your physical assessment to confirm the pulse ox value.

5. *How would you describe Howard's cardiac rhythm?*

   There is no discernible P wave; the QRS = 0.12, the rate is slightly irregular and rapid at about 140 to 150. This meets the criteria for either VT or SVT with aberrant conduction.

6. *Is there a relationship between Howard's rhythm and his BP? Dyspnea?*

   Yes, Howard's rhythm is either too fast for his heart to keep up, or his rhythm is VT and is too inefficient for the needs of his body, or it is a combination of the both.

7. *How bad is Howard?*

   He may seem relatively stable; however, if his rhythm is VT, that is an unstable rhythm and may deteriorate any moment.

8. *What is Howard at risk for?*

   Either v-fib or rapid decompensation and arrest.

9. *Is there a recognizable pattern to Howard's signs and symptoms? What are the possibilities?*

   Yes, rhythm induced cardiogenic shock. Other possibilities include a "silent" MI with associated dysrhythmia.

10. *Would you treat Howard's rhythm and when?*

    Yes, after oxygenation.

11. *What is your first priority of care and why?*

    The first priority is oxygen by non-rebreather mask at 15 lpm with a reservoir. If this dysrhythmia is triggered by a hypoxic heart, oxygen may be the only necessary treatment.

12. *After your first priority is taken care of, what are your choices for treatment?*

    Your options include lidocaine if you are sure the rhythm is ventricular in origin, adenosine if you have reason to believe it is atrial in origin, or cardioversion if he would deteriorate. Lidocaine and adenosine should not be used interchangeably. If you are confident the rhythm is VT then use lidocaine.

13. *What is your field impression?*

    Even though Howard's ECG shows a QRS that is borderline, his general physical condition highly suggests VT.

14. How would you treat?

After oxygen is applied and an IV is started, lidocaine at 1 to 1.5 mg/kg IVP or sedation and car-dioversion are the options. Even though he is hypotensive, he is alert and oriented. Some systems would sedate and cardiovert, while other systems would weigh his mental status against possible side effects of sedation. In either case you will follow local protocols.

15. In this case, lidocaine was chosen to treat Howard. What is the most likely explanation?

Cardioversion is extreme in this case because Howard was alert and oriented. Even though his BP was low, his brain was perfusing enough for a GCS of 15. To sedate for cardioversion is unnecessary at this point. When a rhythm has no P waves, is regular and tachycardic with a QRS that is exactly 0.12 sec in width, assume the worst and the worst is VT. If lidocaine has no effect, then try adenosine. If at any point the patient deteriorates, then sedate and cardiovert.

16. Would there have been any harm in trying adenosine first?

Adenosine only works in the atria, and with such a short half-life there are relatively few side effects. The harm would have been in terms of time. VT is an unstable rhythm and can deteriorate into v-fib without warning so why waste time giving a drug that may not work? In comparison, SVT is considered relatively stable.

17. When a lidocaine bolus is successful, a lidocaine drip is often started but not always. Why?

A lidocaine drip is used to maintain a therapeutic blood level established by the bolus. Because the initial lidocaine bolus can maintain a therapeutic blood level for approximately 15 minutes, a repeat bolus of half the initial dose, 8 to 10 minutes later will maintain a therapeutic level for another 10 to 15 minutes, enough time in many systems to get to the hospital. In some systems with short transport times, it is easier to bolus than to hang a drip. The preferred way is usually up to the program medical director. Some systems leave it up to the medic, based on transport times.

18. Is the potential for side effects of lidocaine increased when repeat boluses are used?

Only if too much is given or the lidocaine is given too fast. That can also happen with the initial bolus or if a drip gets away from a medic. Side effects include circumoral numbness and tingling, drowsiness, bradycardia, and hypotension or patients may complain of a "funny" feeling. Seizures are rare but may also occur when lidocaine is given too fast or if too much is given.

19. How does this patient compare to the patient in Case 1?

Both patients are in cardiogenic shock, with similar signs and symptoms. However, the similarity stops there. Fred in Case 1 has ventricular muscle failure, whereas Howard has failure caused by an ineffective rhythm, ventricular tachycardia. The type of shock is the same but the difference in cause requires different initial pharmacologic treatment. The ECG is a valuable assessment tool to determine appropriate pharmacologic intervention.

OUTCOME

After high flow oxygen, medics started an IV kvo and gave lidocaine, 120 mg IVP with no result. After approximately 10 minutes during which they got loaded up and began transport, they gave an additional 60 mg IVP. Howard then converted to a sinus rhythm with an occasional PVC. On arrival at the hospital a lidocaine drip, 3 mg, was added. A 12-lead ECG was done and Howard was admitting to the CCU.

CASE 4

Dispatch: A 54 y/o female with chest pain.

On Arrival: You find 54 y/o Elizabeth, sitting on the floor beside her washing machine. She is awake but drowsy and appears very pale and diaphoretic. Her husband is with her.

Initial Assessment Findings

Mental Status—Awake and oriented but sleepy: GCS 15
Airway—Open and clear
Breathing—RR 22 and shallow, talking in complete sentences; lung sounds clear in upper lobes, diminished in bases
Circulation—Skin pale, cool, and clammy
        Radial pulse unable to feel, carotid thready, unable to count
        BP 60/Palpable
Chief Complaint—Short of breath

Focused History

Events—Elizabeth was sorting the laundry when she suddenly could not catch her breath, then the chest pain started. She got dizzy, sat down, and called for her husband. He called the squad.
Previous Illness—History of PAT (paroxysmal atrial tachycardia); this is different than her previous episodes
Current Health Status—Considers it good, with last episode of PAT several years ago
Allergies—Hay fever, pollen, cats
Medications—None

Focused Physical

Current Set of VS—BP 66/P, HR 214, R 22
Other Pertinent Findings—Chest pain is now an ache, rated as 3 on a scale of 10, no other pertinent findings
Diagnostic Tests—Pulse oximetry reads "ERROR"

ECG

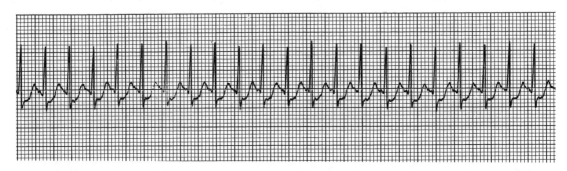

Figure 15-4

QUESTIONS

1. What is significant about Elizabeth's history?

2. What body systems are affected?

3. What is the relationship between Elizabeth's heart rate and her chest pain? Her difficulty breathing?

4. Is there an explanation for Elizabeth's pulse oximetry reading?

5. How would you describe Elizabeth's cardiac rhythm?

6. How serious is Elizabeth's condition?

7. What is Elizabeth at risk for?

8. Would you treat Elizabeth's rhythm, and when?

9. What is your first priority of care, and why?

10. What is your field impression?

11. How would you treat?

12. What criteria should be present before deciding to cardiovert a patient with symptomatic SVT?

13. When sedating a patient with diazepam (Valium), how do you know what dose to use?

14. What makes the delivery of adenosine unusual when compared to other IV push medications?

15. What are the criteria for the use of adenosine?

16. Are there any times when adenosine will probably not work?

17. What are the side effects of adenosine?

18. How does Elizabeth compare to the patients in Cases 1 and 3?

QUESTIONS AND ANSWERS

1. What is significant about Elizabeth's history?

Sudden onset of chest pain, then shortness of breath and dizziness with no definite precipitating factor, history of PAT but this episode is different, no meds.

2. What body systems are affected?

Cardiovascular—chest pain, tachycardia, severe hypotension, pallor, cyanotic lips
Respiratory—sensation of shortness of breath

3. What is the relationship between Elizabeth's heart rate and her chest pain? Her difficulty breathing?

Elizabeth's heart rate is too fast to allow for adequate ventricular filling leading to decreased cardiac output and severe hypotension, severe hypoperfusion and myocardial ischemia. Adequate oxygen and carbon dioxide exchange is not occurring leading to hypoxia and, with a drop in cardiac output, cellular ischemia is present. Pulmonary edema has a strong probability of developing.

4. Is there an explanation for Elizabeth's pulse oximetry reading?

With severe hypotension and/or peripheral vasoconstriction, pulse oximetry readings are inaccurate. It may be that the device cannot get a reading.

5. How would you describe Elizabeth's cardiac rhythm?

SVT. The QRS is < 0.10, the rhythm is regular but extremely fast with no identifiable P waves. This meets the criteria for SVT.

6. How serious is Elizabeth's condition?

Her condition is very serious because she is unstable.

7. What is Elizabeth at risk for?

Sudden loss of existing pressure leading to an arrest and/or acute myocardial infarct.

8. Would you treat Elizabeth's rhythm, and when?

Yes, her rapid rate is the cause of her severe hypotension and should be treated immediately.

9. What is your first priority of care and why?

High flow oxygen, because she is extremely hypoxic. Treatment will have a better chance of success and greater chance of preventing further damage if she is well oxygenated.

10. What is your field impression?

Symptomatic SVT.

11. How would you treat?

She meets the criteria for sedation and immediate cardioversion.

12. What criteria should be present before deciding to cardiovert a patient with symptomatic SVT?

The American Heart Association states that a person who is symptomatic and hypotensive or with pulmonary edema should be sedated and cardioverted. However, there are situations where opinions may differ. In some systems medical directors give the additional criteria of altered mental status regardless of the blood pressure. Sedation carries the risk of airway compromise and aspiration, though when done carefully that risk is minimized. Most systems would sedate and cardiovert a patient like Elizabeth to avoid the risk of further myocardial damage from ischemia.

13. When sedating a patient with diazepam (Valium), how do you know what dose to use?

Diazepam is the most common method for field sedation outside of air transport systems. Diazepam is useful because it interferes with memory, causing amnesia of the event; however, it also has the additional side effect of respiratory depression.

Respiratory depression can be avoided if the drug is given slow IV push. There is a dose range; start with 5 mg slow IV push, and work up to 10 mg. To assess for the presence of the amnestic effect, instruct the patient to remember a vegetable or a color, change the subject for a sentence or two then ask if they remember what you requested. If they can't, memory isn't being laid down and you can cardiovert.

14. *What makes the delivery of adenosine unusual when compared to other IV push medications?*

Adenosine must be given very rapidly, IVP, in the port as close to the patient as possible and followed by a bolus of fluid. Adenosine is very short acting. Its half life is less than 5 seconds.

15. *What are the criteria for use of adenosine?*

Adenosine is useful for SVT caused by reentry phenomenon (most frequent cause of SVT) even when caused by Wolff-Parkinson-White syndrome (short P-R interval and delta wave preceding R).

16. *Are there any times when adenosine will probably not work?*

Yes, adenosine is not known to be successful when the SVT is *not* a result of reentry involving the AV node or sinus node, such as atrial fibrillation or atrial flutter. However, it may produce a transient AV block that may slow the rhythm enough to determine the origin.

17. *What are side effects of adenosine?*

As field providers and hospitals are using adenosine more frequently, more side effects are being documented. The patient may complain of dizziness, a sensation in his or her chest (sometimes described as a pain), a flushing of the face or just a sudden feeling similar to being in a elevator that descends too quickly. These effects are transient. Other common side effects, however, involve a period of asystole, ventricular ectopy, or sinus bradycardia. The asystolic pause may be as long as 15 seconds and can be startling, but the rhythm starts spontaneously. There is no documented instance of the rhythm not returning.

18. *How does Elizabeth compare to the patients in Cases 1 and 3?*

All three patients are in cardiogenic shock, with similar signs and symptoms. However, the similarity stops there. Fred in Case 1 has ventricular muscle failure, whereas Howard in Case 3 and Elizabeth have failure resulting from tachycardia, ventricular and atrial. All three require different medications. The ECG is a valuable assessment tool to determine appropriate intervention. Do not confuse treating the rhythm with treating the patient. *Always treat the patient.*

OUTCOME

After high flow oxygen was on, IV access was established and 6 mg adenosine was given rapid IVP. See Figure 15-5 for the resulting rhythm.

After the adenosine, several short bursts of VT occur before the rhythm dropped to an irregular rate of 178 that appeared to be caused by atrial fibrillation. Some complexes appear to be either ventricular in origin or aberrantly conducted. However, her systolic pressure increased to 78. Another bolus of adenosine, 12 mg was given rapid IVP. The resulting heart rate dropped to 120 with frequent PACs. Elizabeth's color improved markedly, she became more alert, and her skin was dry. Vital signs were: BP 136/84, P 120 irregular, R 18. On arrival at the ED a 12-lead EKG was done. During the ECG she had another episode of SVT with a precipitous drop in BP. She was rapidly sedated and cardioverted to an irregular sinus rhythm of 110. Elizabeth was given Cardizem IV and admitted to CCU with a heart rate of 88 and BP of 124/82.

ECG

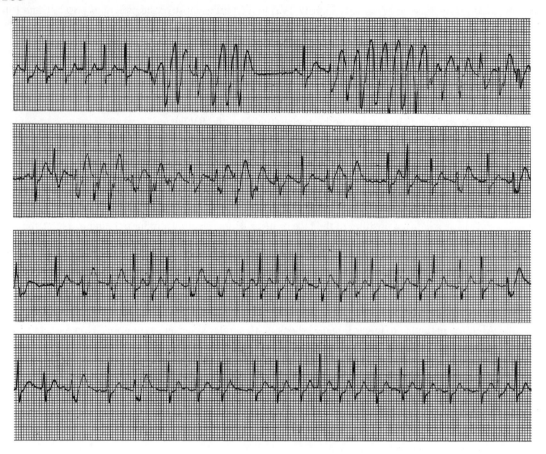

Figure 15-5

CASE 5

Dispatch: A 78 y/o female, weakness, possible stroke

On Arrival: You find 78 y/o Matilda, lying on her sofa. She is awake and appears pale.

Initial Assessment Findings

Mental Status—Alert, oriented, and obeys command; GCS 15
Airway—Open and clear
Breathing—RR 16 and shallow, lung sounds clear to all lobes
Circulation—Skin pale, cool, and dry with poor turgor
      Radial pulse irregular at 44
      BP 80/56
Chief Complaint—"Too weak to walk"

Focused History

Events—Matilda couldn't get up off the couch without getting so dizzy she was afraid she would fall.
Previous Illness—Hypertension, "heart problems," and "too much water"
Current Health Status—"Not too good," described lack of appetite, general abdominal discomfort, diarrhea, and weakness for last 3 to 4 days
Allergies—None known
Medications—"BP pill," "heart pill," and "water pill." Matilda identifies her pills by color and has them all in a sugar bowl on the kitchen table; the prescription bottles are not available. She takes them when she remembers; she took them today.

Focused Physical

Current Set of VS—BP 80/56, P 44, R 16
Other Pertinent Findings—Skin "tents," no edema noted, no other abnormalities
Diagnostic Tests—Pulse oximetry is 98%, blood sugar 88, 300 ml bolus of NS improved BP to 90/64 with clear lung sounds bilaterally, there is no pitting edema noted, stools are once every 2 to 3 days, denies melena

ECG

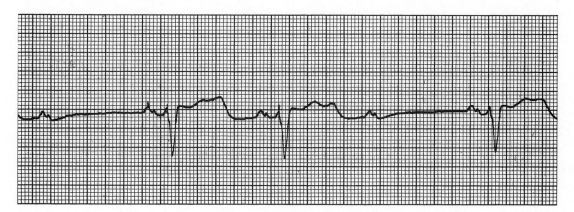

Figure 15-6

QUESTIONS

1. What is significant about Matilda's history?

2. What body systems are affected?

3. What is the significance of Matilda's poor skin turgor?

4. Is there a relationship between Matilda's pulse and her hypotension?

5. How would you describe Matilda's cardiac rhythm?

6. Is there a recognizable pattern to Matilda's signs and symptoms? What are the possibilities?

7. How serious is Matilda's condition?

8. What is Matilda at risk for?

9. Would you treat Matilda's rhythm? Why or why not?

10. What is your first priority of care?

11. What is your field impression?

12. How would you continue treatment?

13. Would Ringer's lactate have helped Matilda more than normal saline?

14. If Matilda has a history of congestive heart failure, why are her lungs sounds clear?

15. Since she is prone to pulmonary edema, yet is dehydrated, how much fluid is enough?

16. Are there any risk factors, specific for the geriatric population group, that have contributed to Matilda's current problem?

QUESTIONS AND ANSWERS

1. **What is significant about Matilda's history?**

   Vague, diffuse symptoms have had a gradual onset over several days; irregular medication use, poor historian

2. **What body systems are affected?**

   Cardiovascular—bradycardia, irregular pulse; hypotension; poor turgor

3. **What is the significance of Matilda's poor skin turgor?**

   This strongly suggests dehydration.

4. **Is there a relationship between Matilda's pulse and her hypotension?**

   Yes, cardiac output is determined by stroke volume and heart rate. In the field, cardiac output is roughly measured by BP. If either the stroke volume (amount of blood in the left ventricle) or the heart rate decrease, cardiac output falls. If compensatory mechanisms fail, hypotension results. In Matilda's case her heart rate is too slow and her stroke volume is decreased (poor skin turgor). The combination is enough to overwhelm compensatory mechanisms and cause hypotension.

5. **How would you describe Matilda's cardiac rhythm?**

   An intermittent second-degree block, type II (the P-R interval is consistent when present) with a notched, prolonged P wave and a U wave. A notched, prolonged P wave is sometimes termed "P mitrale" and may be seen when the left atria is dilated and hypertrophied, as found in hypertension, mitral and aortic valvular disease, AMI, and congestive heart failure. A "U" wave may be present in hypokalemia, cardiomyopathy, left ventricular hypertrophy, and diabetes.

6. **Is there a recognizable pattern to Matilda's signs and symptoms? What are the possibilities?**

   Yes, Matilda's description of her pills suggests congestive heart failure: digitalis (heart pill), furosemide (water pill), and antihypertensive (blood pressure pill). The typical medications prescribed for CHF "waste" potassium. Her cardiac rhythm is consistent with congestive failure and a lack of potassium. Digitalis, when taken in excess, can result in dysrhythmias such as a block. Hypokalemia can also result in dysrhythmias such as this one. Her physical symptoms are consistent with hypokalemia, too much digitalis, and dehydration. The results of the fluid challenge helps to confirm the presence of dehydration. There is another associated possibility with Matilda and that is the potential for anemia.

7. **How serious is Matilda's condition?**

   Matilda is stable right now. She needs evaluation for fluid and potassium replacement, adjustment of medication, and social service referral.

8. **What is Matilda at risk for?**

   Further dehydration, falling with the risk of associated fractures, worsening of dysrhythmia, stroke, and myocardial infarction.

9. **Would you treat Matilda's rhythm? Why or why not?**

   Not at this point. The fluid bolus currently has her pressure up to 90 systolic; she is alert and oriented with good respiratory effort, and is tolerating her condition. Her rhythm is most likely caused by either too much or too little digitalis or an electrolyte imbalance (too little potassium). A problem with digitalis and the potassium imbalance cannot be effectively managed in the field. If, however, her pressure could not be maintained with fluid, then consider atropine or pacing. Other pharmacologic intervention would be overkill and could potentially cause other problems.

10. **What is your first priority of care?**

    Apply oxygen. Matilda is alert and oriented; there is no cyanosis and no other indicators of hypoxia. Adjust oxygen delivery to maintain pulse oximetry between 98% to 100%.

11. **What is your field impression?**

    Dehydration with associated electrolyte imbalance and cardiac dysrhythmia.

12. ***How would you continue treatment?***

Further treatment may include an additional fluid bolus. Unless she starts to deteriorate, treatment of her rhythm is unnecessary.

13. ***Would Ringer's lactate have helped Matilda more than normal saline?***

Probably not. Even though Ringer's lactate has several electrolytes including potassium, the concentration of potassium is only 4 mEq/L, whereas calcium is 3 mEq/L, sodium is 130 mEq/L, and chloride is 109 mEq/L (lactate is 28). On the other hand, normal saline (0.9% NaCl) has 154 mEq/L sodium and 154 mEq/L chloride. Ringer's lactate will not hurt her and, as long as she has a healthy liver, will be just as effective. If the status of her liver is in doubt (lactate is processed by the liver and changed into bicarbonate) give normal saline.

14. ***If Matilda has a history of congestive heart failure, why are her lungs sounds clear?***

She is dehydrated. Dehydration increases the concentration of particles, or solute, in the blood. An increased concentration of particles increases the osmotic pressure of the blood, pulling fluid into the vascular space, thus preventing formation of pulmonary edema.

15. ***Since she is prone to pulmonary edema, yet is dehydrated, how much fluid is enough?***

Enough to maintain perfusion and not interfere with her respiratory effort or exchange. This involves careful monitoring of fluid. For this reason, many systems advocate repeated fluid boluses with reassessment instead of a maintaining a constant IV drip.

16. ***Are there any risk factors, specific for the geriatric population group, that have contributed to Matilda's current problem?***

Yes. As people grow older, the thirst mechanism becomes depressed and changes occur in the drinking response, which makes it easier for the elderly to become dehydrated. Drug compliance is frequently very poor, leading to adverse reactions that may go unrecognized or misdiagnosed. Decreased renal function, a result of the aging process, can lead to unintentional overdose with medication such as digitalis. The half-life of digoxin increases from 40 to 70 hours with age.

OUTCOME

After the nasal cannula was applied, medics started an IV of normal saline and administered a bolus of 300 ml. The bolus improved her BP to 90 systolic and Matilda stated she felt so much better that she didn't want to go to the hospital. After much convincing, she agreed to go. In the ED Matilda admitted to doubling her next dose of medication whenever she forgot to take her meds. Matilda had a serum potassium level of 2.0 and significantly elevated serum digitalis levels. Her IV was changed and 80 mEq potassium chloride added. Digibind (antidigoxin Fab fragments) was also administered to excrete excess digitalis. Matilda was admitted to the hospital with severe dehydration, digitalis overdose, and hypokalemia.

CASE 6

Dispatch: 56 y/o with chest pain

On Arrival: You find 56 y/o Thomas, sitting on his living room couch. He is awake, appears slightly pale and his wife is with him.

Initial Assessment Findings

Mental Status—Alert and oriented; GCS 15
Airway—Open and clear
Breathing—RR 16 and shallow, speaks in complete sentences; lung sounds clear in all lobes
Circulation—Skin pale, warm, and dry
      Radial pulse regular at 90
      BP 118/78
Chief Complaint—Chest pain

Focused History

Events—Thomas got up this morning with an ache in his chest that has not improved (it is now noon). He called his doctor and his doctor told him to go to the hospital so he called you. His ache is located in the upper chest bilaterally, but more on the left, and has stayed constant. He denies radiation, ranked the pain as a 4 on a scale of 10, and states that it worsens with deep breaths.
Previous Illness—Thomas had a heart transplant 3 years ago for viral cardiomyopathy
Current Health Status—Was told 2 weeks ago that he had early nephrotoxic effect from cyclosporine and hypertension, has had a runny nose for 2 days, no cough
Allergies—Morphine
Medications—Cyclosporine, prednisone, timolol, furosemide, Nitro-Bid, and aspirin. He also has muscle relaxants, vitamins, stool softeners, and an iron supplement.

Focused Physical

Current Set of VS—BP 118/78, P 90, and regular, R 16
Other Physical Findings—Sternal scar, edema of ankles but no pitting edema
Diagnostic Tests—Blood sugar 106

ECG

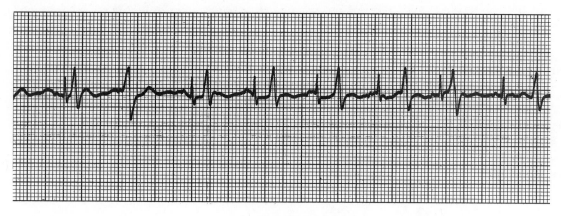

Figure 15-7

QUESTIONS

1. What is significant about Thomas's history?

2. What body systems are affected?

3. Is there anything else, either from history or physical assessment that would help?

4. What is significant about Thomas's "ache" in his chest?

5. How would you describe Thomas's cardiac rhythm?

6. How serious is Thomas's condition?

7. What is Thomas at risk for?

8. How would organ rejection probably present?

9. Is there anything in Thomas's history or physical examination that would support the possibility of infection?

10. Are there any of the traditional cardiac medications used in the field (e.g., nitro, lidocaine, atropine, epinephrine) that would be contraindicated or rendered ineffective by the transplant process?

11. What is your field impression?

12. How would you treat?

13. Thomas tells you he has an early nephrotoxic effect from the cyclosporin. What does that mean?

14. Thomas has edema in his ankles. Is there anything in his history that is consistent with this type of edema?

QUESTIONS AND ANSWERS

1. What is significant about Thomas's history?

Chest pain, described as an "ache," woke up with it, worsens with deep breath, history of heart transplant, early kidney failure as side effect from medication.

2. What body systems are affected?

No obvious ones. Though the suspicion of cardiac involvement from his history (heart transplant) and description of pain (an ache in his chest) is present, there is no other finding that would confirm that cardiac involvement is present.

3. Is there anything else, either from history or physical assessment, that would help?

Ask what activity he did yesterday; has this ever happened before? Has he done anything for his complaint?

4. What is significant about Thomas's "ache" in his chest?

It doesn't sound like typical cardiac pain. Pain that does not radiate and worsens with a deep breath may also be pleuritic in nature.

5. How would you describe Thomas's cardiac rhythm?

At first glance it looks like a bigeminy of some sort. The very narrow complexes are perfusing. On closer inspection, both types of QRS complexes have P waves, the narrow complexes are more consistent. There are two rhythms superimposed on each other. This gentleman still has his original heart. The transplanted heart is generating the complexes that perfuse.

6. How serious is Thomas's condition?

Thomas appears stable at the moment.

7. What is Thomas at risk for?

Infection, organ rejection, a more acute problem with his transplanted heart.

8. How would organ rejection probably present?

This is something that is not routinely taught in paramedic class. Onset is usually insidious. In mild cases ECG changes may be the first sign. In other cases vague, diffuse discomfort, often described as "flu-like" symptoms occur. Fever, malaise, tachycardia, hypotension, and right sided heart failure follow. Pain at the site of transplant may or may not be present.

9. Is there anything in Thomas's history or physical that would support the possibility of infection?

He has had a runny nose. If he does have an upper respiratory infection, normal signs and symptoms of infection would be masked by the immunosuppressive drugs he is taking for his transplant.

10. Are there any of the traditional cardiac medications used in the field (e.g., nitro, lidocaine, atropine, epinephrine) that would be contraindicated or rendered ineffective by the transplant process?

Yes, atropine, a parasympathetic blocker that works on the vagal nerve, would be ineffective in a heart transplant patient. The vagal nerve is cut and not reattached. Symptomatic, hypotensive bradycardias would need to be treated by a pacer or dopamine.

11. What is your field impression?

Chest pain, pleuritic in nature, origin unknown.

12. How would you treat?

Administer oxygen to maintain pulse oximetry between 98% to 100% and consider an IV in case pharmacologic intervention would be necessary. Consider administering nitroglycerine in case this is cardiac in origin and monitor the effect.

13. Thomas tells you he has an early nephrotoxic effect from the cyclosporin. What does that mean?

Cyclosporin is toxic to his kidneys. An early nephrotoxic effect, combined with his ankle edema suggests early kidney failure. If in doubt, ask the patient what it means to him or her.

14. ***Thomas has edema in his ankles. Is there anything in his history that is consistent with this type of edema?***

Standing for long periods of time can cause this. Early kidney failure as a result of the nephro-toxicity can also be a cause. If allowed to continue without relief, pitting edema may occur.

OUTCOME

Thomas was put on oxygen by a nasal cannula at 2 to 4 liters, a precautionary IV was started at kvo, and he was transported with his sack of medications. At the hospital he told the staff that he supposed that helping his wife move the furniture the day before was something he probably shouldn't have done. After notifying his physician, Thomas was diagnosed with costochondritis and dismissed.

BIBLIOGRAPHY

Cummins R. O. (Ed.). (1994). *Advanced cardiac life support textbook.* Dallas, TX: American Heart Association.

Bradway, C. W. (1996). *Nursing care of geriatric emergencies.* New York: Springer Publishing.

Fulmer, T. T., & Walker, M. K. (Eds.). (1992). *Critical care nursing of the elderly.* New York: Springer Publishing.

Haak, S. W., Richardson, S. J., & Davey, S. S. (1994). Alterations of cardiovascular function. In K. L. McCance & S. E. Huether (Eds.). *Pathophysiology: The biologic basis for disease in adults and children* (2nd ed.). St. Louis, MO: Mosby.

Kane, R. L., Ouslander, J. G., & Abrass, I. B. (1994). *Essentials of clinical geriatrics* (3rd ed.). Philadelphia: McGraw-Hill.

Kelly, R. A., & Smith, T. W. (1996). Pharmacological treatment of heart failure. In J. G. Hardman & L. E. Limbird (Eds.). *Goodman & Gilman's: The pharmacological basis of therapeutics* (9th ed.). Philadelphia: McGraw-Hill.

Mistovich, J. J., Benner, R. W., & Margolis, G. S. (1998). *Advanced cardiac life support.* Upper Saddle River, NJ: Prentice Hall.

Roden, D. M. (1996). Antiarrhythmic drugs. In j. G. Hardman & L. E. Limbird (Eds.). *Goodman & Gilman's: The pharmacological basis of therapeutics* (9th ed.). Philadelphia: McGraw-Hill.

Roush, W., & Fontanarosa, P. (1997). Palpitations and dysrhythmias. In P. T. Pons & D. Cason (Eds.). *Paramedic field care: A complaint-based approach.* St. Louis, MO: Mosby.

Schwartz, J. B. (1994). Clinical pharmacology. In W. R. Chaptin, E. L. Bierman, J. P. Blass, W. H. Ettinger, & J.B. Halter (Eds.). *Principles of geriatric medicine and gerontology,* (3rd ed.). Philadelphia: McGraw-Hill.

A

Geriatric and Pediatric Cases

GERIATRIC CASES

Chapter	Case	Name and Chief Complaint
1	1	Fred, 67 y/o, c/o difficulty breathing
1	4	Margaret, 76 y/o, unconscious, possible stroke
2	1	Harold, elderly male, unconscious
2	2	Mavis, 67 y/o, c/o dizziness
2	3	Ivan, 76 y/o, possible stroke
3	3	Mildred, 78 y/o, unconscious
3	5	Phyllis, 72 y/o, unconscious
10	2	Cleo, 72 y/o heat related illness
14	7	Karl, 81 y/o, trauma
15	1	Fred, 68 y/o, c/o difficulty breathing
15	3	Howard, 76 y/o, c/o difficulty breathing
15	5	Matilda, 78 y/o, c/o weakness

PEDIATRIC CASES

Chapter	Case	Name and Chief Complaint
1	2	Bob, 16 y/o, c/o difficulty breathing
3	2	Jeffery, 8 month old, unconscious infant
4	1	Jarrell, 8 y/o, c/o abdominal pain
5	2	Jimmy, 3 y/o, c/o possible allergic reaction
6	1	Tonya, 13 y/o, unconscious child
6	4	Sammy, 2 y/o, unconscious child
6	5	16 y/o son, c/o flu-like symptoms
7	1	Normal gestation newborn
7	2	Premature newborn
8	6	Connie, 18 y/o, c/o headache
10	1	Nathan, 3 y/o, heat related illness
10	4	Callie, 4 y/o, cold exposure
12	1	Julio, 13 y/o, c/o seizure
12	2	Darin, 3 y/o, c/o seizure
13	1	Sean, 8 month old, trauma
14	4	Muhallah, 16 y/o, trauma
14	8	Yurba, 5 y/o, trauma

Index

355